T0325463

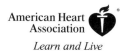

American Heart Association

Learn and Live

The AHA Clinical Series

SERIES EDITOR ELLIOTT ANTMAN

Pacing to Support the Failing Heart

Dedication

To all my colleagues at Fondazione Cardiocentro Ticino, for their support, dedication, understanding and quest for excellence.

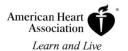

American Heart
Association
Learn and Live

Pacing to Support the Failing Heart

EDITED BY

Kenneth A. Ellenbogen, MD
Kontos Professor of Cardiology
Medical College of Virginia
Richmond, VA, USA

Angelo Auricchio, MD, PhD
Director, Heart Failure Service
Fondazione Cardiocentro Ticino
Lugano, Switzerland

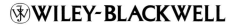

WILEY-BLACKWELL

A John Wiley & Sons, Ltd., Publication

This edition first published 2008, © 2008 American Heart Association
American Heart Association National Center, 7272 Greenville Avenue, Dallas, TX 75231, USA
For further information on the American Heart Association:
www.americanheart.org

Blackwell Publishing was acquired by John Wiley & Sons in February 2007. Blackwell's publishing program has been merged with Wiley's global Scientific, Technical and Medical business to form Wiley-Blackwell.

Registered office: John Wiley & Sons Ltd, The Atrium, Southern Gate, Chichester, West Sussex, PO19 8SQ, UK

Editorial offices: 9600 Garsington Road, Oxford, OX4 2DQ, UK
The Atrium, Southern Gate, Chichester, West Sussex, PO19 8SQ, UK
111 River Street, Hoboken, NJ 07030-5774, USA

For details of our global editorial offices, for customer services and for information about how to apply for permission to reuse the copyright material in this book please see our website at www.wiley.com/wiley-blackwell

Library of Congress Cataloging-in-Publication Data
Pacing to support the failing heart / edited by Kenneth Ellenbogen and Angelo Auricchio.
    p. ; cm. – (AHA clinical series)
    Includes bibliographical references.
    ISBN 978-1-4051-7534-0
    1. Heart failure–Treatment.   2. Cardiac pacemakers.   3. Cardiac pacing.
I. Ellenbogen, Kenneth A.   II. Auricchio, Angelo.   III. American Heart Association.
IV. Series.
    [DNLM: 1. Heart Failure–therapy.   2. Cardiac Pacing, Artificial.   3. Heart Failure–diagnosis.
4. Heart Failure–physiopathology. 5. Pacemaker, Artificial. WG 370 P118 2009]
    RC685.C53P33 2009
    616.1′280645–dc22

                                                                            2008030328

ISBN: 9781405175340

A catalogue record for this book is available from the British Library.

Set in 9.25/12 pt Minion by Aptara® Inc., New Delhi, India
Printed & bound in Singapore by Fabulous Printers Pte Ltd

1   2008

Contents

Contributors

Angelo Auricchio, MD, PhD
Fondazione Cardiocentro Ticino
Lugano, Switzerland

S. Serge Barold, MD
Arrhythmia Service and Division of Cardiology
Tampa General Hospital and University of South Florida
Tampa, FL, USA

Dan Blendea, MD, PhD
Cardiac Arrhythmia Service
Massachusetts General Hospital
Harvard Medical School
Cambridge, MA, USA

Martin Borggrefe, MD
Medical Director
Departement of Cardiology
University Hospital of Mannheim
Mannheim, Germany

Przemyslaw P. Borek, MD
Cardiovascular Medicine
Cleveland Clinic
Cleveland, OH, USA

Daniel Burkhoff, MD, PhD
Department of Cardiology
Columbia University
New York, NY, USA and IMPULSE Dynamics
Orangeburg, NY, USA

Christian Butter, MD
Heart Center Brandenburg Bernau/Berlin
Bernau, Germany

Livio Dei Cas, MD
Section of Cardiovascular Diseases,
Department of Experimental and Applied Medicine
University of Brescia
Brescia, Italy

Khalid Chakir, PhD
Division of Cardiology, Department of Medicine
Johns Hopkins Medical Institutions
Baltimore, MD, USA

Kenneth A. Ellenbogen, MD
Kontos Professor of Cardiology
Medical College of Virginia
Richmond, VA, USA

Patrick W. Fisher, DO, PhD
Associate Medical Director
UTAH (Utah Transplantation Affiliated Hospitals) Cardiac Transplant Program
Associate Cardiology Director
Utah Artificial Heart Program
Assistant Medical Director
Heart Failure Prevention and Treatment Program
Cardiology Director
Pulmonary Hypertension Center
Intermountain Medical Center
Murray, Utah

Richard A. Grimm, DO
Cardiovascular Medicine
Cleveland Clinic
Cleveland, OH, USA

Robert H. Helm, MD
Division of Cardiology
Department of Medicine
Johns Hopkins Medical Institutions
Baltimore, MD, USA

Bengt Herweg, MD
Arrhythmia Service and Division of Cardiology
Tampa General Hospital and University of South Florida
Tampa, FL, USA

Arzu Ilercil, MD
Arrhythmia Service and Division of Cardiology
Tampa General Hospital and University of South Florida
Tampa, FL, USA

C. W. Israel, MD
Dept. of Cardiology - Div. of Clinical Electrophysiology
J. W. Goethe University
Frankfurt, Germany

David A. Kass, MD
Abraham and Virginia Weiss Professor of Cardiology
Division of Cardiology
Department of Medicine
Johns Hopkins Medical Institutions
Baltimore, MD, USA

AG. Kfoury, MD, FACC
Medical Director
UTAH (Utah Transplantation Affiliated Hospitals) Cardiac Transplantation Program
Cardiology Director
Utah Artificial Heart Program
Intermountain Medical Center
Murray, UT, USA

Dusan Kocovic, MD
Chief of Electrophysiology
Lankenau Hospital
Main Line Health
Lankenau Medical Center
Wynnewood, PA, USA

Marco Metra, MD
Section of Cardiovascular Diseases
Department of Experimental and Applied Medicine
University of Brescia
Brescia, Italy

Savina Nodari, MD
Section of Cardiovascular Diseases
Department of Experimental and Applied Medicine
University of Brescia
Brescia, Italy

Dale G. Renlund, MD, FACC
Medical Director
Heart Failure Prevention and Treatment Program
Intermountain Medical Center
Professor of Medicine
Division of cardiology
University of Utah School of Medicine
Murray, UT, USA

Jagmeet P. Singh MD, DPhil
Cardiac Arrhythmia Service
Massachusetts General Hospital
Harvard Medical School
Cambridge, MA, USA

David D. Spragg, MD
Division of Cardiology
Department of Medicine
Johns Hopkins Medical Institutions
Baltimore, MD, USA

Kenneth M. Stein, MD
Associate Professor of Medicine
Maurice and Corinne Greenberg Division of Cardiology
Department of Medicine
Weill Medical College of Cornell University
New York, NY, USA

Christian Sticherling, MD, FESC
Director of the Cardiac Electrophysiology Laboratory
Division of Cardiology
Department of Medicine
University Hospital Basel
Basel, Switzerland

Valerio Zacà, MD
Section of Cardiovascular Diseases, Department of Experimental and Applied Medicine
University of Brescia
Brescia, Italy

Preface

Over the past five decades pacing has been regarded as the only non-pharmacological therapy for many life-threatening bradycardias or tachycardias. We are now moving into a new conceptual phase of pacing which could be called the "electrical-mechanical era". It is the application of an electrically-based, highly effective therapy, cardiac resynchronization therapy (CRT), which opens up new areas of potential mechanisms, diagnostic capabilities and treatments.

It has been known for long time that heart failure is often associated with abnormal electrical activation which may lead to regional mechanical dyssynchrony. The ability to correct electrical and mechanical dyssynchrony via simultaneous pacing of the left and right ventricles has had to await the development of technology to place leads into the coronary sinus and into the left ventricular lateral cardiac vein; this requires high skill and great confidence in pacing lead manipulation using coronary angioplasty-like tools. CRT improves symptoms, reduces mortality and reverses maladaptive remodeling processes. Indications for CRT and other electrically-based therapies of heart failure are rapidly evolving, including application of this technology to less sick heart failure patients and more traditional pacing populations. However, it is equally clear that not all patients benefit and there is a subset who fail to show the expected improvement. Much effort has been expended recently in trying to characterize these patients. Studies have been designed to identify different potential predictors of lack of response to CRT therapy, but not routinely implemented yet into clinical practice. Novel technologies enable us to provide continuous, device-based, heart failure monitoring and management resulting in an unprecedented integration of medical know-how, and imposing novel strategies for health care professionals managing heart failure patients.

We are making progress in the treatment of what was considered to be a progressive and highly lethal disease and pacing to support the failing heart is another big step forward. This book intends to share with students, allied health care professionals, and physicians interested in the management of heart failure the most updated knowledge in the field of pacing for heart failure. We are extremely grateful to the American Heart Association and to Series Editor, Dr. Elliott Antman, for the opportunity to collect and to edit the view of several world-class experts in device therapy and heart failure.

Kenneth Ellenbogen
Angelo Auricchio

Foreword

The strategic driving force behind the American Heart Association's mission of reducing disability and death from cardiovascular diseases and stroke is to change practice by providing information and solutions to healthcare professionals. The pillars of this strategy are Knowledge Discovery, Knowledge Processing, and Knowledge Transfer. The books in the AHA Clinical Series, of which *Pacing to Support the Failing Heart* is included, focus on high-interest, cutting-edge topics in cardiovascular medicine. This book series is a critical tool that supports the AHA mission of promoting healthy behavior and improved care of patients. Cardiology is a rapidly changing field, and practitioners need data to guide their clinical decision making. The AHA Clinical Series serves this need by providing the latest information on the physiology, diagnosis, and management of a broad spectrum of conditions encountered in daily practice.

Rose Marie Robertson, MD, FAHA
Chief Science Officer, American Heart Association

Elliott Antman, MD, FAHA
Director, Samuel A. Levine Cardiac Unit,
Brigham and Women's Hospital

Integrated heart failure management in the patient with heart failure caused by left ventricular systolic dysfunction

Marco Metra, Valerio Zacà, Savina Nodari, and Livio Dei Cas

Key Points

1. The increasing burden of heart failure is a result of the aging population and improvements in cardiac care. It is estimated that 660,000 new cases of heart failure are diagnosed every year in the United States.
2. Heart failure with normal ejection fraction (HFNEF) is part of a single entity of heart failure that includes also heart failure with decreased ejection fraction. The prognosis of HFNEF is similar to the prognosis of patients with low ejection fraction.
3. Sustained activation of the renin angiotensin aldosterone system as well as the sympathoadrenergic system is one of the main causes of progression of this disease, if not the most important one,.
4. ACE (angiotensin converting enzyme) inhibitors result in beneficial effects on hemodynamics, exercise capacity and improve outcomes, reducing the mortality and hospitalizations rates, of the patients with heart failure.
5. Angiotensin receptor blockers (ARBs) are similar beneficial effects as ACE inhibitors so that they are valid alternatives to ACE inhibitors in patients who do not tolerate them. When added to ACE inhibitors, ARBs provide a further improvement in outcomes.
6. Aldosterone antagonists are recommended in patients with severe symptoms of heart failure and reduced left ventricular ejection fraction in addition to ACE inhibitors, beta-blockers and diuretics.
7. Overwhelming evidence supports the long term efficacy of beta blocker therapy on all cause and cardiovascular mortality in patients with mild to severe heart failure.

Pacing to Support the Failing Heart, 1st edition. Edited by K. Ellenbogen and A. Auricchio.
© 2008 American Heart Association, ISBN: 978-1-4051-7534-0

8. Hydralazine and isorbide dinitrate are useful for the treatment of heart failure in African-American patients. Treatment with these agents in combination improves symptoms and outcomes.
9. Antiarrhythmic agents are not indicated for sudden cardiac death prophylaxis in heart failure patients.
10. QRS prolongation is an independent predictor of poor prognosis in various heart failure populations.

Introduction

Definitions and epidemiology

Heart failure (HF) has been defined as a syndrome in which a patient has symptoms, typically breathlessness or fatigue, either at rest of during exertion, and/or ankle swelling, and objective evidence of cardiac dysfunction at rest [1].

Heart failure is the final stage of virtually all cardiac diseases and represents a major public health problem for Western countries[1–3]. The prevalence of HF has risen to epidemic levels in both North America and Europe [4]. It is estimated there are approximately 5,300,000 adults with HF in the United States with 660,000 new cases diagnosed every year—these cases have been increasing steadily over the past 20 years [5, 6]. Due to the aging population and the improvement of acute cardiac care, the burden of HF is expected to grow further, with one projection showing an increase in prevalence of HF of 31% and 17%, in males and females, respectively by the year 2020. [7] The number of hospitalizations has also risen—1,084,000 hospital discharges (a 171% increase as compared to 1979) were recorded in 2005 in the United States [4]. Similar data have been obtained in Europe with a prevalence of 0.4– 2% of the general European population, which shows acute HF as the main cause of hospitalization in patients >65 years of age [8, 9]. The overall economic cost of HF is expected to reach US$34.8 billion in 2008 [4] with HF causing 2–3% of the total healthcare expenditure in European countries

Mortality rates have significantly decreased over the last 10 years [10–13]. New drugs and cardiac resynchronization therapy (CRT) have further reduced annual mortality to rates of approximately 8–10% [14–16]. However, the prognosis for patients with HF remains worse in an in-hospital mortality rate of 4–9%, with postdischarge 6-month mortality and rehospitalization rates of 9%–15% and 30–45%. One-year and 5-year mortality rates remain at 20–30% and about 50%, respectively [10–13].

Asymptomatic and symptomatic, systolic and diastolic left ventricular dysfunction

Heart failure is the final outcome of a process initiated by risk factors and, then, a cardiovascular disease causing myocardial damage, followed by left ventricular (LV) remodeling, LV dysfunction, and progression to symptomatic HF [2, 3]. As a result, the first step of an integrated HF management strategy is prevention with effective treatment of known risk factors (hypertension, diabetes, hyperlipidemia) and early diagnosis and treatment of LV dysfunction in subjects at high risk (e.g. families of patients with dilated cardiomyopathy, patients on chemotherapy) [2, 3]. Either systolic and/or diastolic LV dysfunction or, more frequently, their combination may be the underlying mechanism of HF. Systolic dysfunction is usually defined on the basis of the LV ejection fraction (EF). In general, 38–54% of patients with HF have preserved left ventricular ejection fraction (LVEF) [21]. As these patients may have other, more subtle, abnormalities of LV systolic function (e.g. a depressed LV long-axis shortening) and as abnormalities of diastolic function are present also in the patients with a low LVEF (in whom the abnormalities may actually be more related to symptoms than abnormalities of systolic function), the definition of HF with preserved EF (HFPEF) or HF with normal EF is preferred, over that of diastolic HF [1, 21].

The hypothesis underlying this preferred definition is that HF is a single-entity characterized by a progressive decline in LV systolic performance so that there is a progression from HFPEF to HF with reduced LVEF. Actually, LV volumes, measured by three-dimensional echocardiography, are often increased in HFPEF patients, compared to normal subjects after matching for age, gender, and body size, which suggests an earlier stage of LV remodeling in these patients [21]. In addition, LVEF has shown a unimodal distribution in large studies including HF patients independent of their LVEF values. This definition is in agreement with the "single entity hypothesis" for HFPEF and HF with reduced LVEF [9,22,23]. Lastly, despite demographic differences (HFPEF patients are more likely to be females, older, and with a history of hypertension), the prognosis of HFPEF is similar to the prognosis of the patients with low LVEF with respect of both hospitalization and mortality [21].

Once the diagnosis of HF is established, treatment is aimed at the improvement of symptoms, quality of life, and/or survival [1–3]. Several pharmacological and nonpharmacological tools have consistently been shown to be effective in reducing mortality and morbidity [1–3]. However, treating HF remains an extremely challenging task. We will summarize the optimal medical management of chronic HF. We will focus mainly on patients with evidence of LV systolic dysfunction. There are no major differences in the medical treatment of patients with HFPEF, compared to those with reduced LVEF [24]. We will not discuss the treatment of these patients (HFPEF) or of the patients with acute HF in this chapter.

Medical management of chronic heart failure

General considerations

Medical treatment of HF is based on the combination of different agents administered with the aim of improving prognosis (mainly through neurohormonal inhibition) and/or relieving symptoms. Combination of an ACE inhibitor and a beta-blocker constitute the background therapy for virtually all HF patients, the addition of agents, such as angiotensin receptor blockers (ARBs), aldosterone antagonists, hydralazine, and isosorbide dinitrate, may provide, additional survival benefits [1–3]. As a rule, only agents with proven efficacy in large randomized controlled trials are recommended for clinical practice, and these agents should be administered at the doses shown to be effective in controlled trials [1–3]. Failure to reach the target dose may translate into lower clinical benefits or no benefits at all. To be effective, medical therapy of HF with neurohumoral antagonists has to be optimal with regard to drug choice, as well as include up-titration to the recommended dose [1–3]. Other agents are critical in the management of HF not for prognosis but rather for their effect on symptoms. Diuretics are of crucial importance in the control of the volume status and for improving symptoms due to fluid retention and congestion, while digoxin ameliorates the clinical status and reduces the need for hospitalization due to HF [1–3].

Angiotensin converting enzyme inhibitors

The introduction of angiotensin converting enzyme (ACE) inhibitors into clinical practice has radically changed treatment of HF. Their use is based on numerous placebo-controlled trials showing their beneficial effects on outcome [25, 26]. Their effects were also shown to be different and of greater magnitude, with respect to outcome, compared to those of direct vasodilators [27]. Based on these data, ACE inhibitors have become, and still remain, the drugs of first choice for the treatment of chronic HF [1–3]. Their efficacy has also indirectly proven the hypothesis that neurohormonal mechanisms, namely the rnin-angioteusin aldosterone system (RAAS), play a pivotal role in the progression of LV dysfunction and the poor outcome of the patients with HF [28–33].

Mechanisms

Sustained activation of the RAAS, as well as of the sympathoadrenergic system, although initially acting as a compensatory mechanism, is a major determinant of the development and progression of HF ultimately leading to LV dysfunction and maladaptive remodeling. Modulation of these neurohormonal systems plays a pivotal role in the management of HF and inhibitors of the RAAS and beta-adrenergic receptor blockers are the keystones of current medical therapy of HF[28–33]. The RAAS is activated in patients with HF and has multiple effects contributing to the progression of this disease [31, 32, 34]. Angiotensin II (AII) causes constriction of the peripheral vasculature with increased LV afterload, is implicated in the development of atherosclerosis, and causes salt and water retention at the renal level. In the long-term, AII stimulation causes hypertrophy of smooth muscle vascular cells, which contributes further to peripheral vasoconstriction, and myocardial hypertrophy. Myocardial pathological hypertrophy and fibrosis are the mechanisms causing LV remodeling and dysfunction.

In addition, AII stimulates sympathetic drive through increased norepinephrine release from nerve terminals, increased ganglionic transmission, and heightened sympathetic central drive. It also stimulates aldosterone secretion, and aldosterone further contributes to renal salt and water retention, potassium loss, myocardial fibrosis, and increased sympathetic drive.

Clinical effects

Angiotensin converting enzyme inhibitors act upstream in the RAAS inhibiting the conversion of Ang I to Ang II and the degradation of bradykinin [1–3]. It has become clear, however, that ACE inhibitors provide only an incomplete inhibition of the RAAS so that concomitant administration of angiotensin receptor blockers and/or aldosterone antagonists is warranted in many patients with HF [14, 35].

As early as 30 years ago, ACE inhibitors were shown to exert many beneficial effects on hemodynamic parameters and exercise capacity [36, 37]. More importantly, these agents were shown to inhibit or reverse LV remodeling with stable or reduced LV volumes during long-term treatment [38, 39].

The effects on outcomes of long-term therapy with ACE inhibitors have been assessed in several randomized controlled clinical trials in different clinical conditions, including chronic HF [25, 26], postmyocardial infarction HF and/or LV systolic dysfunction [40–43], and asymptomatic LV systolic dysfunction [44] (Table 1.1). In patients with chronic HF, long-term administration of ACE inhibitors is associated with a significant reduction in mortality and hospitalizations for HF [25–27]. In the post-MI setting, ACE inhibition has been shown to favorably affect LV remodeling, reduce HF hospitalizations, as well as recurrent ischemic events, and improve survival [40–43].

The role of ACE inhibitors in patients with asymptomatic LV systolic dysfunction was assessed for the first time in the Studies of Left Ventricular Dysfunction (SOLVD)-Prevention study. This trial included 4,228 patients with asymptomatic LV systolic dysfunction (EF <35%), randomized to enalapril 10 mg b.i.d. or a placebo, and showed a significant reduction in the number of deaths and HF hospitalizations, but not of mortality alone, with the ACE-inhibitor (20% risk reduction; 95% confidence interval [CI], 9–30%; $p < 0.001$) [44]. The lack of effects on mortality alone in the original study is explained by the low number of events. Accordingly, Jong et al. reported an improvement of the 12-year survival in the SOLVD-Prevention study population randomized to enalapril as compared to those on a placebo in a longer-term follow-up [45]. Persistence of the beneficial effects of ACE-inhibitor therapy has been shown also in the 10-year follow-up of the patients randomized in CONSENSUS (risk reduction of 30%, 95%CIs 11–46%; $p = 0.008$). This long-term follow-up study showed that the beneficial effects of enalapril, compared to a placebo, was sustained for at least 4 years

Table 1.1 Selection of landmark controlled trials of medical therapy in heart failure and asymptomatic and symptomatic left ventricular dysfunction.

Trial	Agent	Inclusion criteria		Patients No.	Target dose	Follow-up	Overall mortality[−]
		NYHA Class	LVEF				
ACE-Inhibitors							
Chronic HF							
Captopril Multicenter Research Group	Captopril	II–III	≤40%	92	100 mg t.i.d.	12 weeks	n/a
CONSENSUS	Enalapril	IV	n/a	253	20 mg b.i.d.	188 days	−40%
SOLVD-Treatment	Enalapril	II–III	≤35%	2,569	10 mg b.i.d.	41.4 months	−16%
Post-MI							
SAVE	Captopril	–	≤40%	2,231	25–50 mg t.i.d.	42 months	−19%
AIRE	Ramipril	Clinical HF		2,006	5 mg b.i.d.	15 months	−27%
TRACE	Trandolapril	–	≤35%	1,749	4 mg s.i.d.	24–50 months	−22%
Asymptomatic LV dysfunction							
SOLVD-Prevention	Enalapril	–	<35%	4,228	10 mg b.i.d.	37.4 months	N.S.
ARBs							
Chronic HF							
CHARM-Added	Candesartan	II–IV	≤40%	2,548	32 mg s.i.d.	41 months	N.S.
CHARM-Alternative	Candesartan		≤40%	2,028	32 mg s.i.d.	33.7 months	−23%*
Post-MI							
VALIANT	Valsartan vs. Captopril	–	<40%	14,703	320 mg s.i.d. vs. 80 mg t.i.d.	24.7 months	noninferiority

Aldosterone Antagonists								
Chronic HF	RALES	Spironolactone	III–IV	≤35%	1,633	25 s.i.d.	24 months	–30%
Post-MI	EPHESUS	Eplerenone	–	≤40%	6,632	50 mg s.i.d.	16 months	–15%*
Beta-Blockers								
Chronic HF	US Carvedilol Heart Failure Study	Carvedilol	II–IV	<35%	1,094	25–50 mg b.i.d.	7 months	–65%
	CIBIS II	Bisoprolol	III–IV	<35%	2,647	10 mg s.i.d.	15.6 months	–34%
	MERIT-HF	Metoprolol CR/XL	II–IV	<40%	3,991	200 mg s.i.d.	15 months	–34%
	COPERNICUS	Carvedilol	III–IV	<25%	2,289	25 mg b.i.d.	10.4 months	–35%
Post-MI	CAPRICORN	Capricorn	–	≤40%	1,959	25 mg b.i.d.		–23%

*cardiovascular death or hospital admission for HF. ACE = angiotensin converting enzyme; AIRE = Acute Infarction Ramipril Efficacy; ARBs = angiotensin receptor blockers; CAPRICORN = Carvedilol Post Infarct Survival Control in Left Ventricular Dysfunction; CHARM = Candesartan in Heart Failure: Assessment of Reduction in Mortality and Morbidity; CIBIS = Cardiac Insufficiency Bisoprolol Trial; CONSENSUS = Cooperative North Scandinavian Enalapril Survival Study; COPERNICUS = Carvedilol Prospective Randomized Cumulative Survival; EF = ejection fraction; EPHESUS = Eplerenone Post-Acute Myocardial Infarction Heart failure Efficacy and Survival Study; HF = heart failure; MERIT = Metoprolol Controlled-Release Randomized Intervention Trial in Congestive Heart Failure; MI = myocardial infarction NYHA = New York Heart Association; RALES = Randomized Aldactone Evaluation Study; SAVE = Survival and Ventricular Enlargement; SOLVD = Studies of Left Ventricular Dysfunction; TRACE = Trandolapril Cardiac Evaluation; VALIANT = Valsartan in Acute Myocardial Infarction Trial.

(–) a reduction in overall mortality of (minus)...

with a 50% average prolongation of life duration (from 521 days to 781 days) [46]. These data, therefore, also show that the beneficial effects of ACE inhibition are limited in time, and ACE inhibitors cannot be considered the only treatment of patients with chronic HF both with respect to inhibition of the RAAS and, more generally, with the aim of improving outcomes.

Recommendations for clinical practice

All current guidelines recommend the use of an ACE inhibitor as first-line therapy for all patients with reduced LVEF ($\leq$40–45%) with or without current or prior symptoms of HF. Doses of ACE inhibitors indicated for the treatment of HF (i.e. captopril, enalapril, lisinopril, ramipril, and trandolapril) should be those that have been shown to be effective in clinical trials [1–3].

Angiotensin receptor blockers

Angiotensin receptors blockers (ARBs) block the action of AII on AII type I receptors (AT1) [1, 2, 14, 47]. ARBs do not interfere with the degradation of bradykinin as ACE inhibitors do. ARBs are different than ACE inhibitors in two ways: first, lack of the favorable effects of increased kinin levels on peripheral vasodilation and LV remodeling; second, lack of the kinin-mediated side effects of ACE inhibitors, namely, cough and angioneurotic edema. In addition, administration of ARBs is associated with increased AII levels with greater stimulation of AII type II receptors, which seem to mediate mainly beneficial effects on peripheral vasodilation and myocardial hyper- trophy.

Clinical effects

The hemodynamic and antiremodeling effects of ARBs are similar to those of ACE inhibitors [48]. A II levels tend to progressively increase after months to years of ACE-inhibition therapy [35] (the so-called escape phenomenon) and, as a consequence, the effects of ACE inhibitors on cardiac remodeling attenuate after 1 year of treatment. These observations, along with the biologic rationale of a more complete inhibition of the RAAS, have led to the development of strategies combining the use of ARBs and ACE inhibitors.

Clinical trials

Trials have been specifically designed to assess the effects of candesartan, losartan, and valsartan, the only ARBs currently recommended for use in HF patients, as alternatives to [49–52], or in combination with, [53–55] ACE inhibitors.

Among the trials in patients with post-MI LV systolic dysfunction or HF, Optimal Trial in Myocardial Infarction with Angiotensin II Antagonist Losartan (OPTIMAAL) showed similar effects on outcomes of losartan, compared to captopril. The Valsartan in Acute Myocardial Infarction (VALIANT) trial demonstrated the noninferiority of valsartan, compared to captopril, with respect to all-cause mortality, the combined cardiovascular endpoints, and all of the secondary endpoints [49].

In the Valsartan in Heart Failure Trial (Val-HeFT) trial, 5,010 patients with chronic HF were randomized to valsartan, titrated up to dosage of 160 mg b.i.d., or a placebo, on top of optimal medical treatment for HF, including ACE inhibitors in 93% of patients and beta-blockers in 35% of patients [54]. Candesartan administration was associated with a reduction in the primary endpoint of morbidity and mortality and in HF hospitalization but not a reduction in mortality alone [54]. In the Candesartan in Heart Failure: Assessment of Reduction in Mortality and Morbidity (CHARM)-Added trial, 2,548 patients with NYHA Class II–IV HF and LV dysfunction (EF<40%) already treated with ACE inhibitors (all patients), beta-blockers (55%), and aldosterone antagonists (17%) were randomized to a candesartan 32 mg, once daily dosage, or a placebo. Addition of candesartan reduced the incidence of the primary endpoint (risk reduction, 15%, 95% CIs, 4–15%; $p = 0.011$), as well as its individual components: cardiovascular deaths ($p = 0.029$) and HF hospitalizations ($p = 0.014$)[55]. An important result showed that the association of ACE inhibitors and ARBs in patients on beta-blockers and/or on high doses of ACE inhibitors was associated with a reduction in cardiac events. These results differ from the results in the Val-HeFT [54, 55]. These differences are likely explained by the larger number of patients on beta-blocker treatment and by greater severity of HF in the patients who were randomized in the CHARM trial compared to those in Val-HeFT (e.g. patients in Class II randomized in the CHARM-Added trial had to have hospital admission for a cardiac reason in the previous 6 months, more patients were on beta-blockers, and the event rate was higher).

The CHARM-Alternative trial specifically tested the hypothesis of the efficacy of ARBs as an alternative to ACE-inhibitor–intolerant patients [52]. Among the 2,028 patients enrolled in the study, treatment with a candesartan 32 mg daily dosage was associated with a significant reduction of cardiovascular mortality and HF hospitalizations as compared to placebo (unadjusted risk reduction 23%; 95% CI, 11– 33%; $p<0.0004$; covariate adjusted risk reduction 30%; 95% CI, 19– 40%; $p<0.0001$), with similar discontinuation rates compared to placebo (30% vs. 29%). Similar effects were also found with respect to clinical endpoints [52]. Consistently with what was shown by a retrospective analysis of Val-HeFT [56], the magnitude of the beneficial effects of ARBs administration, compared to a placebo, were larger than when these agents are added to ongoing ACE-inhibitor treatment.

Recommendations for clinical practice
ARBs of proven efficacy in HF trials is recommended as a first-line therapy in patients intolerant to ACE inhibitors. An association of ARBs and ACE inhibitors appears reasonable in patients with reduced LVEF who remain symptomatic despite background treatment with conventional agents [1–3,57].

Aldosterone antagonists

Activation of the RAAS causes an increase in plasma aldosterone levels. These remain elevated despite treatment with ACE inhibitors and/or ARBs (aldosterone escape phenomenon) [35,58]. Aldosterone has many untoward effects including salt and water retention, increased potassium loss with hypokalemia, increased sympathetic drive, myocardial hypertrophy, and fibrosis. These changes are consistent with the increase in cardiovascular events in the patients with higher aldosterone plasma levels [59–61] and constitute the rationale for concomitant administration of aldosterone receptor blockers in patients with HF on optimal medical therapy. This hypothesis has been formally tested in the Randomized Aldactone Evaluation Study (RALES) [62] and the Eplerenone Post-Acute Myocardial Infraction Heart Failure Efficacy and Survival Study (EPHESUS) trials [63].

The RALES trial assessed the effects of a spironolactone 25 mg daily dosage, as an adjunct to ACE inhibitors and diuretics, in 1,633 patients with severe HF (LVEF <35% and NYHA Class IV or Class III but Class IV in the previous 6 months). Spironolactone treatment was associated with a 30% (95% CI, 18–40%; $p<0.001$) relative risk reduction in mortality and a 35% risk reduction (95% CI, 33–46%; $p<0.001$) in HF hospitalizations paralleled by an improvement in functional class [62]. The selective aldosterone antagonist eplerenone was evaluated in the EPHESUS trial in 6,632 patients with recent MI, LV systolic dysfunction, and either symptomatic HF or diabetes. Therapy with an eplerenone 50 mg daily dosage resulted in a 15% reduction in all-cause mortality (95% CI, 4–25%; $p = 0.008$), with a significant reduction in cardiovascular death (including sudden death), and in hospitalizations for HF and cardiovascular causes [63].

Recommendations for clinical practice

Administration of an aldosterone antagonist is recommended in patients with severe symptoms of HF (NYHA Class III–IV) and reduced LVEF in addition to ACE inhibitors, beta-blockers, and diuretics. The adjunct of these agents is also recommended in post-MI patients with evidence of LV systolic dysfunction and HF. Careful monitoring of serum potassium and creatinine is necessary [1–3, 57]. Current guidelines do not give any indication with respect to which drug (e.g. an ARB or an aldosterone antagonist) should be added first when a patient is still symptomatic and is still receiving on ongoing treatment with ACE inhibitors and beta-blockers [1–3].

Quadruple combination of neurohormonal antagonists

Although fascinating from a biologic standpoint, a complete inhibition of the RAAS with a combination of ACE inhibitors, ARBs, and aldosterone antagonists, on top of beta-blockers, is used infrequently because of its low tolerability. A retrospective analysis from the CHARM trials has, however, shown no change in the beneficial effects on outcomes with candesartan, compared to a placebo, when added to triple therapy with neurohormonal antagonists, including ACE inhibitors, aldosterone antagonists, and beta-blockers, compared to the results in the overall study population [64]. Increased risk of hypotension, renal dysfunction and hyperkalemia must, however, be taken into account when administering all four neurohormonal anatgonists [1–3, 20, 57].

Beta- blockers

Sympathoadrenergic stimulation has long-term untoward effects on the failing heart. These include beta-1 receptor downregulation and desensitization, increased heart rate, increased wall stress and myocardial oxygen consumption, abnormal sarcoplasmic reticulum calcium cycling, induction of fetal gene program with downregulation of alpha-myosin heavy chains and upregulation of beta-myosin heavy expression with decreased myosin ATPase enzyme velocity, and slow speed of contraction, induction of cell necrosis and apoptosis[30, 33, 65–68]. These mechanisms constitute the rationale basis for beta-blocker treatment of patients with HF.

Effects on LV function and symptoms

Beta-blocker administration has short-term negative inotropic effects. For many years, this has represented a contraindication to their administration to patients with HF. However, it may be safely avoided by starting treatment with very low doses followed by their gradual and slow up-titration to target doses [1–3, 57, 69]. In selected patients with severe and hemodynamically unstable HF, concomitant administration of inotropic agents acting independently from beta-receptors may be useful [8, 70].

Long-term therapy with beta-blockers produces an increase in stroke volume and cardiac output along with a reduction in pulmonary capillary wedge pressure, right atrial pressure, and systemic vascular resistance [71–73]. These favorable hemodynamic changes are generally not associated with significant improvement in exercise capacity because blunting of the heart rate response to exercise does not allow a sufficient increase in exercise cardiac output. An improvement in symptoms may be more easily shown by direct patient assessment, questionnaires, and, above all, in single center studies by submaximal exercise capacity assessment [74,75]. An exception may be represented by nebivolol, as shown in a study in patients with HF and preserved LVEF [76].

All of the beta-blockers currently approved for the treatment of HF, have been shown to induce a significant improvement in cardiac function and a true global and structural reverse remodeling of the LV [77–79]. The profound changes in LV structure and function associated with beta-blocker therapy (more elliptical shape of the LV, reduction in mitral regurgitation and LV volumes) show the importance of sympathetic activation in the pathogenesis of myocardial dysfunction and the ability of beta-blockers to interfere with the intrinsic mechanisms leading to HF [65, 66, 80]. The observed benefits on LV function, as well as those on outcomes, are maintained or magnified over time and are superior to those obtained with any other agent available for treating HF [65, 66].

Nonischemic aetiology of HF, higher blood pressure, and reversible contractile dysfunction at dobutamine echocardiography (as indexes of reversibility of myocardial damage) are predictors of greater improvement in LVEF and function during long-term beta-blocker therapy [81, 82]. Marked improvement in LVEF may be observed in approximately 25% of patients with chronic HF and is associated with an excellent long-term outcome [81]. Beta-blockers were the first agents for which such a tight link between improvement in LV function and outcome could be shown. Similar results were going to be later shown with CRT [83–85].

Effects on outcomes

There is overwhelming evidence supporting the beneficial effects of long-term beta-blocker therapy on all-cause and cardiovascular mortality as well as all-cause, cardiovascular, and HF hospitalizations. These beneficial effects have been shown across a broad range of severity of LV systolic dysfunction and NYHA classes [86–90]. The reduction in mortality with beta-blockers, compared to placebo, is about 35% and is greater in magnitude compared to that obtained with other neurohormonal antagonists [65]. There is also a significant percent reduction in sudden death (41–44%), all-cause hospitalizations (18–20%) and HF hospitalizations (32–35%) [86–90].

Differences between beta-blockers with respect to their effects on outcome, consistent with what has been previously shown with respect to their effects on LV function [67, 73], have been shown[91]. Although differences in doses and degrees of beta-blockade may have influenced these results [92], it is likely that peculiar characteristics of carvedilol (as compared to metoprolol tartrate), yield a more stable and persistent blockade of beta-1 adrenergic receptors [70, 93], and have ancillary effects on other mechanisms (beta-2 receptor blockade, antioxidant activity, metabolic effects, protection from ischemic events), which may account for differences in outcomes [94–96].

The efficacy of beta-blockers has been more recently shown in groups of patients that were not included in the initial trials. The Carvedilol Post-Infarct Survival Control in LV Dysfunction (CAPRICORN) study showed the beneficial effects on mortality of carvedilol in patients with post-MI LV dysfunction on optimal medical treatment including ACE inhibition and reperfusion [97]. The recent Study of the Effects of Nebivolol Intervention on Outcomes and Rehospitalisation in Seniors with Heart Failure (SENIORS) pointed out the potential effects of beta-blockade therapy in elderly patients ($\geq$ 70 years) with a broad spectrum of LV systolic dysfunction.[98] This trial included 2,128 patients with a mean age of 76 years, history of HF regardless of LVEF, who were randomized to either nebivolol (target dose 10 mg) or placebo. Patients were followed for a mean of 21 months [98]. Nebivolol was associated with a 14% relative risk reduction (95% CI 1–%; $p = 0.039$) for the occurrence of the primary endpoint of all-cause mortality and cardiovascular hospitalizations [98].To overcome the potential bias, due to the differences in the studied populations and compare to previous HF trials, a non-prespecified analysis of a subgroup of patients aged <75 years and with LVEF ≤35% was performed. In this subgroup of patients, more similar to those from the other major mortality trials, there was a 27% (95% CI, 4–44%) relative risk reduction for the primary endpoint and a 38% (95% CI, 11–37%) relative risk reduction for all-cause mortality alone[98], which is similar to that found in previous HF trials.

It has been recently proposed that, at least with some beta-blockers (e.g. bucin-dolol), assessment of gene polymorphisms may help to better select patients more likely to show a favorable response to treatment. The influence of polymor-phisms of the genes encoding for the beta-1 adrenergic receptors was assessed in 1,040 patients enrolled in the Beta-Blocker Evaluation of Survival Trial (BEST). Bucindolol had a neutral effect on mortality compared to placebo, in this trial. However, homozygotes for the Arg-389 allele, associated with a three-fold increase in sensitivity to adrenergic stimulation *in vitro*, had an age-adjusted, sex-adjusted, and race-adjusted 38% reduction in mortality ($p = 0.03$) and 34% reduction in mortality or hospitalization ($p = 0.004$) when randomized to bucin-dolol versus a placebo. In contrast, Gly-389 carriers had no clinical response to bucindolol compared with the placebo [99].

Recommendations for clinical practice

Bisoprolol, carvedilol, and sustained release metoprolol succinate, are recom-mended for the treatment of all patients with mild-to-severe HF and reduced LVEF [1–3,57]. European guidelines include also nebivolol among the beta-blockers indicated for HF treatment [1]. Beta-blockers should always be used in association with ACE inhibitors (although the recent CIBIS-III trial showed no difference in outcomes when beta-blockers are started first) [100]. As mentioned earlier, beta-blockade therapy should be initiated with very low doses followed by gradual titration up to doses achieved in clinical trials. Doses are shown in the guidelines [1–3,57]. If possible, beta-blockers should not be discontinued in patients with acute decompensation of HF as this may be associated with increased mortality [8, 101].

Diuretics

Fluid retention, with systemic and/or pulmonary congestion, accounts for the vast majority of symptoms in HF patients [102, 103]. Diuretics are, therefore, the mainstay of treatment of symptoms of the patients with HF. Diuretics promote the urinary excretion of salt and water by acting at different levels in the nephron: the Henle loop for loop diuretics (furosemide, torasemide, bumetanide, etacrinic acid) and the distal convoluting tubule for thiazides, metolazone and potassium-sparing diuretics [102, 104] Loop diuretics are the preferred agents for most of the patients with the possible exception of only patients with mild symptoms [1, 2].

Diuretics promptly ameliorate symptoms, reduce signs of congestion, and treat and prevent salt and water retention[1–3]. Their effect on symptoms has always prevented any randomized controlled trial to assess their effects on outcomes. However, diuretic therapy [105–107], as well as treatment with high furosemide doses [108, 109], have been associated with a poor outcome (mortality, hospitalizations, incidence of worsening renal function). These associations persist after adjustment for other baseline variables, including those related to HF severity. This suggests, although it does not prove, that diuretic treatment may contribute to the progression of LV dysfunction and HF [110]. The potential mechanisms that may be involved include neurohormonal activation, namely RAAS [111], electrolyte abnormalities (with increased arrhythmic risk) [105, 106, 112], and worsening renal function [109]. Long-term treatment with loop diuretics is also associated with the development of resistance (e.g. the need of increasing doses to achieve diuresis and the increase of maximal diuretic response). This is a hallmark of advanced HF and one of the major problems in these patients [20].

Concerns regarding the long-term effects of diuretic therapy have fostered research to look for potential alternatives (e.g. ultrafiltration) [113] or concomitant agents (e.g. adenosine antagonists, RAAS inhibitors) [114], which may counteract the untoward effects of diuretic treatment. To date, it is universally recommended to administer diuretics at the lowest doses that are effective to correct and prevent salt and water retention and combine them with ACE inhibitors and beta-blockers[1–3].

Digitalis

Cardiac glycosides are among the oldest medications still used in current medical practice. Digitalis exerts positive inotropic effects via inhibition of Na-K-ATPase and stimulation of Na+-Ca2+ exchange with a secondary increase in intracellular calcium [115]. Furthermore, digitalis modulates the autonomic nervous system activity by partially restoring the responsiveness of the baroreflex system, possibly at blood concentrations lower than those necessary to achieve an inotropic effect [115]. Digitalis is useful for symptom control as it may improve clinical status and exercise tolerance, and decrease HF hospitalization rate. No effect on mortality has been shown in the same large multicenter trial in the overall study group [116]. Retrospective analyses of the Digitalis Investigators Study have shown opposite effects on mortality depending on the serum digoxin levels achieved during treatment. Mortality was reduced with digoxin, compared to a placebo, only in the patients who achieved low serum digoxin concentration (SDC) (0.5–0.9 pg/ml) during treatment whereas HF hospitalizations were reduced independently from SDC [117]. Similar results were obtained in a previous analysis, which also showed an increase in mortality in the patients with SDC >1.2 ng/ml [118].

Recommendations for clinical practice

Digitalis glycosides can be recommended for the prevention of HF hospitalizations in the patients with HF and severe, NYHA Class III–IV, HF and/or previous HF hospitalizations. It should be administered at low doses targeting SDC less than 1 ng/ml. Digitalis remains indicated in the patients with HF and atrial fibrillation for heart rate control [1].

Hydralazine-isosorbide dinitrate

Vasodilating agents, such as isosorbide dinitrate, theoretically could be useful in the treatment of chronic HF as they may improve dyspnea through a reduction in LV preload [119]. The association of hydralazine and isosorbide dinitrate has been shown to be less effective in improving outcomes, compared to enalapril therapy [27]. However, it has been more recently shown to further improve outcome, compared to a placebo, in African-American patients already treated with neurohormonal antagonists [120]. Accordingly this association is indicated in the HFSA guidelines as part of standard therapy in African-Americans with reduced LVEF [3]. This combination may be useful for symptomatic treatment in patients with LV systolic dysfunction persistently symptomatic despite optimal therapy.

Antiarrhythmic agents

The use of antiarrhythmic agents for the prevention of sudden cardiac death has been investigated in several randomized controlled trials. The results of these studies have led to the absolute contraindication to the use of Class I antiarrhythmic drugs and d-sotalol because of a significant increase in mortality associated with administration of these agents [121, 122]. Amiodarone and dofetilide have been shown to exert neutral effects on overall mortality and sudden cardiac death so that their administration for primary prevention of sudden cardiac death prophylaxis is not recommended [1–3].

Statins

Statins have a plethora of nonlipid-lowering properties that are, theoretically, useful for the treatment of HF. Evidence from experimental and observational studies suggest that statin therapy may improve cardiac function and LV remodeling along with clinical status mainly through modulation of the systemic inflammatory process [123, 124]. The Controlled Rosuvastatin Multinational Trial in Heart Failure (CORONA) investigated the effects of rosuvastatin added on top of optimal medical therapy in elderly patients with ischemic systolic HF [125]. Rosuvastatin had a neutral effect on the primary composite outcome of death from cardiovascular causes, nonfatal myocardial infarction, and nonfatal stroke ($p = 0.12$). However, patients in the rosuvastatin group had lower all-cause ($p<0.001$) and HF ($p = 0.01$) hospitalizations rate. The GISSI-HF trial, including patients with ischemic and nonischemic HF, will study the effects of rosuvastatin treatment on outcomes in HF [126].

Disease management programs

Disease management has been initially defined as "a comprehensive, integrated system for managing patients by using best practices, clinical practice improvement and other resources and tools to reduce overall cost and improve measurable outcomes in the quality of care" [127]. Disease management programs encompass three major levels of intervention: HF clinics, in which assistance is provided essentially in an outpatient clinic home-delivered care services, and telemedicine [128]. Available evidence on disease management programs suggests that such models of care may significantly reduce hospital re-admission rates and costs while improving patients' clinical status and quality of life with a positive effect on overall survival [128, 129].

From medical treatment to devices: The role of dyssynchrony in heart failure outcomes

Current medical treatment has allowed an impressive improvement in the natural history of HF caused by LV systolic dysfunction. However, as outlined in the introductory section, the quality of life and prognosis of patients with HF remains poor. Despite the benefits obtained with RAAS inhibitors and beta-blockers, the neurohormonal model of HF has not worked out as expected when other agents, acting on seemingly important mechanisms, have been tested [130]. The current model of multicenter randomized controlled trials (e.g. large trials targeting the widest study group as possible, with a single new treatment added on top of a more-and-more complex pharmacologic therapy, and with no knowledge of the main pathogenetic mechanisms acting in that single patient) seems to have reached its limits. Thus, the poor prognosis and quality of life of HF patients, the failure of the neurohormonal model with the new agents tested, and the failure of recent multicenter trials targeting a noncharacterized HF population have paved the way to device therapy, namely, CRT. This treatment, differently from neurohormonal antagonists, acts on a specific well characterized mechanical defect leading to LV remodeling and HF. The selection of patients based on a simple criterion (e.g. QRS duration) and its direct correction through a device, (e.g. without some of the limitations of medical treatment (pharmacokinetics variability, need of compliance, etc)) may explain the success of this treatment, which is, actually, the most beneficial treatment recently shown for patients with HF.

The presence of a QRS duration >120 ms on the surface electrocardiogram (ECG) is an index of mechanical dyssynchroncy [131]. Although this association is not absolute, it is estimated that approximately 70% of patients with left-sided conduction delay have evidence of mechanical dyssynchroncy [132]. The delay in LV electrical activation causing prolonged QRS duration has an important pathophysiological significance because it is associated to an abnormal and mechanically disadvantageous pattern of LV contraction with an impairment of LV pump performance and increased severity of mitral regurgitation [133]. These changes are consistent with the prognostic significance of QRS prolongation as well as with the beneficial effects of CRT on symptoms and prognosis of the HF patients with LV conduction delay.

Epidemiology and prognosis

A prolongation of the QRS complex, defined as a duration ≥120 ms, has been shown in 14–47% of patients with HF, with proportions close to 30% in most studies [134–137]. Intraventricular conduction delay with left bundle branch block (LBBB) morphology is five-fold to seven-fold more frequent than right bundle branch block (RBBB) [137]. QRS prolongation is directly correlated with LV end-diastolic and end-systolic volumes and hence severity of LV dysfunction (Figure 1.1) [138–140]. A QRS duration >120 ms has been shown to have a 99% specificity for LV dysfunction [141]. QRS prolongation is also related with severity of symptoms as assessed through the NYHA functional class [142, 143]. In contrast, it is not related to other factors, such as etiology of HF or concomitant medication. Longitudinal studies have also shown a progressive prolongation of QRS duration during long-term follow-up in HF patients [144].

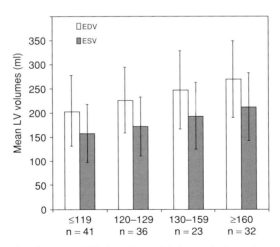

Fig. 1.1 Relationship between QRS duration and left ventricular volumes. A significant increase in LV endiastolic (EDV) and endsystolic (ESV) volumes is noted according to QRS duration. De Winter et al. *Eur J Heart Fail.* 2006;8:275–77.

QRS prolongation has been identified as an independent predictor of poor prognosis in various HF populations [137]. Its potential role was first proposed in the early 1960s [145]. Further studies have shown that QRS prolongation is associated with a higher risk of all-cause death and sudden cardiac death [134–137]. Iuliano et al.[134] retrospectively analyzed data from 669 patients with HF secondary to ischemic and nonischemic cardiomyopathy subdivided into two groups according to QRS duration[134]. Over the course of a median follow-up of 45 months, 129 deaths (34%) and 143 deaths (49.3%) occurred in patients with QRS <120 ms and in patients with QRS ≥120 ms, respectively [134]. Sudden death occurred in 17.4% of patients with QRS <120 ms as compared to 24.8% in patients with QRS ≥120[134]. The role of QRS prolongation was additive to that of LVEF (Figure 1.2) [134]. A recent subgroup analysis from the Val-HeFT trial confirmed the prognostic impact of QRS widening, indicating a gradual increase in mortality rate with increasing duration of QRS, with a 1.8% mortality rate in patients with a QRS <120 ms, 8% in patients with a QRS duration of 120–159 ms, and 17% in patients with a QRS duration ≥160 ms during a median observation

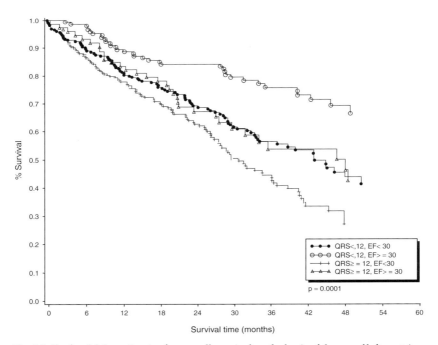

Fig. 1.2 Kaplan-Meier estimates for overall survival on the basis of degree of left ventricular dysfunction and and QRS Duration. Among the four groups, patients with both severe cardiomyopathy (EF<30%) and QRS prolongation (>120 ms) have a significant increase in overall mortality. Iuliano S et al. *Am Heart J.* 2002;143:1085-91.

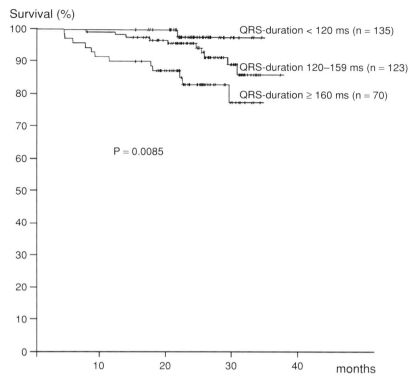

Survival (%)

QRS-duration < 120 ms (n = 135)

QRS-duration 120–159 ms (n = 123)

QRS-duration ≥ 160 ms (n = 70)

P = 0.0085

months

Fig. 1.3 Kaplan-Meier survival curves of patients categorized according to QRS duration <120 ms, 120–159 ms and ≥160 ms. Hofmann M et al. *J Card Fail*. 2005;7:523–8.

period of 25.8 ± 5 months [146] (Figure 1.3). Prolonged QRS duration has been shown to be related to prognosis with a two-fold increase in mortality in patients with a prolonged QRS admitted for acutely decompensated HF [147].

Cardiac resynchronization therapy

A device able to perform atrial-synchronized biventricular pacing (e.g. CRT) was first successfully implanted by Cazeau in 1994, in a 54-year-old man with NYHA Class IV HF and QRS duration of 200 ms [148]. The clinical status of the patient dramatically improved in the first 6 weeks postimplantation. Following this initial experience, the effects of CRT have been extensively investigated in many observational studies and several randomized controlled trials for a total of approximately 15,000 patients with HF and LV systolic dysfunction [149]. Inclusion criteria in major clinical trials of CRT were NYHA Class III–IV, sinus rhythm, QRS duration ≥120 ms and LVEF ≤35% [149]. A recent systematic meta-analysis of 14 randomized controlled trials indicated that CRT improves LVEF (weighted mean difference, 3.0%; 95% CI, 0.9%–5.1%), quality of life (weighted mean reduction in Minnesota Living With Heart Failure Questionnaire, 8.0 points; 95% CI, 5.6–10.4 points), and functional status (improvements of ≥ 1 NYHA class were observed in 59% of CRT recipients in the randomized trials) [149]. More importantly, CRT is associated with a significant reduction in hospitalizations by 37% (95% CI, 7–57%), and in all-cause mortality by 22% (95% CI, 9%–33%) [149]. The positive impact of CRT on morbidity and mortality in HF patients is additional to that provided by polypharmacy as it has been demonstrated in subjects already treated with optimal evidence-based medical therapy [149]. Based on this compelling evidence of the beneficial effects of CRT, current international guidelines recommend the implantation of a CRT, alone or in combination with an implantable cardioverter defibrillator (ICD), device in all eligible HF patients. Accordingly, subjects with persistently symptomatic HF, NYHA functional Class III or ambulatory Class IV, in spite of optimal medical therapy, sinus rhythm, severe LV systolic function (EF $\leq 35\%$), and QRS duration ≥ 120 ms should be implanted with a biventricular pacemaker. It is estimated that approximately 1–3% of all patients discharged alive after their index HF hospitalization, and 15–20% of patients observed in dedicated HF clinics meet CRT trials' eligibility criteria [150], while approximately 50% of these subjects also met trials' eligibility criteria for an ICD [151].

Conclusions

Effective options are now available for the treatment of HF patients. However, despite recent advances in pharmacological and nonpharmacological therapy, morbidity and mortality of HF patients remain unacceptably high [2]. Thus, any effort is necessary to optimize treatment of our patients. Nowadays, this requires an integrated management approach combining medical treatment and devices. On the other hand, the benefits of device treatment have been shown on top of optimal medical management. Such a complex management can not be afforded by a single expert but rather requires the integrated effort of a well-organized team, able to furnish thorough diagnostic assessment, medical therapy, device implantation, and in-hospital and out-of-hospital patient's monitoring, treatment, and follow-up.

References

1. Swedberg K, Cleland J, Dargie H, et al. Guidelines for the diagnosis and treatment ochronic heart failure: executive summary (2005 update). The Task Force for the Diagnosis and Treatment of Chronic Heart Failure of the European Society of Cardiology. *Eur Heart J*. 2005;26:1115–40.
2. Hunt SA, Abraham WT, Chin MH, et al. ACC/AHA 2005 guideline update for the diagnosis and management of chronic heart failure in the adult: a report of the

American College of Cardiology / American Heart Association Task Force on Practice Guidelines. (Writing Committee to Update the 2001 Guidelines for the Evaluation and Management of Heart Failure). *Circulation.* 2005;112:1825–52.

3. Arnold JMO, Baker DW, Barnard DH, et al. HFSA 2006 comprehensive heart failure practice guideline. *J Card Fail.* 2006;1:E1–E122.

4. Rosamond W, Flegal K, Furie K, et al. Heart disease and stroke statistics—2008 update: a report from the American Heart Association Statistics Committee and Stroke Statistics Subcommittee. *Circulation.* 2008;117:E25–E146.

5. McCullough PA, Philbin EF, Spertus JA, et al. Confirmation of a heart failure epidemic: findings from the Resource Utilization Among Congestive Heart Failure (REACH) study. *J Am Coll Cardiol.* 2002;23:60–9.

6. Roger VL, Weston SA, Redfield MM, et al. Trends in heart failure incidence and survival in a community-based population. *JAMA.* 2004;292:344–50.

7. Stewart S, MacIntyre K, Capewell S, McMurray JJ. Heart failure and the aging population: an increasing burden in the 21st century? *Heart.* 2003;89:49–53.

8. Nieminen MS, Bohm M, Cowie MR, et al. Executive summary of the guidelines on the diagnosis and treatment of acute heart failure: the Task Force on Acute Heart Failure of the European Society of Cardiology. *Eur Heart J.* 2005;26:384–416.

9. Nieminen MS, Brutsaert D, Dickstein K, et al. EuroHeart Failure Survey II (EHFS II): a survey on hospitalized acute heart failure patients: description of population. *Eur Heart J.* 2006; 27, 2725–36.

10. Blackledge HM, Tomlinson J, Squire IB. Prognosis for patients newly admitted to hospital with heart failure: survival trends in 12 220 index admissions in Leicestershire 1993–2001. *Heart.* 2003;89:615–20.

11. MacIntyre K, Capewell S, Stewart S, et al. Evidence of improving prognosis in heart failure: trends in case fatality in 66,547 patients hospitalized between 1986 and 1995. *Circulation.* 2000;102:1126–31.

12. Levy D, Kenchaiah S, Larson MG, et al. Long-term trends in the incidence of and survival with heart failure. *N Engl J Med.* 2002;347:1397–1402.

13. Schaufelberger M, Swedberg K, Koster M, Rosen M, Rosengren A. Decreasing one-year mortality and hospitalization rates for heart failure in Sweden; data from the Swedish Hospital discharge registry 1988 to 2000. *Eur Heart J.* 2004;25:300–7.

14. McMurray JJ, Pfeffer MA, Swedberg K, Dzau VJ. Which inhibitor of the renin-angiotensin system should be used in chronic heart failure and acute myocardial infarction? *Circulation.* 2004;110:3281–8.

15. Cleland JG, Daubert JC, Erdmann E, et al. The effect of cardiac resynchronization on morbidity and mortality in heart failure. *N Engl J Med.* 2005;352:1539–49.

16. Cleland JG, Daubert JC, Erdmann E, et al. Longer-term effects of cardiac resynchronization therapy on mortality in heart failure [the CArdiac REsynchronization-Heart Failure (CARE-HF) trial extension phase]. *Eur Heart J.* 2006;27:1928–32.

17. Lee DS, Mamdani MM, Austin PC, et al. Trends in heart failure outcomes and pharmacotherapy: 1992–2000. *Am J Med.* 2004;116:581–9.

18. Baker DW, Einstadter D, Thomas C, et al. Mortality trends for 23,505 Medicare patients hospitalized with heart failure in Northeast Ohio, 1991– 1997. *Am Heart J.* 2003;146:258–64.

19. Bursi F, Weston SA, Redfield MM, et al. Systolic and diastolic heart failure in the community. *JAMA.* 2006;296:2209–16.

20. Metra M, Ponikowski P, Dickstein K, et al. Advanced chronic heart failure: a position statement from the Study Group on Advanced Heart Failure of the Heart Failure Association of the European Society of Cardiology. *Eur J Heart Fail*. 2007;9: 684–94.
21. Paulus WJ, Tschöpe C, Sanderson JE, et al. How to diagnose diastolic heart failure: a consensus statement on the diagnosis of heart failure with normal left ventricular ejection fraction by the Heart Failure and Echocardiography Associations of the European Society of Cardiology. *Eur Heart J*. 2007;28:2539–50.
22. Lenzen MJ, Scholte OP, Reimer WJ, et al. Differences between patients with a preserved and a depressed left ventricular function: a report from the EuroHeart Failure Survey. *Eur Heart J*. 2004; 25:1214–20.
23. Flather MD, Shibata MC, Coats AJ, et al. Randomized trial to determine the effect of nebivolol on mortality and cardiovascular hospital admission in elderly patients with heart failure (SENIORS). *Eur Heart J*. 2005;26:215–25.
24. Metra M, Brutsaert D, Dickstein K, et al. Treatment of advanced chronic heart failure with normal left ventricular ejection fraction. Response to the letter by Dr. Martinez-Selles. *Eur J Heart Fail*. 2007;9:1224–5.
25. The CONSENSUS Trial Study Group Effects of enalapril on mortality in severe congestive heart failure. Results of the Cooperative North Scandinavian Enalapril Survival Study (CONSENSUS). *N Engl J Med*. 1987;316:1429–35.
26. The SOLVD Investigators. Effect of Enalapril on survival in patients with reduced left ventricular ejection fractions and congestive heart failure. *N Engl J Med*. 1991;325:293–302.
27. Cohn JN, Johnson G, Ziesche S, et al. A comparison of enalapril with hydralazine-isosorbide dinitrate in the treatment of chronic congestive heart failure. *N Engl J Med*. 1991;325:303–10.
28. Francis GS, Goldsmith SR, Levine TB, Olivari MT, Cohn JN. The neurohumoral axis in congestive heart failure. *Ann Intern Med*. 1984;101:370–7.
29. Swedberg K. Is neurohormonal activation deleterious to the long-term outcome of patients with congestive heart failure? II. Protagonist's viewpoint. *J Am Coll Cardiol*. 1988;12:550–4.
30. Bristow MR. The adrenergic nervous system in heart failure. *N Engl J Med*. 1983;311:850–1.
31. Cody RJ. Neurohormonal influences in the pathogenesis of congestive heart failure. *Cardiol Clin*. 1989;7:73–86.
32. Packer M. The neurohormonal hypothesis: a theory to explain the mechanism of disease progression in heart failure. *J Am Coll Cardiol*. 1992;20:248–54.
33. Mann DL. Mechanisms and models in heart failure: a combinatorial approach. *Circulation*. 1999;100:999–1008.
34. Givertz MM. Manipulation of the renin-angiotensin system. *Circulation*. 2001;104: E14–E8.
35. MacFayden RJ, Lee AF, Morton JJ, et al. How often are angiotensin II and aldosterone concentration raised during chronic ACE inhibitor treatment in cardiac failure? *Heart*. 1999;82:57–61.
36. Massie B, Kramer BL, Topic N, et al. Hemodynamic and radionuclide effects of acute captopril therapy for heart failure: changes in left and right ventricular volumes and function at rest and during exercise. *Circulation*. 1982;65:1374–81.

37. DiCarlo L, Chatterjee K, Pamley WW, et al. Enalapril: a new angiotensin-converting enzyme inhibitor in chronic heart failure: acute and chronic hemodynamic evaluation. *J Am Coll Cardiol.* 1983;2:865–71.
38. Greenberg B, Quinones MA, Koilpollai C, et al. Enalapril therapy on cardiac structure and function in patients with left ventricular dysfunction: results of the SOLVD echocardiography substudy. *Circulation.* 1995;91:2573–81.
39. Pfeffer MA, Lamas GA, Vaughan DE, et al. Effect of captopril on progressive left ventricular dilatation after anterior myocardial infarction. *N Engl J Med.* 1988;319: 80–6.
40. Pfeffer MA, Braunwald E, Moye LA, et al. on behalf of the SAVE investigators. Effect of captopril on mortality and morbidity in patients with left ventricular dysfunction after myocardial infarction: results of the Survival and Ventricular Enlargement Trial. *N Engl J Med.* 1992;327:669–77.
41. The Acute Infarction Ramipril Efficacy (AIRE) Study Investigators. Effect of ramipril on mortality and morbidity of survivors of acute myocardial infarction with clinical evidence of heart failure. *Lancet.* 1993;342:821–8.
42. Ambrosioni E, Borghi C, Magnani B. The effect of the angiotensin-converting enzyme inhibitor zofenopril on mortality and morbidity after anterior myocardial infarction: the Survival of Myocardial Infarction Long-Term Evaluation (SMILE) Study Investigators. *N Engl J Med.* 1995;332:80–5.
43. Kober L, Torp-Pedersen C, Carlsen JE, et al. For the Trandolapril Cardiac Evaluation (TRACE) Study Group. A clinical trial of the angiotensin-converting enzyme inhibitor trandolapril in patients with left ventricular dysfunction after myocardial infarction. *N Engl J Med.* 1995;333:1670–6.
44. The SOLVD Investigators. Effect of enalapril on mortality and the development of heart failure in asymptomatic patients with reduced left ventricular ejection fraction. *N Engl J Med.* 1992;327:685–91.
45. Jong P, Yusuf S, Rousseau MF, et al. Effect of enalapril on 12-year survival and life expectancy in patients with left ventricular systolic dysfunction: a follow-up study. *Lancet.* 2003;361:1843–8.
46. Swedberg K, Kjekshus J, Snapinn S. Long-term survival in severe heart failure in patients treated with enalapril. Ten year follow-up of CONSENSUS I. *Eur Heart J.* 1999;20:136–9.
47. Burnier M. Angiotensin II type 1 receptor blockers. *Circulation.* 2001;103:904-12.
48. Opie LH, Sack MN. Enhanced angiotensin II activity in heart failure: reevaluation of the counter regulatory hypothesis of receptor subtypes. *Circ Res.* 2001;88:654–8.
49. Dickstein K, Kjekshus J; OPTIMAAL Steering Committee of the OPTIMAAL Study Group. Effects of losartan and captopril on mortality and morbidity in high-risk patients after acute myocardial infarction: the OPTIMAAL randomised trial. Optimal Trial in Myocardial Infarction with Angiotensin II Antagonist Losartan. *Lancet.* 2002;360:752–60.
50. Pfeffer MA, McMurray JJ, Velazquez EJ, et al. Valsartan, captopril, or both in myocardial infarction complicated by heart failure, left ventricular dysfunction or both. *N Engl J Med.* 2003;349:1893–906.
51. Konstman MA, Riegger G, Klinger GH, et al. Randomised trial of losartan versus captopril on mortality in patients with symptomatic heart failure: the losartan heart failure survival study, ELITE II. *Lancet.* 2000;355:1582–7.

52. Granger CB, McMurray JJ, Yusuf S, et al. Effects of candesartan in patients with chronic heart failure and reduced left-ventricular systolic function intolerant to angiotensin-converting-enzyme inhibitors: the CHARM-Alternative trial. *Lancet.* 2003;362:772–6.

53. McKelvie RS, Yusuf S, Pericak D, et al. Comparison of candesartan, enalapril, and their combination in congestive heart failure: randomized evaluation of strategies for left ventricular dysfunction (RESOLVD) pilot study. The RESOLVD Pilot Study Investigators. *Circulation.* 1999;100:1056–64.

54. Cohn JN, Tognoni G for the Valsartan Heart Failure Trial Investigators. A randomized trial of the angiotensin receptor blocker valsartan in chronic heart failure. *N Engl J Med.* 2001;345:1667–75.

55. McMurray JJ, Ostergren J, Swedberg K, et al. Effects of candesartan in patients with chronic heart failure and reduced left-ventricular systolic function taking angiotensin-converting-enzyme inhibitors: the CHARM-Added trial. *Lancet.* 2003;362:767–71.

56. Maggioni AP, Anand I, Gottlieb SO, et al. Effects of valsartan on morbidity and mortality in patients with heart failure not receiving angiotensin-converting enzyme inhibitors. *J Am Coll Cardiol.* 2002;40:1414–21.

57. McMurray J, Cohen-Solal A, Dietz R, et al. Practical recommendations for the use of ACE inhibitors, beta-blockers, aldosterone antagonists and angiotensin receptor blockers in heart failure: putting guidelines into practice. *Eur J Heart Fail.* 2005;7:710–21.

58. Jorde UP, Vittorio T, Katz SD, et al. Elevated plasma aldosterone levels despite complete inhibition of the vascular angiotensin-converting enzyme in chronic heart failure. *Circulation.* 2002;106:1055–7.

59. Vantrimpont P, Rouleau JL, Ciampi A, et al. Two-year time course and significance of neurohumoral activation in the Survival and Ventricular Enlargement (SAVE) Study. *Eur Heart J.* 1998;19:1552–63.

60. Rastogi S, Mishra S, Zacà V, et al. Effect of long-term monotherapy with the aldosterone receptor blocker eplerenone on cytoskeletal proteins and matrix metalloproteinases in dogs with heart failure. *Cardiovasc Drugs Ther.* 2007;21:415–22.

61. Zannad F, Alla F, Dousset B, et al. for the RALES Investigators. Limitation of excessive extracellular matrix turnover may contribute to survival benefit of spironolactone therapy in patients with congestive heart failure. *Circulation.* 2000;102:2700–6.

62. Pitt B, Zannad F, Remme WJ, et al. The effect of spironolactone on morbidity and mortality in patients with severe heart failure. Randomized Aldactone Evaluation Study Investigators. *N Engl J Med.* 1999;341:709–17.

63. Pitt B, Remme W, Zannad F, et al. Eplerenone, a selective aldosterone blocker, in patients with left ventricular dysfunction after myocardial infarction. *N Engl J Med.* 2003;348:1309–21.

64. Weir RAP, McMurray JJV, Puu M, et al. Efficacy and tolerability of adding an angiotensin receptor blocker in patients with heart failure already receiving an angiotensin-converting inhibitor plus aldosterone antagonist, with or without a beta blocker: findings from the Candesartan in Heart failure: Assessment of Reduction in Mortality and morbidity (CHARM)-Added trial. *Eur J Heart Fail.* 2008;10:157–63.

65. Bristow MR. Beta-adrenergic receptor blockade in chronic heart failure. *Circulation.* 2000;101:558–69.

66. Metra M, Nodari S, D'Aloia A, Bontempi L, Boldi E, Dei Cas L. A rationale for the use of beta-blockers as standard treatment for heart failure. *Am Heart J*. 2000;139: 511–21.

67. Metra M, Dei Cas L, di Lenarda A, Poole-Wilson P. Beta-blockers in heart failure: are pharmacological differences clinically important? *Heart Fail Rev*. 2004;9: 123–30.

68. Sabbah HN. Biologic rationale for the use of beta-blockers in the treatment of heart failure. *Heart Fail Rev*. 2004;9:91–7.

69. Metra M, Nodari S, D'Aloia A, Cagnazzi E, Fiorina C, Verde S, Dei Cas L. Beta blockers in heart failure: issues in the management of individual patients. *Heart Fail Rev*. 1999; 4:65–77.

70. Metra M, Nodari S, D'Aloia A, et al. Beta-blocker therapy influences the hemo-dynamic response to inotropic agents in patients with heart failure: a randomized comparison of dobutamine and enoximone before and after chronic treatment with metoprolol or carvedilol. *J Am Coll Cardiol*. 2002;40:1248–58.

71. Waagstein F, Caidhal K, Wallentin I, et al. Long-term β-blockade in dilated cardiomy-opathy. *Circulation*. 1989;80:551–63.

72. Metra M, Nardi M, Giubbini R, Dei Cas L. Effects of short- and long-term carvedilol administration on rest and exercise hemodynamic variables, exercise capacity and clinical conditions in patients with idiopathic dilated cardiomyopathy. *J Am Coll Cardiol*. 1994;24: 1678–87.

73. Metra M, Giubbini R, Nodari S, et al. Differential effects of beta-blockers in patient with heart failure: a prospective, randomized, double-blind comparison of the long-term effects of metoprolol versus carvedilol. *Circulation*. 2000;102:546–51.

74. Metra M, Nodari S, D'Aloia A, et al. Effects of neurohormonal antagonism on symp-toms and quality-of-life in heart failure. *Eur Heart J*. 1998;19 Suppl B:B25–B35.

75. Metra M, Nodari S, Raccagni D, et al. Maximal and submaximal exercise testing in heart failure. *J Cardiovasc Pharmacol*. 1998;32 Suppl 1:S36–S45.

76. Nodari S, Metra M, Dei Cas L. Beta-blocker treatment of patients with diastolic heart failure and arterial hypertension. A prospective, randomized, comparison of the long-term effects of atenolol vs. nebivolol. *Eur J Heart Fail*. 2005;621–7.

77. Lowes BD, Abraham WT, Larrain JR, et al. Effects of carvedilol on left ventricular mass, chamber geometry, and mitral regurgitation in chronic heart failure. *Am J Cardiol*. 1999;83:1201–5.

78. Dubach P, Myers J, Bonetti P, et al. Effects of bisoprolol fumarate on left ventricu-lar size, function and exercise capacity in patients with heart failure: analysis with magnetic resonance myocardial tagging. *Am Heart J*. 2002;143:676–83.

79. Waagstein F, Strombald O, Andersson B, et al. Increase exercise ejection fraction and reverse remodeling after long-term treatment with metoprolol in congestive heart failure: a randomized, stratified, double-blind, placebo-controlled trial in mild to moderate heart failure due to ischemic or idiopathic dilated cardiomyopathy. *Eur J Heart Fail*. 2003;5:679–91.

80. Eichhorn EJ, Bristow MR. Medical therapy can improve the biological properties of the chronically failing heart. A new era in the treatment of heart failure. *Circulation*. 1996;94:2285–96.

81. Metra M, Nodari S, Parrinello G, Giubbini R, Manca C, Dei Cas L. Marked improve-ment in left ventricular ejection fraction during long-term beta-blockade in patients

with chronic heart failure: clinical correlates and prognostic significance. *Am Heart J.* 2003;145:292–9.

82. Eichhorn EJ, Grayburn PA, Mayer SA, et al. Myocardial contractile reserve by dobutamine stress echocardiography predicts improvement in ejection fraction with beta-blockade in patients with heart failure: the Beta-Blocker Evaluation of Survival Trial (BEST). *Circulation.* 2003;108:2336–41.

83. Mann DL, Bristow MR. Mechanisms and models in heart failure: the biomechanical model and beyond. *Circulation.* 2005;111:2837–49.

84. Auricchio A, Fantoni C, Steinberg JS. Acute and chronic sequelae of ventricular dyssynchrony. *Prog Cardiovasc Dis.* 2006;48:227–31.

85. Auricchio A, Metra M, Gasparini M, et al. Long-term survival of patients with heart failure and ventricular conduction delay treated with cardiac resynchronization therapy. *Am J Cardiol.* 2007;99:232–8.

86. Packer M, Bristol MR, Cohn JN, et al. The effect of carvedilol on morbidity and mortality in patients with chronic heart failure. U.S. Carvedilol Heart Failure Study Group. *N Engl J Med.* 1996;334:1349–55.

87. CIBIS II Investigators and Committees. The Cardiac Insufficiency Bisoprolol Study II (CIBIS II): a randomised trial. *Lancet.* 1999;353:9–13.

88. The MERIT-HF Investigators. Effect of metoprolol CR/XL in chronic heart failure: Metoprolol CR/XL Randomised Intervention Trial in Congestive Heart Failure (MERIT-HF) *Lancet.* 1999;353:2001–7.

89. Hjalmarson A, Goldstein S, Fagerberg B, et al. for the MERIT-HF Study Group. Effects of controlled-release metoprolol on total mortality, hospitalizations, and well-being in patients with heart failure: the Metoprolol CR/XL Randomized Intervention Trial in Congestive Heart Failure (MERIT-HF). *JAMA.* 2000;283: 1295–302.

90. Packer M, Coats AJ, Fowler MB, et al. for the Carvedilol Prospective Randomized Cumulative Survival Study Group. Effect of carvedilol on survival in severe chronic heart failure. *N Engl J Med.* 2001;344:1652–8.

91. Poole-Wilson PA, Swedberg K, Cleland JG, et al. Comparison of carvedilol and metoprolol on clinical outcomes in patients with chronic heart failure in the Carvedilol Or Metoprolol European Trial (COMET): randomised controlled trial. *Lancet.* 2003;362:7–13.

92. Bristow MR, Feldman AM, Adams KF Jr, Goldstein S. Selective versus nonselective beta-blockade for heart failure therapy: are there lessons to be learned from the COMET trial? *J Card Fail.* 2003;9:444–53.

93. Kindermann M, Maack C, Schaller S, et al. Carvedilol but not metoprolol reduces beta-adrenergic responsiveness after complete elimination from plasma in vivo. *Circulation.* 2004;109:3182–90.

94. Torp-Pedersen C, Metra M, Charlesworth A, et al. Effects of metoprolol and carvedilol on pre-existing and new onset diabetes in patients with chronic heart failure: data from the Carvedilol Or Metoprolol European Trial (COMET). *Heart.* 2007;93:968–73.

95. Remme WJ, Torp-Pedersen C, Cleland JG, et al. Carvedilol protects better against vascular events than metoprolol in heart failure: results from COMET. *J Am Coll Cardiol.* 2007;49:963–71.

96. Metra M, Dei Cas L, Cleland JG. Pharmacokinetic and pharmacodynamic characteristics of beta-blockers: when differences may matter. *J Card Fail.* 2006;12: 177–81.

97. Dargie HJ. Effect of carvedilol on outcome after myocardial infarction in patients with left-ventricular dysfunction: the CAPRICORN randomised trial. *Lancet.* 2001;357:1385–90.

98. Flather MD, Shibata MC, Coats AJ, et al. Randomized trial to determine the effect of nebivolol on mortality and cardiovascular hospital admission in elderly patients with heart failure (SENIORS). *Eur Heart J.* 2005;26:215–25.

99. Liggett SB, Mialet-Perez J, Thaneemit-Chen S, et al. A polymorphism within a conserved beta(1)-adrenergic receptor motif alters cardiac function and beta-blocker response in human heart failure. *Proc Natl Acad Sci USA.* 2006;103:11288–93.

100. Willenheimer R, van Veldhuisen DJ, Silke B, et al. Effect on survival and hospitalization of initiating treatment for chronic heart failure with bisoprolol followed by enalapril, as compared with the opposite sequence: results of the randomized Cardiac Insufficiency Bisoprolol Study (CIBIS) III. *Circulation.* 2005;112:2426–35.

101. Metra M, Torp-Pedersen C, Cleland JG, et al. Should beta-blocker therapy be reduced or withdrawn after an episode of decompensated heart failure? Results from COMET. *Eur J Heart Fail.* 2007;9:901–9.

102. Cody RJ, Covit AB, Schaer GL, Laragh JH, Sealey JE, Feldschuh J. Sodium and water balance in chronic congestive heart failure. *J Clin Invest.* 1986;77:1441–52.

103. Metra M, Dei Cas L, Bristow MR. The pathophysiology of acute heart failure—it is a lot about fluid accumulation. *Am Heart J.* 2008;155:1–5.

104. Puschett JB. Physiologic basis for the use of new and older diuretics in congestive heart failure. *Cardiovasc Med.* 1977;2:119–34.

105. Domanski M, Norman J, Pitt B, et al. Diuretic use, progressive heart failure, and death in patients in the Studies Of Left Ventricular Dysfunction (SOLVD). *J Am Coll Cardiol.* 2003;42(4):705–8.

106. Domanski M, Tian X, Haigney M, Pitt B. Diuretic use, progressive heart failure, and death in patients in the DIG study. *J Card Fail.* 2006;12:327–32.

107. Ahmed A, Husain A, Love TE, et al. Heart failure, chronic diuretic use, and increase in mortality and hospitalization: an observational study using propensity score methods. *Eur Heart J.* 2006;27:1431–9.

108. Eshaghian S, Horwich TB, Fonarow GC. Relation of loop diuretic dose to mortality in advanced heart failure. *Am J Cardiol.* 2006;Jun 15;97(12):1759–64.

109. Metra M, Nodari S, Parrinello G, et al. Worsening renal function in patients hospitalised for acute heart failure: clinical implications and prognostic significance. *Eur J Heart Fail.* 2008; 10:188–95.

110. McCurley JM, Hanlon SU, Wei SK, et al. Furosemide and the progression of left ventricular dysfunction in experimental heart failure. *J Am Coll Cardiol.* 2004;44:1301–7.

111. Francis GF, Benedict C, Johnstone DE, et al. for the SOLVD Investigators. Comparison of neuroendocrine activation on patients with left ventricular dysfunction with and without congestive heart failure: a substudy of the Studies of Left Ventricular Dysfunction (SOLVD). *Circulation.* 1990;82:1724–9.

112. Leier CV, Dei Cas L, Metra M. Clinical relevance and management of the major electrolyte abnormalities in congestive heart failure: hyponatremia, hypokalemia, and hypomagnesemia. *Am Heart J.* 1994;128:564–74.

113. Costanzo MR, Guglin ME, Saltzberg MT, et al. Ultrafiltration versus intravenous diuretics for patients hospitalized for acute decompensated heart failure. *J Am Coll Cardiol.* 2007;49:675–83.

114. Givertz MM, Massie BM, Fields TK, Pearson LL, Dittrich HC. CKI-201 and CKI-202 Investigators. The effects of KW-3902, an adenosine A1-receptor antagonist, on diuresis and renal function in patients with acute decompensated heart failure and renal impairment or diuretic resistance. *J Am Coll Cardiol.* 2007;50:1551–60.

115. Gheorghiade M, Ferguson D. Digoxin: a neurohormonal modulator in heart failure? *Circulation.* 1991;84:2181–6.

116. The effect of digoxin on mortality and morbidity in patients with heart failure. The Digitalis Investigation Group. *N Engl J Med.* 1997;336:525–33.

117. Ahmed A, Rich MW, Love TE, et al. Digoxin and reduction in mortality and hospitalization in heart failure: a comprehensive post hoc analysis of the DIG trial. *Eur Heart J.* 2006;27:178–86.

118. Rathore SS, Curtis JP, Wang Y, Bristow MR, Krumholz HM. Association of serum digoxin concentration and outcomes in patients with heart failure. *JAMA.* 2003;Feb 19;289(7):871–8.

119. Leier CV, Hass P, Magorien RD, et al. Improved exercise capacity and differing arterial and venous tolerance during chronic isosorbide dinitrate therapy for congestive heart failure. *Circulation.* 1983;67:817–22.

120. Taylor AL, Ziesche S, Yancy C, et al. Combination of isosorbide dinitrate and hydralazine in blacks with heart failure. *N Engl J Med.* 2004;351:2049–57.

121. Echt DS, Liebson PR, Mitchell B, et al. and the CAST investigators. Mortality and morbidity in patients receiving encainide, flecainide, or placebo: the Cardiac Arrhythmias Suppression Trial. *N Engl J Med.* 1991;324:781–8.

122. Waldo AL, Camm AJ, De Ruyter H, et al. for the SWORD Investigators. Effect of d-sotalol on mortality in patients with left ventricular dysfunction after recent and remote myocardial infarction. *Lancet.* 1996;348:7–12.

123. Zacà V, Rastogi S, Imai M, et al. Chronic monotherapy with rosuvastatin prevents progressive left ventricular dysfunction and remodeling in dogs with heart failure. *J Am Coll Cardiol.* 2007;50:551–7.

124. Ramasubbu K, Estep J, White DL, et al. Experimental and clinical basis for the use of statins in patients with ischemic and nonischemic cardiomyopathy. *J Am Coll Cardiol.* 2008;51:412–26.

125. Kjekshus J, Apetrei E, Barrios V, et al. for the CORONA Group. Rosuvastin in older patients with systolic heart failure. *N Engl J Med.* 2007;357:2248–61.

126. Tavazzi L, Tognoni G, Franzosi MG, et al. on behalf of the GISSI-HF Investigators. Rationale and design of the GISSI heart failure trial: a large trial to assess the effects of n-3 polyunsaturated fatty acids and rosuvastatin in symptomatic congestive heart failure. *Eur J Heart Fail.* 2004;6:635–41.

127. Bernard S. Disease management: a pharmaceutical industry perspective. *Pharmaceutical Exec.* 1995;16:48–50.

128. Rich MW. Heart failure disease management: a critical review. *J Card Fail.* 1999;5:64–75.

129. Stewart S, Horowitz JD. Home-based intervention in congestive heart failure: long-term implications on readmission and survival. *Circulation.* 2002;105:2861–6.

130. Mehra MR, Uber PA, Francis GS. Heart failure therapy at a crossroad: are there limits to the neurohormonal model? *J Am Coll Cardiol*. 2003;41:1606–10.

131. Kass DA. An epidemic of dissynchrony: but what does it mean? *J Am Coll Cardiol*. 2008;51:12–7.

132. Bleeker GB, Schalij MJ, Molhoek SG, et al. Relationship between QRS duration and left ventricular dyssinchrony in patients with end-stage heart failure. *J Cardiovasc Electrophysiol*. 2004;15:544–9.

133. Leclercq C, Cazeau S, Le Breton H, et al. Acute hemodynamic effects of biventricular DDD pacing in patients with end-stage heart failure. *J Am Coll Cardiol*. 1998;32:1825–31.

134. Iuliano S, Fish SG, Karasik PE, et al. QRS duration and mortality in patients with congestive heart failure. *Am Heart J*. 2002;143:1085–91.

135. Shamin W, Francis DP, Yousufuddin M, et al. Intraventricular conduction delay : a prognostic marker in chronic heart failure. *Int J Cardiol*. 1999;70:171–8.

136. Baldasseroni S, Gentile A, Gorini M, et al. Intraventricular conduction defects in patients with congestive heart failure: left but not right bundle branch block is an independent predictor of prognosis. A report from the Italian Network on Congestive Heart Failure (IN-CHF database). *Ital Heart J*. 2003;4:607–13.

137. Kashani A, Barold SS. Significance of QRS complex duration in patients with heart failure. *J Am Coll Cardiol*. 2005;46:2183–92.

138. De Winter O, Van de Veire N, Van Heuverswijn F, et al. Relationship between QRS duration, left ventricular volumes and prevalence of nonviability in patients with coronary artery disease and severe left ventricular dysfunction. *Eur J Heart Fail*. 2005;8:275–7.

139. Kearney MT, Zaman A, Eckberg Dl, et al. Cardiac size, autonomic function, and 5-year follow-up of chronic heart failure patients with severe prolongation of ventricular activation. *J Card Fail*. 2003;9:93–9.

140. Sandhu R, Bahler RC. Prevalence of QRS prolongation in a community hospital cohort of patients with heart failure and its relation to left ventricular systolic dysfunction. *Am J Cardiol*. 2004;93:244–6.

141. Murkofsky RL, Dangas G, Diamond JA, et al. A prolonged QR duration on surface electrocardiogram in a specific indicator of left ventricular dysfunction. *J Am Coll Cardiol*. 1998;32:476–82.

142. Baldasseroni S, Opasich C, Gorini M, et al. Left bundle-branch block is associated with increased 1-year sudden and total mortality rate in 5,517 patients with congestive heart failure: a report from the italian network on congestive heart failure. *Am Heart J*. 2002;143:398–405.

143. Stellbrink C, Auricchio A, Diem B, et al. Potential benefit of biventricular pacing in patients with congestive heart failure and ventricular tachyarrhythmia. *Am J Cardiol*. 1999;83:143D–50D.

144. Xiao HB, Roy C, Fujimoto S, Gibson DG. Natural history of abnormal conduction and its relation to prognosis in patients with dilated cardiomyopathy. *Int J Cardiol*. 1996;53:163–70.

145. Dye CL, Rosenbaum D, Lowe JC, et al. Primary myocardial disease part I: clinical features. *Ann Intern Med*. 1963;58:426–41.

146. Hofmann M, Bauer R, Handrock R, Weidinger G, Goedel-Meinen L. Prognostic value of the QRS duration in patients with heart failure: a subgroup analysis from 24 centers of Val-HeFT. *J Card Fail.* 2005;11:523–8.

147. Breidthardt T, Christ M, Matti M, et al. QRS and QTc interval prolongation in the prediction of long-term mortality of patients with acute destabilised heart failure. *Heart.* 2007;93:1093–7.

148. Cazeau S, Ritter P, Bakdach S, et al. Four chamber pacing in dilated cardiomyopathy. *Pacing Clin Electrophysiol.* 1994;17:1974–9.

149. McAlister FA, Ezekowitz J, Hooton N, et al. Cardiac resynchronization therapy for patients with left ventricular dysfunction: a systematic review. *JAMA.* 2007;297:2502–14.

150. McAlister FA, Tu JV, Newman A, et al. How many patients with heart failure are eligible for cardiac resynchronization? Insights from two prospective cohorts. *Eur Heart J.* 2006;27:323–9.

151. Toma M, McAlister FA, Ezekowitz J, et al. Proportion of patients followed in a specialized heart failure clinic needing an implantable cardioverter defibrillator as determined by applying different trial eligibility criteria. *Am J Cardiol.* 2006; 97:882–5.

Chapter 2

Pathobiology of left ventricular dyssynchrony and resynchronization

Robert H. Helm, David D. Spragg, Khalid Chakir, and David A. Kass

Key Points

1. Heart failure is characterized by neurohormonal activation and marked molecular and cellular remodeling, which alters excitation–contraction coupling, myofilament function, and energetics.
2. Left ventricular dyssynchrony due to left bundle branch block (LBBB) results in regionally delayed myocardial activation and heterogeneous ventricular wall stress. This depresses systolic function and prolongs relaxation.
3. Dyssynchrony results in a decline in net pump function, myocardial inefficiency, regional molecular activation of stress-response proteins in the late contracting wall, and global reduction in cell survival signaling.
4. Transmural changes in conduction velocity and repolarization are induced, notably in the late activated wall. This is associated with Connexin-43 remodeling in the myocyte.
5. Cardiac resynchronization therapy (CRT) acutely re-coordinates regional contraction improving chamber function and energetic efficiency, and chronic therapy reverses cellular gene expression and molecular remodeling changes and improves rate-dependent contractility.
6. A broad region of optimal left ventricular stimulation during cardiac resynchronization exists over the lateral wall. More anterior and posterior positions do not provide much CRT effect. Improvement in regional coordinated contraction correlates with global functional benefit.
7. CRT not only reduces regional heterogeneity of stress response signaling but also enhances global cell survival signaling.

Pacing to Support the Failing Heart, 1st edition. Edited by K. Ellenbogen and A. Auricchio.
© 2008 American Heart Association, ISBN: 978-1-4051-7534-0

8. Although resynchronization results in cellular and cellular/molecular reverse remodeling, it remains is unclear if provides direct improvement of arrhythmia susceptibility.

9. CRT can benefit the failing heart with a RBBB, although the impact is less than in a heart with a LBBB-type delay, and the effect from RV pacing is similar to that achieved by biventricular stimulation.

Introduction: Heart failure and resynchronization therapy

Heart failure (HF) is a systemic disease that typically starts with a cardiac insult but is rapidly accompanied by the activation of multiple cascades triggered to offset reduced pump function. The latter includes neurohormonal stimulation, loading changes, and complex chamber structural, cellular, and molecular remodeling [1,2]. Neurohumoral stimulation occurs at both the systemic and local myocardial level, and myocardial responses can be induced by hormone-receptor interactions, or mechanical loading [3]. Catecholamines play a major role in stimulating the heart to contract more vigorously, working though cAMP-PKA pathways. However, when sustained, they result in abnormal calcium handling and activation of stress kinases that worsening cell survival [4]. Myocytes are certainly not the only cell types involved, and vascular insufficiency, fibroblast activation and generation of interstitial fibrosis, matrix remodeling proteins (metalloproteinase) activation, and other factors all contribute to the HF phenotype [1].

A key functional consequence of this chronic maladaptive remodeling is that both rest and reserve functions of the heart become compromised. This is manifest by blunted responses to neurohumoral stimulation (i.e. sympathetic stimulation), loading, and increases in heart rate. Many factors contribute to this behavior, including down-regulation of G-coupled receptor pathways, abnormal calcium cycling [5,6], activation of multiple stress response signaling pathways [7,8], depressed energetics [9], and sarcomere changes. Calcium cycling into and out of the sarcoplasmic reticulum is blunted, reducing Ca^{2+} available for systolic activation while delaying its re-uptake to prolong relaxation. Activation of many stress kinases, phosphatases, and associated transcription factors alter everything from contractile function and calcium handling to growth remodeling and cell survival. Bio-energetics is also abnormal, with the heart rendered inefficient and its relative use of glucose versus free fatty acids also altered. Lastly, myofilament proteins are altered also in the failure state, involving changes in the type of myosin, posttranslational modifications of regulatory and structural proteins such as troponin I and titin [1,10].

On this backdrop of overall cardiac failure, a quarter or more of HF patients develop electrical conduction delays resulting in marked discoordinate contraction. Such dyssynchrony reduces chamber function and efficiency even in normal hearts, and its superimposition in HF worsens an already compromised state. Furthermore, the effects of dyssynchrony may not simply be additive but reflect a complex interaction with the HF substrate to generate a particular form of heart failure. As such, dyssynchrony and, correspondingly, resynchronization can influence molecular and cellular signaling in unique ways and understanding how and what is being achieved is increasingly important as cardiac resynchronization (CRT) has taken hold as a clinical therapy for groups of heart failure patients. In this chapter, we update current understanding of the mechanical and molecular/cellular changes brought about by cardiac dyssynchrony and what CRT is imparting to the failing heart.

Left ventricular dyssynchrony

Mechanics of dyssynchrony

Electrical activation of the heart normally occurs in a rapid and coordinated manner as electrical impulses conduct through the His–Purkinje system to activate both ventricles within approximately 50–80 ms. Excitation propagates from endocardium to epicardium and apex to base allowing for coordinated and efficient contraction as all walls simultaneously help to develop pressure. This also provides for appropriate temporal activation of papillary muscles to optimize mitral valve function and prevent regurgitation.

In heart failure, electrical impulse propagation can be diffusely impaired by abnormal His-Purkinje activation and slowed intramyocardial conduction [11]. More marked regional delays (as from conduction block) cause regional delay in contraction and thus dyssynchrony. Both left bundle branch block (LBBB) and right ventricular (RV) pacing results in a phase delay in regional stiffening in the lateral wall, and are the most common mechanisms for LV dyssynchrony. The septal region is activated first via the intact right bundle (or RV pacing) followed by delayed activation of the lateral LV free wall as excitation occurs through relatively slow intramyocardial conduction. The forces from early septal contraction do not translate into a rise in chamber pressure. Rather, these forces are largely converted into prestretch of the still-quiescent lateral wall. This results not only in the observed delay in intracavitary pressure rise (dP/dt_{max}) but also increased lateral wall stress. Conversely, late-systolic activation of the lateral free wall generates forces that are dissipated in part by stretching the early relaxing septal region, reducing net cardiac output. Furthermore, delayed papillary muscle activation results in suboptimal stiffening of the mitral valve apparatus, causing mitral regurgitation.

This most common pattern of mechanical dyssynchrony is demonstrated in Figure 2.1a. Tagged magnetic resonance imaging was used to assess regional strain in a canine model of dyssynchronous heart failure (LBB ablation with 3 weeks of atrial tachypacing) [12]. Strain is plotted as a function of LV region. In early systole (dashed line), the septum contracts whereas the lateral wall stretches (positive strain). In late systole (solid line), this biphasic pattern is

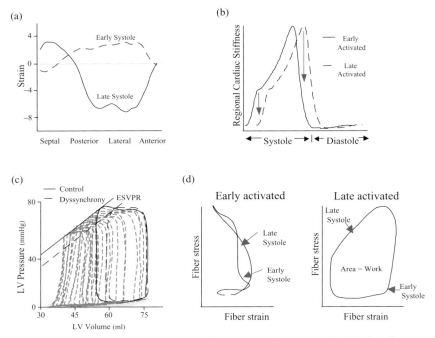

Fig. 2.1 (a) Cardiac dyssynchrony is revealed in circumferential strain (relative shortening) at different regions across a short-axis section of the mid-LV. Data for early (dashed) and late (solid) systole are shown, and reveal septal and lateral regions are out-of-phase with each other. (b) Model of generating dyssynchrony based on a time-delay of ventricular activation (stiffening) between early versus late-stimulated myocardium. Vertical distance between the curves would mean one wall pushing on the other, and the arrows highlight two times—early contraction and late systole where this disparity is greatest and discoordinate motion most manifest. (c) Pressure–volume loops showing effect of LV dyssynchrony on end-systolic pressure–volume relation (ESPVR) and resting cardiac cycle (loop). The ESPVR shifts rightward, end-systolic volume increases, and stroke volume and work decline. (d) Stress-strain loops from early activated versus late-activated regions in a dyssynchronous heart. Whereas these regions would normally appear the same, with dyssynchrony, the early-activated region first contracts at a low load, and then it is stretched and generates a figure-8 shaped loop with little area (reduced work). In contrast, the late contracting lateral wall operates at higher preload and stress, requiring greater work. This correlates with disparate blood flow, energy consumption, and stress molecular signaling in the two regions. (See color plate section).

reversed as the lateral wall now contracts and the septum stretches. Conceptually, left ventricular dyssynchrony may be portrayed as two time-varying elastance curves representing regional activation of myocardium, one phase delayed relative to the other (Figure 2.1b). The vertical difference between the curves indicates disparities in wall stiffening due to the phase delay, and is marked in early systole (i.e. during isovolumic contraction) reducing the peak rate of pressure development (dP/dt_{max}), and even greater in late systole-early diastole. The latter is typically when echo-Doppler measures of dyssynchrony are observed. Such mechanical dyssynchrony has been documented in humans using magnetic resonance imaging [13,14], contrast echocardiography [15], tissue-Doppler imaging [16,17], gated myocardial perfusion SPECT [18], and other methods [19].

Although most dyssynchrony is due to delay in lateral wall excitation, the converse (right-sided delay) certainly exists, and is most typically coupled to a right-bundle block. As discussed later (e.g. Fig. 2.8), this produces less-effective dyssynchrony to the chamber overall [12], highlighting the fact that the heart is not perfectly symmetric and that both the size of the delay-activated region and its location are important factors to determining its net impact.

Effect of dyssynchrony on global function and efficiency

One of the important consequences of ventricular dyssynchrony is that chamber pump function becomes inefficient. Work performed on one side of the heart is wasted by its stretching of the alternative side both in early and later systole. The result is a decline in net cardiac output despite similar energy requirements for the contraction. The global effect is displayed in Figure 2.1c by sets of pressure–volume loops, first reported by the laboratory of Little and colleagues in the mid 1980s [20]. The slope of the end-systolic pressure–volume relationship (ESPRV) shifts to the right, indicating a decline in net systolic function due to dyssynchrony. Stroke volume (loop width) and stroke work (loop area) declines as well, without a fall in end-diastolic volume. End-systolic wall stress, however is increased as the end-systolic volume rises [21,22] Pre-ejection dP/dt_{max} declines by approximately 20%, stroke work falls by 10–15%, and the time constant of relaxation is increased by approximately 10–15% [23,24].

Chamber efficiency also declines. Using a canine model of ventricular dyssynchrony induced with right ventricular (RV) pacing, Prinzen and colleagues [25] assessed regional myocardial strain and work by tagged MRI imaging. With RA pacing, regional work was fairly homogeneous, whereas with RV pacing, there were marked differences in local work with the lateral wall being increased by 125% and early activated septum reciprocally decreased. Local stress-strain plots illustrate these findings (Figure 2.1d). In the early-activated region, workload (loop area) is low coupled to a figure-8-shaped loop due to early low load shortening and subsequent stretch. It is much greater in the late contracting lateral wall which operates at higher initial stretch and contracts against higher stress. These regional differences in work correlate with regional blood flow and metabolic demands [26–28]. Owen and colleagues [22] compared myocardial oxygen consumption (MVO_2) during RA versus RV pacing in the dog heart, by invasively measuring coronary blood flow and coronary sinus O_2

saturation. Despite a striking decline in LV stroke work and external work associated with RV pacing, MVO_2 consumption remained the same indicating a marked decrease in LV efficiency (work/MVO_2 consumption). Other investigators have shown similar findings [29,30].

Dyssynchrony, relaxation, and loading

Dyssynchrony of contraction is also a mechanism for delay in muscle relaxation. This occurs as one region shortens against a still inactivated part of the wall [31]. Relaxation delay and concomitant dyssynchrony can be induced by increasing ventricular afterload as occurs with a pressure rise. An example is shown in Figure 2.2(a,b), taken from a 1994 paper by Yano et al. [32]. Here, regional shortening became dyssynchronous and relaxation time constant prolonged by clamping on the aorta to increase afterload in an otherwise normal canine ventricle. It is important to be reminded of this earlier work—although

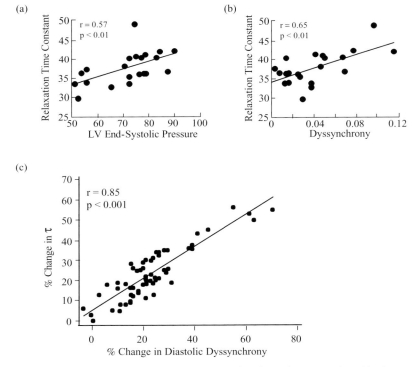

Fig. 2.2 (a,b) Cardiac dyssynchrony and delay in chamber relaxation induced by increasing afterload (systolic end-systolic pressure) by aortic occlusion. (Adapted from Yano et al. [32].) (c) Lowering loading in human heart failure improves both relaxation and regional wall motion dyssynchrony assessed during early diastole. (Adapted from Wang et al. [33].)

most current attention has been on cardiac dyssynchrony due to conduction delay (typically LBB pattern)—loading is abnormal in heart failure and can contribute to dyssynchrony. Support for this was provided by Wang et al. [33] who showed that vasodilators and diuretics could improve dyssynchrony (measured during the diastolic period) and relaxation in HF patients (Figure 2.2c). Importantly, this cause for dyssynchrony is far less likely to be amenable to electrical resynchronization [34].

Gross pathologic changes associated with LV dyssynchrony

Chronic dyssynchrony leads to further changes in maladaptive ventricular remodeling. Vernooy and colleagues assessed structural and functional changes 16 weeks after ablation of the left bundle branch in a canine model of cardiac dyssynchrony. A decline in LV EF (−25%) paralleled an increase in chamber diameter by (+23%) [27]. In a model of dyssynchronous heart failure (LBB ablation with 3 weeks of atrial tachypacing), Helm et al. [35] showed regional changes in wall thickness: thinning of the early activated septum and increased thickness in late-activated lateral wall despite marked chamber dilatation consistent with myocyte hypertrophy in this high-stress territory (Figure 2.3). These data are

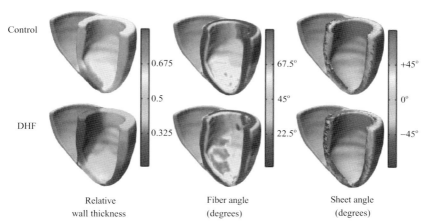

Fig. 2.3 Computational/anatomic rendering of normal hearts (top row) and the dyssynchronous failing heart (DHF, bottom row) color coded to show mean relative wall thickness (RWT = wall thickness/ chamber radius), fiber angle, and myocardial fiber sheet angle. Normal hearts have fairly homogeneous thickness, somewhat greater at the apex (smaller radius of curvature). The DHF heart has wall thinning overall, but significantly more thinning in the early activated septum. Myocardial fiber angle did not significantly change between groups. However, muscle fiber sheet angles (blue-downward, red-upward angle relative to circumferential orientation) were altered, with a more positive orientation in the septum (+15°; p<0.01) (Data courtesy of Dr. Patrick Helm, based on study reported by the author, Ref 35.) (See color plate section).

consistent with changes observed clinically. As previously discussed, standard RV pacing also creates mechanical dyssynchrony similar though not identical to that from a LBBB. Thambo et al. [36] studied the long-term effects of RV pacing (at physiologic heart rates) in 23 patients with congenital heart block who underwent dual-chamber pacemaker implantation with a RV apical lead. They observed thinning of the early-activated septum and thickening in late-activated posterior wall with a 30% increase in the ratio of posterior to septal wall thickness. Furthermore, LV chamber diameter increased by 20%.

Left ventricular dyssynchrony also results in regional changes in underlying myocardial fiber structure. Using high-resolution magnetic resonance and computational anatomical registering, Helm et al. also [35] found that although primary fiber orientation (epicardium downward, endocardium upward relative to circumferential angle) was not significantly altered, the transmural fiber gradient was given wall thinning in the septal region. Furthermore, they showed that the orientation of laminar sheets (planes of muscle fibers that constitute the myocardium) were oriented more vertically in the early-activated septum but not changed in the lateral wall (Figure 2.3). Such regional alterations in fiber architecture could affect the biophysical/mechanical properties of tissue locally and impact propagation of electrical excitation.

Biochemical consequences of dyssynchrony

Regional disparities of wall stress in the dyssynchronous failing heart further impacts the expression and activity of various proteins beyond that observed with heart failure alone. In the first study to test for such effects, Spragg et al. [37] contrasted regional molecular changes in hearts with HF induced by tachypacing with dyssynchrony (LBBB) or without (atrial pacing). In dyssynchronous HF, calcium-handling proteins including SR Ca^{2+}-ATPase and phospholamban were down-regulated ($\sim$20–30%) in the lateral endocardium versus other territories. The former actively transfers Ca^{2+} from the cytosol into the sarcoplasmic reticulum, while the latter is a key coregulator of this uptake process. Another protein examined was the extracellular response kinase (ERK1/2), a mitogen-activated kinase that was highly activated in the lateral endocardium versus other regions. ERK1/2 is associated with stress stimulation pathways involving cell survival and differentiation. Lastly, the investigators showed marked down-regulation of the gap-junction protein connexin-43. Connexin-43 allows for rapid, coordinated, cell-to-cell depolarization. None of these regional changes in the lateral endocardium were not observed in failing myocardium without dyssynchrony. In a recent investigation by the same laboratory, Chakir et al. [38] further revealed differential activation of stress response proteins such as tumor necrosis factor-alpha, Ca^{2+}-calmodulin dependent kinase II, and p38 MAP kinase. Interestingly, in a model of dyssynchrony (LBBB) without cardiac failure, these changes were not observed [39] – indicating that dyssynchrony interacts specifically with underlying heart failure to trigger these abnormalities.

In mice, 7–10 days of LV dyssynchrony induced by RV pacing resulted in regional expression of genes involved with growth and hypertrophy, stress signaling, and matrix remodeling [40]. Thus, regional molecular polarization in the dyssynchronous failing heart may contribute to heterogeneous electromechanical coupling and enhanced arrhythmia susceptibility.

Dyssynchrony alters regional electrical heterogeneity and arrhythmia susceptibility

Spragg et al. [39] studied regional myocardial conduction in canine hearts with chronic mechanical dyssynchrony (LBB ablation) without superimposed heart failure, and compared this to behavior in normal dogs. Myocardial conduction is anisotropic with more rapid cell-to-cell conduction occurring along the myocardial fiber direction owing to gap junction protein coupling at intercalated discs. Dogs with synchronous contraction had faster endocardial conduction versus epicardial conduction in both anterior and lateral territories (Figure 2.4a). However, in hearts with a chronic LBBB, the transmural pattern of conduction speed was flipped in the lateral wall (epicardium faster then endocardium), but maintained normally in the anterior wall. This was accompanied by reduced expression of Connexin-43 in lateral epicardium (Figure 2.4b) and a redistribution of the protein away from intercalated discs to the lateral wall of the myocyte (Figure 2.4c). Both lateral wall myocardial layers had similar Connexin-43 redistribution so, altered Connexin-43 trafficking was unlikely the only basis for reduced endocardial conduction velocity. Finally, significant reductions in action potential duration and relative refractory period were observed in the lateral compared to anterior wall, whereas both time periods were regionally similar in normal (synchronous) controls. The combination of shortened refractoriness but slowed conduction would seem a potential substrate for arrhythmia.

Acute effects from cardiac resynchronization therapy

Mechanics and energetics

The chamber mechanical and hemodynamic effects of cardiac resychronization therapy (CRT) occur rapidly-essentially within a beat. This is depicted by the time tracings from a patient with HF and a LBBB (Figure 2.5a), which shows abrupt increases in dP/dt_{max} and aortic pulse pressure when pacing is turned on. The pressure–volume loop (Figure 2.5b) shows a corresponding increase in stroke volume and decline in end-systolic stress, with little change in end-diastolic volume or pressure. Improved chamber contraction is accompanied by enhanced efficiency [41]. Figure 2.5c shows the change in myocardial oxygen consumption (per beat) induced by dobutamine infusion versus CRT; the latter increased dP/dt_{max} similar to the drug, but with a fall in O_2 consumption versus a rise with the former. The finding of negligible energetic cost despite improved

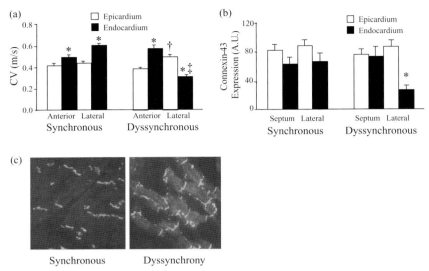

Fig. 2.4 (a) Epicardial and endocardial conduction velocity in normal and dyssynchronous (LBBB) canine ventricular wedge preparations isolated from anterior and lateral regions. The normal pattern shows faster endocardial conduction throughout. However, with chronic dyssynchrony, there is reversal of this pattern in the lateral wall, but maintenance of the pattern in the early activated septum (*p <0.001 vs. corresponding epicardial value; $^{†}p = 0.001$ vs. other epicardial values; $^{‡}P = 0.001$ vs. all other endocardial values. (b) Expression of connexin-43 in synchronous controls is slightly reduced in endocardium overall, though these changes were not statistically significant. However, with chronic LBBB, expression fell markedly solely in the lateral epicardium, with a marked transmural gradient in this territory (*p <0.001). (c) Confocal imaging of connexin-43 in myocytes from normal synchronous versus dyssynchronous hearts. Normal localization at the terminal intercalated discs was altered, as connexin-43 appeared more prevalent in the lateral margins of the cells (remodeling). (Data from Spragg et al. [39].) (See color plate section).

systolic function from CRT has been supported by other studies [42,43], and is a particularly unique feature of CRT among current HF therapies. To date, pharmacologic treatments that enhance systolic function acutely (without lowering afterload as the mechanism) have been associated with chronic increases in mortality. CRT is different, and the enhancement of energetics may play a key role. CRT also enhances the functional reserve response associated with increasing heart rate. This behavior, known as the force–frequency relation, is related to enhanced calcium cycling coupled to beat frequency. As shown in Figure 2.5d, the augmentation of cardiac function with LV only or BiV pacing compared to RV pacing (the latter modeling LBBB) is greater at faster heart rates. This was subsequently explored in more detail by Vollmann et al. [44], and has been recently further investigated following chronic treatment [45,46] (discussed below, c.f. Figure 2.9).

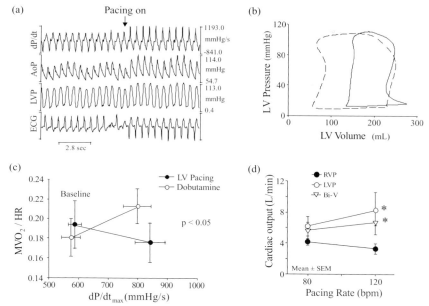

Fig. 2.5 (a) Acute hemodynamic effects of CRT in a patient, assessed by peak rate of pressure rise (dP/dt$_{max}$), aortic pressure (AoP) pulse–indicating enhanced cardiac output), and LV pressure (LVP). Changes occur abruptly upon initiating CRT (note change in QRS morphology). (b) Pressure–volume loops showing the acute effect of CRT (dashed line) compared with baseline dyssynchronous contraction (solid line). Resynchronization induces a left shift of the entire loop, with increased stroke volume and reduced end-diastolic filling pressures. (From Kass et al. [48].) (c) CRT improves LV energetics. Data shows comparison to intravenous dobutamine. Both interventions raised dP/dt$_{max}$ over baseline, but dobutamine increased myocardial oxygen consumption (MV0$_2$), whereas CRT reduced it.) From Nelson et al. [41].) (d) CRT enhances cardiac output more at faster heart rates. Patients with atrial fibrillation and complete AV block received RV, LV, or BiV pacing. Output was lowest with RV pacing (LBBB-type dyssynchrony) and improved by either LV only or BiV pacing. These disparities became enhanced at the faster pacing rate, and shown due to improved diastolic filling with CRT. (From Hay et al. [51].)

Chamber effects from CRT are accompanied by improved synchrony of regional wall contraction. This has been best captured in using three-dimensional cardiac MR tagged imaging analysis displayed in Figures 2.6a and 2.6b using a canine model [14], though this method has yet to be applied clinically to patients post-CRT implantation. The regional circumferential strain maps show how CRT reduces the out-of-phase reciprocal stretch and shortening in anterior versus lateral walls, measured in multiple short axis slices of the ventricle. These data were also used to compile the first temporal plot of

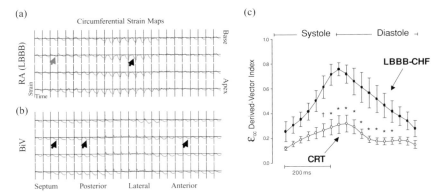

Fig. 2.6 (a) Regional circumferential strain plots from tagged MRI for a heart with failure and LBBB dyssynchrony, and (b) the same heart with biventricular CRT. Marked heterogeneity of strain, with reciprocal shortening/stretch of septal and then lateral walls was reduced by CRT. (c) Time course of dyssynchrony development and recovery throughout a cardiac cycle in HF ventricle with LBBB. Dyssynchrony peaks near end-systole, and CRT markedly reduces both systolic and diastolic dyssynchrony in concert. (From Helm et al. [14].)

the generation and recovery of chamber dyssynchrony. This is shown in Figure 2.6c, employing a vector index that increases not only if regions of the heart are contracting out of phase, but particularly if they are geographically clustered together (i.e. lateral wall) [14]. A color cine of this metric is available on line[14]. Dyssynchrony increases throughout systole peaking shortly after end-systole and then declining. CRT reduces both systolic and diastolic dyssynchrony.

Optimizing CRT

Several parameters determine the efficacy of CRT, including timing intervals between atrial-ventricular and right–left ventricular stimulation, the location of the left ventricular lead, and whether one stimulates both ventricles or only stimulates the LV. The last issue attracted attention early on, when it was found that LV only pacing could enhance systolic function as well if not slightly better than Bi-V modes [47-49]. Both modes similarly enhanced LV function as reflected in parameters such as dP/dt_{max}, stroke work, and cardiac output [48], yet the former does not typically shorten the QRS duration nor generate electrical synchrony [49,50]. This was also revealed in studies in which there was no possibility of a fusion complex as patients had complete AV blockade [51] (Figure 2.5), leading to the conclusion that mechanical synchrony was more important to achieve CRT effects [14,15,23,49,52]. Biventricular stimulation may better impact diastolic relaxation and early filling [51].

AV timing delay influences both the interaction of atrial systole on cardiac preload and mitral valve function, as well as determines if sufficient pre-excitation has been achieved for BiV stimulation. Although many studies have examined how this delay can be optimized [53,54], clinical findings indicate that it has only minor impact in most patients and that a standard delay of near 120 ms is generally effective [48,52]. The RV–LV delay similarly has been shown to be a parameter that can influence CRT efficacy in some subjects, with LV advanced being the usually preferred mode. However, the phase delay is short ($\leq$20 ms in most patients) and simultaneous stimulation results in similar effects on average [51]. Furthermore, optimization of these delays has been always performed in subjects at rest, and it remains unclear if these values remain "optimal" under stress.

One factor that clearly makes a difference is where the LV lead is placed. This was first reported by Butter [55] in patients, and more comprehensively by Helm et al. [23] in a canine model of dyssynchronous heart failure. For the latter, dogs with dilated HF and a LBBB were subjected to CRT where the LV pacing site was randomly varied across the entire LV wall by means of a multi-electrode epicardial sock. Three-dimensional maps of global functional response were generated where the percent change in a given parameter was color coded and placed on the map where the LV pacing lead was located. Figures 2.7a–i show representative maps for systolic (dP/dt_{max} and stroke work) and diastolic (relaxation time constant) in both dyssynchronous, nonfailing and failing dogs. The region where CRT was efficacious ($\geq$70% of the maximal response; dark orange/red) was similarly localized independent of which chamber index was being represented, and was fairly broad, covering approximately 40% of the lateral free wall. The anatomical extent and location of this region was not influenced by heart failure despite the underlying myocardial abnormalities in the latter, suggesting the result was more dependent on the geographic location of LV stimulation than electrical dispersion.

To define the optimal zone for lead placement, we developed a cost-function based on the ratio of mean CRT response to the size of region involved. This way, a region that yielded a big response but was very small (i.e. would be hard to hit) would be less advantageous than one that might have a somewhat ower response but was larger in geographic scope. An overly broad territory would include sites that yielded little CRT effect. The result (Figure 2.7j) shows that the 70% response territory was optimal. We then determined if this region was similar if a chamber mechanical measurement (i.e. stroke work) was used as the output variable, or if we separately determined how much mechanical resynchronization had been achieved. The latter maps were generated from MRI-tagged images generated as pacing site was varied, and then the strain maps were analyzed using a CURE index for dyssynchrony (CURE = 1 for pure synchrony, 0 for pure dyssynchrony) [14,49]. An example is shown in Figure 2.7k, and the overlap map in Figure 2.6l. The latter suggested rather good concordance. The same study examined the impact of altering pacing site (base to apex; anterior-lateral-posterior) for function (stroke work) and wall motion

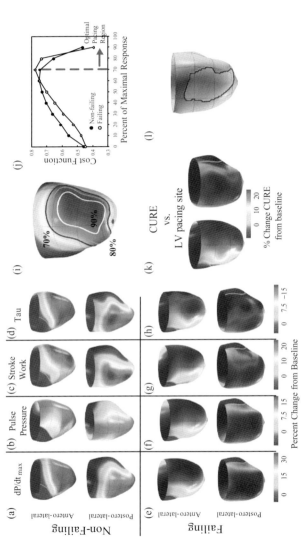

Fig. 2.7 (a)–(h) Representative global heart function maps showing percent change in chamber mechanical parameters from CRT, with color coding mapped according to the site of the LV stimulation electrode used. Dark orange/red indicates the most optimal response to CRT. Data are shown for nonfailing and failing dyssynchrony canine models, and anterolateral and posterolateral orientations. The size and relative location of LV pacing lead regions generating optimal chamber function was generally similar between heart types and parameters. (i) Identification of response iso-regions defined by territories achieving 70%, 80%, or 90% of the maximal CRT response. (j) The optimal zone was determined using a cost function calculated as the ratio of the mean functional response for a territory divided by its size (percent of the LV free wall). The peak tradeoff between response and region size was at the less than 70% iso-region, which occupied approximately 40% of the LV free wall. (k) Global functional response (work) maps correlated with mechanical dyssynchrony maps (CURE index) for the various LV pacing sites. This was further demonstrated by their overlay (l) which shows a generally similar pacing region on the LV free-wall that generated optimal synchrony and global work. (From Helm et al. [23].) (See color plate section).

synchrony (CURE). As shown in Figure 2.7, the best results were in the lateral and somewhat more apically located leads for both types of parameter. Anterior pacing particularly at the base could worsen both synchrony and function.

The optimal pacing site certainly depends on the specifics of the conduction delay, and although most patients have late lateral-wall activation, this can vary, and some extent of right-sided blockade is common. Interestingly, dyssynchrony generated from a pure right bundle branch is significantly less than that associated with left bundle branch block [12], and the corresponding impact of CRT is less (Figure 2.8). Furthermore, one achieved the same benefit using a right heart pacing lead alone as from a traditional biventricular activation mode. In this setting LV only pacing had no benefit—but rather depressed function.

Chronic effects of cardiac resynchronization

Reverse chamber remodeling

Chronic CRT induces further changes in LV remodeling [56–59]. Here, the focus has been on chamber end-systolic and end-diastolic volumes that decline in most studies by an average of 10% over a 6-month period. As first indicated by Yu et al.

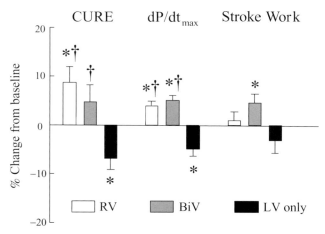

Fig. 2.8 Effect of CRT in canine model of heart failure with a right bundle branch block. Responses for three different pacing modes—RV only, LV only, and BiV stimulation—are shown as percent change relative to right-atrial paced baseline. (*$p<0.007$ compared to baseline; $^{i}<0.047$ compared with baseline; $^{\ddagger}p<0.005$ compared with left ventricular (LV)-only pacing; $p = 0.015$ compared with LV-only pacing. CURE = circumferential uniformity ratio estimate (metric of mechanical synchrony); dP/dt$_{max}$ = maximum time derivative of left ventricular pressure; RV = right ventricle. RV and BiV pacing resulted in similar improvements, and both were quantitatively less than reported in HF and LBBB studies [14,48,49].

[59], this reduction of heart volumes is not an acute effect of CRT, as it persisted even if pacing was temporarily suspended, whereas the rise in dP/dt_{max} associated with resynchronization acutely declined. Reduction of end-systolic volume has been used as a surrogate for mortality in heart failure patients receiving CRT [60], and marker of response [17], whereas acute hemodynamic changes have not generally predicted long-term response to therapy [61].

Altered gene expression

As noted, excitation–contraction coupling and calcium handling is impaired in heart failure, and contributes to blunting of the force frequency response. CRT was shown to acutely enhance function at faster rates, and chronically, this appears to be coupled to improved gene expression of key Ca^{2+} handling proteins. Mullens et al. [45] obtained endomyocardial biopsies from the left interventricular apical septum and contrasted gene expression of calcium-handling proteins at the time of CRT implant to results at the 4-months follow-up. Significant up-regulation in sarcoplasmic reticular ATPase (SERCA2α), phospholamban, and the β1- adrenergic receptor gene expression was found after chronic CRT, with the SERCA2α/PLB ratio rising (Figure 2.9a). The latter is thought associated with improving calcium uptake into the SR and thus the force–frequency response (FFR). There was also a trend toward increased sodium calcium exchange (NCX) gene expression, which has also been associated with an improved FFR [62]. The authors found that these chronic gene expression changes were accompanied by an increase in the FFR (Figure 2.9b).

In another study of CRT effects on gene expression, Iyengar et al. [63] obtained endomyocardial biopsies from the RV septum in 10 patients with nonischemic cardiomyopathy and NYHA Class III–IV symptoms undergoing CRT implantation and repeated this after 6 months of CRT. The investigators found CRT increased the expression of α–myosin heavy chain (MHC) with a trend toward decreasing β–MHC, an isoform switch that is the reversal of that observed in heart failure (fetal gene recapitulation pattern)[64]. The investigators also found a rise in phospholamban and trend toward increased SERCA2α–expression. Most recently, Vanderheyden et al. [46] reported similar changes in gene expression, but further suggested they occurred only in clinical "responders" to the therapy, and not those who were not.

CRT reverses localized molecular remodeling and enhances global cell-survival signaling

To more comprehensively explore the impact of CRT on molecular and cellular remodeling, one must obtain more than the tiny pieces of tissue extracted from endomyocardial biopsies. To approach this, our laboratory developed a canine model combining HF with dyssynchrony and CRT. In this model, dogs first undergo LBB ablation, followed by 3 weeks of atrial tachypacing to develop

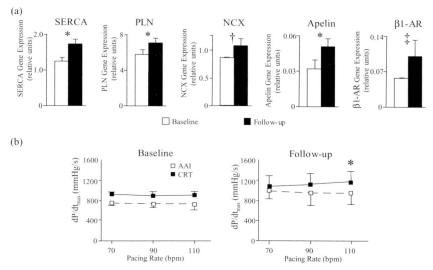

Fig. 2.9 (a) Gene expression pre-CRT and at after 4 months of follow-up (post-CRT) from human left ventricle. SERCA = sarcoplasmic reticulum calcium ATPase 2α; PLN = phospholamban; NCX = sarcolemmal sodium calcium exchanger; β1-AR = β1-adrenoreceptor. $^{*}P = 0.01$, $^{‡}P = 0.03$, and $^{†}P = 0.06$ as compared with baseline, respectively. (b) Force-frequency relationship with AAI versus CRT pacing measured prior to and after 4-month CRT (follow-up). Acute improvement in dP/dt$_{max}$ with CRT was seen initially, though this was not further augmented at faster heart rates. However, after chronic CRT, there was a significant rise in the slope of the FFR, consistent with gene expression changes. $^{*}P = 0.03$. (Adapted from Mullens W et al. [45].)

dyssynchronous HF. They are then randomized to an additional 3 weeks of atrial tachypacing (dyssynchronous HF) or biventricular tachypacing (CRT), both at the same rapid rate. Using this model, Chakir et al. [38] again found regional amplification of stress kinase expression and activation (e.g. p38 MAP kinase and calcium-calmodulin dependant kinase II) in the late activated lateral wall of DHF animals (Figures 2.10a and 2.10b). Both proteins are linked to maladaptive changes in heart failure, contributing to fibrosis and myocyte dysfunction as well as arrhythmia [65,66]. In addition, the cytokine tumor necrosis factor-α (TNF-α) was markedly increased in the lateral wall (Figure 2.10c). Upregulation of TNF-α itself induces dilated cardiomyopathy [67]. In the resynchronized (CRT) failing dogs, however, these regional increases were reduced to re-achieve more homogeneous activation and expression. Although little human data on such kinases have been obtained, D'Ascia et al. [68] have reported similar suppression of TNF-α in LV biopsies from a small group of patients studied before and after receiving CRT.

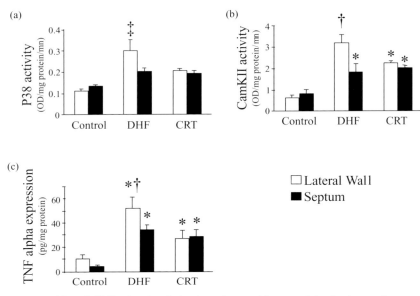

Fig. 2.10 (a) and (b) Regional polarization of stress kinase activity in dyssynchronous failing heart is ameliorated by CRT. Data for p38 mitogen activated kinase and calcium-calmodulin dependant kinase II (CAMKII) in septal and lateral regions are shown. ($\ddagger P<0.001$ vs. control and CRT, $P<0.05$ vs. septum; $*P<0.001$ vs. control; $\dagger P<0.05$ vs septum, $P<0.05$ vs. CRT.) (c) Regional expression of tumor necrosis factor-alpha (TNF-α). Enhanced total and particularly alteral wall expression in DHF hearts was ameliorated by CRT. ($*P<0.05$ vs. control; $\dagger P<0.05$ vs. septum; $P<0.05$ vs. CRT.) (From Chakir et al. [38].)

An even more intriguing finding was global improvement in cell survival signaling associated with CRT. Myocyte apoptosis increased in DHF, confirmed by TUNEL staining (Figure 2.11a), caspase-3 activity (a key pro-apoptotic enzyme; Figure 2.11b) and other assays. This was supported by recent clinical data showing reduced TUNEL positive myocytes in LV myocardial biopsies of patients having received chronic CRT [68]. Unlike stress kinase signaling, however, the decline in apoptosis was global. These findings were further related to global normalization of activated (phosphorylated) Akt kinase, an important regulator of cell survival pathways, with CRT (Figure 2.11b). This was further coupled to the phosphorylation of BAD, inactivating the protein by its dissociation from Bcl-2 to suppress apoptosis.

Electrophysiologic alterations and arrhythmia susceptibility

Several studies have assessed the effect of CRT on arrhythmia susceptibility. In one, Kies et al. [69] examined 19 subjects with advanced heart failure treated with CRT for 6 months and found decreased inducibility of ventricular

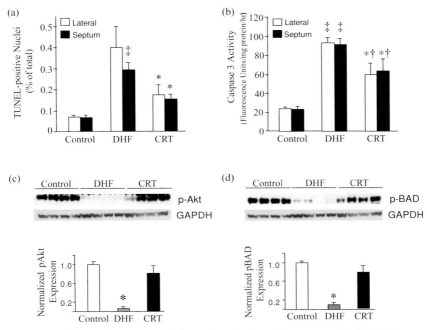

Fig. 2.11 (a) CRT reduces apoptosis throughout the heart. Data summarized TUNEL positive nuclei in myocardium from both DHF and CRT hearts. Positive nuclei were more prevalent in DHF than in CRT or controls. (*$P<0.05$ vs. control and DHF, †$p<0.01$ vs. control). (b) Caspase-3 activity (pro-apoptotic) is globally increased in DHF, and significantly reduced by CRT dogs (*$p \leq 0.05$ vs. DHF, †$p \leq 0.01$ vs. control, ‡$p \leq 0.0003$ vs. control.) (c) and (d) Phosphorylation of AKT and BAD in control, DHF and CRT dogs. Reduced phosphorylation was observed with DHF and essentially normalized by CRT. (*$p<0.001$ vs. control and CRT). (Reproduced from Chakir et al. [38].)

tachycardia (VT) and fibrillation (VF) by programmed stimulation compared to pre-implantation baseline. In another study, Ermis et al. [70] followed 18 patients undergoing an upgrade from a ICD to a CRT-ICD device and found ventricular tachyarrhythmia burden particularly with short-cycle lengths declined, as did the number of appropriate ICD therapies. However, there have also been case reports that VT may increase in patients undergoing CRT [71,72], which some have suggested may relate to the standard use of epicardial LV stimulation [73]. However, overall, meta-analyses of CRT trials indicates the incidence of arrhythmia with CRT does not appear increased [74], and the longer term follow-up analysis of the CARE-HF study suggested improved mortality was due both to reduced heart failure and sudden death [75]. Still, whether this reflects a primary influence on arrhythmia substrate or reduction in heart failure progression remains unclear [76].

The impact of CRT on acute myocardial repolarization is somewhat controversial. Medina-Ravel et al. [73] showed an increase in corrected QT interval with CRT, particularly with LV-only pacing. In rabbit wedge preparations, they further showed epicardial pacing prolonged QT and TDR (peak-to-end of T-wave) intervals. In contrast, Berger and colleagues [77] used a high-resolution 65-lead body surface ECG mapping system on 25 patients undergoing CRT implantation and found BiV pacing significantly decreased all metrics of repolarization including root mean square peak-to-end T-wave interval and inter-lead QT dispersion.

CRT may also affect chronic repolarization changes. In a study of 25 HF patients, Henrikson et al. [78] showed QRS duration declined nearly 10% after 6 months of CRT therapy (with pacing temporarily suspended), suggesting improved intramyocardial conduction. Nishijima et al. [79] assessed a canine model of CRT in which irreversible HF was first generated by subjecting animals to long-term (15 months) tachypacing with the rate gradually lowered, followed by RV or Bi-V (CRT) pacing at slightly above sinus rate for 9 additional months. Cardiac myocytes isolated from hearts in dyssynchronous HF had significantly increased action potential duration (at 50% and 90% repolarization) [80], whereas those receiving CRT had durations similar to controls. In addition, myocyte resting membrane potential was reduced in DHF cells, but similar to controls in CRT. Lastly, CRT also altered intracellular calcium handling, with the peak Ca^{2+} transient amplitude being significantly lower in myocytes from the DHF group, but improved by CRT. Thus, CRT improves myocyte repolarization and Ca^{2+} handling in the failing heart. Ongoing studies aim to dissect the molecular and channel signaling mechanisms responsible for these changes.

Conclusion

Dyssynchronous heart failure is characterized by marked abnormalities of regional and global molecular signaling and cellular dysfunction results in changes in excitation–contraction coupling and myocyte-survival. At the chamber level, dyssynchrony reduces net pump function and energetic efficiency. Data obtained in both human and experimental studies is now revealing CRT not only improves chamber level function and energetics, but has profound beneficial effects on molecular and cellular behavior. The importance of these changes to the clinical response and overall outcome from CRT remains to be clarified, but these findings may help clarify how this device-based treatment can be best integrated with pharmacological approaches to treating HF, and provide insights into who is most likely to benefit from these treatments.

References

1. Mudd JO, Kass DA. Tackling heart failure in the twenty-first century. *Nature.* 2008;451:919–28.
2. Hill JA, Olson EN. Cardiac plasticity. *N Engl J Med.* 2008;358:1370–80.
3. Zou Y, Akazawa H, Qin Y, Sano M, Takano H, Minamino T, Makita N, Iwanaga K, Zhu W, Kudoh S, Toko H, Tamura K, Kihara M, Nagai T, Fukamizu A, Umemura S, Iiri T, Fujita T, Komuro I. Mechanical stress activates angiotensin II type 1 receptor without the involvement of angiotensin II. *Nat Cell Biol.* 2004;6:499–506.
4. Zheng M, Han QD, Xiao RP. Distinct beta-adrenergic receptor subtype signaling in the heart and their pathophysiological relevance. *Sheng Li Xue Bao.* 2004;56:1–15.
5. Bers DM. Altered cardiac myocyte Ca regulation in heart failure. *Physiology Bethesda.* 2006;21:380–7.
6. Bers DM. Calcium cycling and signaling in cardiac myocytes. *Annu Rev Physiol.* 2008;70:23–49.
7. McKinsey TA, Kass DA. Small-molecule therapies for cardiac hypertrophy: moving beneath the cell surface. *Nature Reviews Drug Discovery.* 2007;6:1–18.
8. Heineke J, Molkentin JD. Regulation of cardiac hypertrophy by intracellular signalling pathways. *Nat Rev Mol Cell Biol.* 2006;7:589–600.
9. Neubauer S. The failing heart–an engine out of fuel. *N Engl J Med.* 2007;356:1140–51.
10. Linke WA. Sense and stretchability: The role of titin and titin-associated proteins in myocardial stress-sensing and mechanical dysfunction. *Cardiovasc Res.* 2008;77:637–48.
11. Akar FG, Spragg DD, Tunin RS, Kass DA, Tomaselli GF. Mechanisms underlying conduction slowing and arrhythmogenesis in nonischemic dilated cardiomyopathy. *Circ Res.* 2004;95:717–25.
12. Byrne MJ, Helm RH, Daya S, Osman NF, Halperin HR, Berger RD, Kass DA, Lardo AC. Diminished left ventricular dyssynchrony and impact of resynchronization in failing hearts with right versus left bundle branch block. *J Am Coll Cardiol.* 2007;50:1484–90.
13. Nelson GS, Curry CW, Wyman BT, Kramer A, Declerck J, Talbot M, Douglas MR, Berger RD, McVeigh ER, Kass DA. Predictors of systolic augmentation from left ventricular preexcitation in patients with dilated cardiomyopathy and intraventricular conduction delay. *Circulation.* 2000;101:2703–09.
14. Helm RH, Leclercq C, Faris OP, Ozturk C, McVeigh E, Lardo AC, Kass DA. Cardiac dyssynchrony analysis using circumferential versus longitudinal strain: implications for assessing cardiac resynchronization. *Circulation.* 2005;111:2760–67.
15. Kawaguchi M, Murabayashi T, Fetics BJ, Nelson GS, Samejima H, Nevo E, Kass DA. Quantitation of basal dyssynchrony and acute resynchronization from left or biventricular pacing by novel echo-contrast variability imaging. *J Am Coll Cardiol.* 2002;39:2052–58.
16. Yu CM, Zhang Q, Fung JW, Chan HC, Chan YS, Yip GW, Kong SL, Lin H, Zhang Y, Sanderson JE. A novel tool to assess systolic asynchrony and identify responders of cardiac resynchronization therapy by tissue synchronization imaging. *J Am Coll Cardiol.* 2005;45:677–84.
17. Bleeker GB, Mollema SA, Olman ER, Van Dee Veire N, Ypenburg C, Boersma E, van der Wall EE, Schalij MJ, Bax JJ. Left ventricular resynchronization is mandatory for response to cardiac resynchronization therapy. *Circulation.* 2007; in press.

18. Henneman MM, Chen J, Ypenburg C, Dibbets P, Bleeker GB, Boersma E, Stokkel MP, van der Wall EE, Garcia EV, Bax JJ. Phase analysis of gated myocardial perfusion single-photon emission computed tomography compared with tissue Doppler imaging for the assessment of left ventricular dyssynchrony. *J Am Coll Cardiol*. 2007;49: 1708–14.

19. Bleeker GB, Bax JJ, Steendijk P, Schalij MJ, van der Wall EE. Left ventricular dyssynchrony in patients with heart failure: pathophysiology, diagnosis and treatment. *Nat Clin Pract Cardiovasc Med*. 2006;3:213–19.

20. Park RC, Little WC, O'Rourke RA. Effect of alteration of left ventricular activation sequence on the left ventricular end-systolic pressure–volume relation in closed-chest dogs. *Circ Res*. 1985;57:706–17.

21. Grover M, Glantz SA. Endocardial pacing site affects left ventricular end-diastolic volume and performance in the intact anesthetized dog. *Circ Res*. 1983;53:72–85.

22. Owen CH, Esposito DJ, Davis JW, Glower DD. The effects of ventricular pacing on left ventricular geometry, function, myocardial oxygen consumption, and efficiency of contraction in conscious dogs. *Pacing Clin Electrophysiol*. 1998;21:1417–29.

23. Helm RH, Byrne M, Helm PA, Daya SK, Osman NF, Tunin R, Halperin HR, Berger RD, Kass DA, Lardo AC. Three-dimensional mapping of optimal left ventricular pacing site for cardiac resynchronization. *Circulation*. 2007;115:953–61.

24. Suga H, Goto Y, Yaku H, Futaki S, Ohgoshi Y, Kawaguchi O. Simulation of mechanoenergetics of asynchronously contracting ventricle. *Am J Physiol*. 1990;259:R1075–R1082.

25. Prinzen FW, Hunter WC, Wyman BT, McVeigh ER. Mapping of regional myocardial strain and work during ventricular pacing: experimental study using magnetic resonance imaging tagging. *J Am Coll Cardiol*. 1999;33:1735–42.

26. van Oosterhout MF, Arts T, Bassingthwaighte JB, Reneman RS, Prinzen FW. Relation between local myocardial growth and blood flow during chronic ventricular pacing. *Cardiovasc Res*. 2002;53:831–40.

27. Vernooy K, Verbeek XA, Peschar M, Crijns HJ, Arts T, Cornelussen RN, Prinzen FW. Left bundle branch block induces ventricular remodelling and functional septal hypoperfusion. *Eur Heart J*. 2005;26:91–8.

28. Nowak B, Sinha AM, Schaefer WM, Koch KC, Kaiser HJ, Hanrath P, Buell U, Stellbrink C. Cardiac resynchronization therapy homogenizes myocardial glucose metabolism and perfusion in dilated cardiomyopathy and left bundle branch block. *J Am Coll Cardiol*. 2003;41:1523–8.

29. Baller D, Wolpers HG, Zipfel J, Hoeft A, Hellige G. Unfavorable effects of ventricular pacing on myocardial energetics. *Basic Res Cardiol*. 1981;76:115–23.

30. Baller D, Wolpers HG, Zipfel J, Bretschneider HJ, Hellige G. Comparison of the effects of right atrial, right ventricular apex and atrioventricular sequential pacing on myocardial oxygen consumption and cardiac efficiency: a laboratory investigation. *Pacing Clin Electrophysiol*. 1988;11:394–403.

31. Aoyagi T, Iizuka M, Takahashi T, Ohya T, Serizawa T, Momomura S, Sato H, Mochizuki T, Matsui H, Ikenouchi H. Wall motion asynchrony prolongs time constant of left ventricular relaxation. *Am J Physiol*. 1989;257:H883–H890.

32. Yano M, Kohno M, Konishi M, Takahashi T, Seki K, Matsuzaki M. Influence of left ventricular regional nonuniformity on afterload-dependent relaxation in intact dogs. *Am J Physiol*. 1994;267:H148–H154.

33. Wang J, Kurrelmeyer KM, Torre-Amione G, Nagueh SF. Systolic and diastolic

dyssynchrony in patients with diastolic heart failure and the effect of medical therapy. *J Am Coll Cardiol*. 2007;49:88–96.

34. Kass DA. An epidemic of dyssynchrony: but what does it mean? *J Am Coll Cardiol*. 2008;51:12–17.

35. Helm PA, Younes L, Beg MF, Ennis DB, Leclercq C, Faris OP, McVeigh E, Kass D, Miller MI, Winslow RL. Evidence of structural remodeling in the dyssynchronous failing heart. *Circ Res*. 2006;98:125–32.

36. Thambo JB, Bordachar P, Garrigue S, Lafitte S, Sanders P, Reuter S, Girardot R, Crepin D, Reant P, Roudaut R, Jais P, Haissaguerre M, Clementy J, Jimenez M. Detrimental ventricular remodeling in patients with congenital complete heart block and chronic right ventricular apical pacing. *Circulation*. 2004;110:3766–72.

37. Spragg DD, Leclercq C, Loghmani M, Faris OP, Tunin RS, DiSilvestre D, McVeigh ER, Tomaselli GF, Kass DA. Regional alterations in protein expression in the dyssynchronous failing heart. *Circulation*. 2003;108:929–32.

38. Chakir K, Daya SK, Tunin RS, Helm RH, Byrne MJ, Dimaano VL, Lardo AC, Abraham TP, Tomaselli GF, Kass DA. Reversal of Global Apoptosis and Regional Stress Kinase Activation by Cardiac Resynchronization. *Circulation*. 2008;117:1369–77.

39. Spragg DD, Akar FG, Helm RH, Tunin RS, Tomaselli GF, Kass DA. Abnormal conduction and repolarization in late-activated myocardium of dyssynchronously contracting hearts. *Cardiovasc Res*. 2005;67:77–86.

40. Bilchick KC, Saha SK, Mikolajczyk E, Cope L, Ferguson WJ, Yu W, Girouard S, Kass DA. Differential regional gene expression from cardiac dyssynchrony induced by chronic right ventricular free wall pacing in the mouse. *Physiol Genomics*. 2006;26:109–15.

41. Nelson GS, Berger RD, Fetics BJ, Talbot M, Spinelli JC, Hare JM, Kass DA. Left ventricular or biventricular pacing improves cardiac function at diminished energy cost in patients with dilated cardiomyopathy and left bundle-branch block. *Circulation*. 2000;102:3053–59.

42. Lindner O, Sorensen J, Vogt J, Fricke E, Baller D, Horstkotte D, Burchert W. Cardiac efficiency and oxygen consumption measured with 11C-acetate PET after long-term cardiac resynchronization therapy. *J Nucl Med*. 2006;47:378–83.

43. Ukkonen H, Beanlands RS, Burwash IG, de Kemp RA, Nahmias C, Fallen E, Hill MR, Tang AS. Effect of cardiac resynchronization on myocardial efficiency and regional oxidative metabolism. *Circulation*. 2003;107:28–31.

44. Vollmann D, Luthje L, Schott P, Hasenfuss G, Unterberg-Buchwald C. Biventricular pacing improves the blunted force-frequency relation present during univentricular pacing in patients with heart failure and conduction delay. *Circulation*. 2006;113:953–9.

45. Mullens W, Bartunek J, Wilson Tang WH, Delrue L, Herbots L, Willems R, De BB, Goethals M, Verstreken S, Vanderheyden M. Early and late effects of cardiac resynchronization therapy on force–frequency relation and contractility regulating gene expression in heart failure patients. *Heart Rhythm*. 2008;5:52–9.

46. Vanderheyden M, Mullens W, Delrue L, Goethals M, De BB, Wijns W, Geelen P, Verstreken S, Wellens F, Bartunek J. Myocardial gene expression in heart failure patients treated with cardiac resynchronization therapy responders versus nonresponders. *J Am Coll Cardiol*. 2008;51:129–36.

47. Blanc JJ, Etienne Y, Gilard M, Mansourati J, Munier S, Boschat J, Benditt DG, Lurie KG. Evaluation of different ventricular pacing sites in patients with severe heart failure: results of an acute hemodynamic study. *Circulation*. 1997;96:3273–77.

48. Kass DA, Chen CH, Curry C, Talbot M, Berger R, Fetics B, Nevo E. Improved left ventricular mechanics from acute VDD pacing in patients with dilated cardiomyopathy and ventricular conduction delay. *Circulation.* 1999;99:1567–73.

49. Leclercq C, Faris O, Tunin R, Johnson J, Kato R, Evans F, Spinelli J, Halperin H, McVeigh E, Kass DA. Systolic improvement and mechanical resynchronization does not require electrical synchrony in the dilated failing heart with left bundle-branch block. *Circulation.* 2002;106:1760–3.

50. Bordachar P, Lafitte S, Reuter S, Garrigue S, Sanders P, Roudaut R, Jais P, Haissaguerre M, Clementy J. Biventricular pacing and left ventricular pacing in heart failure: similar hemodynamic improvement despite marked electromechanical differences. *J Cardiovasc Electrophysiol.* 2004;15:1342–47.

51. Hay I, Melenovsky V, Fetics BJ, Judge DP, Kramer A, Spinelli J, Reister C, Kass DA, Berger RD. Short-term effects of right-left heart sequential cardiac resynchronization in patients with heart failure, chronic atrial fibrillation, and atrioventricular nodal block. *Circulation.* 2004;110:3404–10.

52. Auricchio A, Stellbrink C, Block M, Sack S, Vogt J, Bakker P, Klein H, Kramer A, Ding J, Salo R, Tockman B, Pochet T, Spinelli J. Effect of pacing chamber and atrioventricular delay on acute systolic function of paced patients with congestive heart failure. The Pacing Therapies for Congestive Heart Failure Study Group. The Guidant Congestive Heart Failure Research Group. *Circulation.* 1999;99:2993–3001.

53. Vernooy K, Verbeek XA, Cornelussen RN, Dijkman B, Crijns HJ, Arts T, Prinzen FW. Calculation of effective VV interval facilitates optimization of AV delay and VV interval in cardiac resynchronization therapy. *Heart Rhythm.* 2007;4:75–82.

54. Dupuis JM, Kobeissi A, Vitali L, Gaggini G, Merheb M, Rouleau F, Leftheriotis G, Ritter P, Victor J. Programming optimal atrioventricular delay in dual chamber pacing using peak endocardial acceleration: comparison with a standard echocardiographic procedure. *Pacing Clin Electrophysiol.* 2003;26:210–13.

55. Butter C, Auricchio A, Stellbrink C, Fleck E, Ding J, Yu Y, Huvelle E, Spinelli J. Effect of resynchronization therapy stimulation site on the systolic function of heart failure patients. *Circulation.* 2001;104:3026–9.

56. St John Sutton MG, Plappert T, Abraham WT, Smith AL, Delurgio DB, Leon AR, Loh E, Kocovic DZ, Fisher WG, Ellestad M, Messenger J, Kruger K, Hilpisch KE, Hill MR. Effect of cardiac resynchronization therapy on left ventricular size and function in chronic heart failure. *Circulation.* 2003;107:1985–90.

57. Steendijk P, Tulner SA, Bax JJ, Oemrawsingh PV, Bleeker GB, van EL, Putter H, Verwey HF, van der Wall EE, Schalij MJ. Hemodynamic effects of long-term cardiac resynchronization therapy: analysis by pressure–volume loops. *Circulation.* 2006;113:1295–1304.

58. Sutton MG, Plappert T, Hilpisch KE, Abraham WT, Hayes DL, Chinchoy E. Sustained reverse left ventricular structural remodeling with cardiac resynchronization at one year is a function of etiology: quantitative Doppler echocardiographic evidence from the Multicenter InSync Randomized Clinical Evaluation (MIRACLE). *Circulation.* 2006;113:266–72.

59. Yu CM, Chau E, Sanderson JE, Fan K, Tang MO, Fung WH, Lin H, Kong SL, Lam YM, Hill MR, Lau CP. Tissue Doppler echocardiographic evidence of reverse remodeling and improved synchronicity by simultaneously delaying regional contraction after biventricular pacing therapy in heart failure. *Circulation.* 2002;105:438–45.

60. Yu CM, Bleeker GB, Fung JW, Schalij MJ, Zhang Q, van der Wall EE, Chan YS, Kong SL, Bax JJ. Left ventricular reverse remodeling but not clinical improvement predicts long-term survival after cardiac resynchronization therapy. *Circulation*. 2005;112: 1580–6.

61. Stellbrink C, Breithardt OA, Franke A, Sack S, Bakker P, Auricchio A, Pochet T, Salo R, Kramer A, Spinelli J. Impact of cardiac resynchronization therapy using hemodynamically optimized pacing on left ventricular remodeling in patients with congestive heart failure and ventricular conduction disturbances. *J Am Coll Cardiol*. 2001;38:1957–65.

62. Schillinger W, Lehnart SE, Prestle J, Preuss M, Pieske B, Maier LS, Meyer M, Just H, Hasenfuss G. Influence of SR Ca(2+)-ATPase and Na(+)-Ca(2+)-exchanger on the force-frequency relation. *Basic Res Cardiol*. 1998;93 Suppl 1:38–45.

63. Iyengar S, Haas G, Lamba S, Orsinelli DA, Babu GJ, Ferketich AK, Yamokoski L, Periasamy M, Abraham WT. Effect of cardiac resynchronization therapy on myocardial gene expression in patients with nonischemic dilated cardiomyopathy. *J Card Fail*. 2007;13:304–11.

64. Abraham WT, Gilbert EM, Lowes BD, Minobe WA, Larrabee P, Roden RL, Dutcher D, Sederberg J, Lindenfeld JA, Wolfel EE, Shakar SF, Ferguson D, Volkman K, Linseman JV, Quaife RA, Robertson AD, Bristow MR. Coordinate changes in Myosin heavy chain isoform gene expression are selectively associated with alterations in dilated cardiomyopathy phenotype. *Mol Med*. 2002;8:750–60.

65. Liao P, Georgakopoulos D, Kovacs A, Zheng M, Lerner D, Pu H, Saffitz J, Chien K, Xiao RP, Kass DA, Wang Y. The in vivo role of p38 MAP kinases in cardiac remodeling and restrictive cardiomyopathy. *Proc Natl Acad Sci USA*. 2001;98:12283–8.

66. Zhang R, Khoo MS, Wu Y, Yang Y, Grueter CE, Ni G, Price EE, Jr., Thiel W, Guatimosim S, Song LS, Madu EC, Shah AN, Vishnivetskaya TA, Atkinson JB, Gurevich VV, Salama G, Lederer WJ, Colbran RJ, Anderson ME. Calmodulin kinase II inhibition protects against structural heart disease. *Nat Med*. 2005;11:409–17.

67. Kubota T, McTiernan CF, Frye CS, Slawson SE, Lemster BH, Koretsky AP, Demetris AJ, Feldman AM. Dilated cardiomyopathy in transgenic mice with cardiac-specific overexpression of tumor necrosis factor-alpha. *Circ Res*. 1997;81:627–35.

68. D'Ascia C, Cittadini A, Monti MG, Riccio G, Sacca L. Effects of biventricular pacing on interstitial remodelling, tumor necrosis factor-alpha expression, and apoptotic death in failing human myocardium. *Eur Heart J*. 2006;27:201–6.

69. Kies P, Bax JJ, Molhoek SG, Bleeker GB, Zeppenfeld K, Bootsma M, van EL, Steendijk P, van der Wall EE, Schalij MJ. Effect of cardiac resynchronization therapy on inducibility of ventricular tachyarrhythmias in cardiac arrest survivors with either ischemic or idiopathic dilated cardiomyopathy. *Am J Cardiol*. 2005;95:1111–14.

70. Ermis C, Seutter R, Zhu AX, Benditt LC, VanHeel L, Sakaguchi S, Lurie KG, Lu F, Benditt DG. Impact of upgrade to cardiac resynchronization therapy on ventricular arrhythmia frequency in patients with implantable cardioverter-defibrillators. *J Am Coll Cardiol*. 2005;46:2258–63.

71. Di CA, Bongiorni MG, Arena G, Soldati E, Giannola G, Zucchelli G, Balbarini A. New-onset ventricular tachycardia after cardiac resynchronization therapy. *J Interv Card Electrophysiol*. 2005;12:231–5.

72. Guerra JM, Wu J, Miller JM, Groh WJ. Increase in ventricular tachycardia frequency after biventricular implantable cardioverter defibrillator upgrade. *J Cardiovasc Electrophysiol*. 2003;14:1245–7.

73. Medina-Ravell VA, Lankipalli RS, Yan GX, Antzelevitch C, Medina-Malpica NA, Medina-Malpica OA, Droogan C, Kowey PR. Effect of epicardial or biventricular pacing to prolong QT interval and increase transmural dispersion of repolarization: does resynchronization therapy pose a risk for patients predisposed to long QT or torsade de pointes? *Circulation.* 2003;107:740–6.

74. McSwain RL, Schwartz RA, Delurgio DB, Mera FV, Langberg JJ, Leon AR. The impact of cardiac resynchronization therapy on ventricular tachycardia/fibrillation: an analysis from the combined Contak-CD and InSync-ICD studies. *J Cardiovasc Electrophysiol.* 2005;16:1168–71.

75. Cleland JG, Daubert JC, Erdmann E, Freemantle N, Gras D, Kappenberger L, Tavazzi L. Longer-term effects of cardiac resynchronization therapy on mortality in heart failure [the CArdiac REsynchronization-Heart Failure (CARE-HF) trial extension phase]. *Eur Heart J.* 2006;27:1928–32.

76. Rivero-Ayerza M, Theuns DA, Garcia-Garcia HM, Boersma E, Simoons M, Jordaens LJ. Effects of cardiac resynchronization therapy on overall mortality and mode of death: a meta-analysis of randomized controlled trials. *Eur Heart J.* 2006;27:2682–8.

77. Berger T, Hanser F, Hintringer F, Poelzl G, Fischer G, Modre R, Tilg B, Pachinger O, Roithinger FX. Effects of cardiac resynchronization therapy on ventricular repolarization in patients with congestive heart failure. *J Cardiovasc Electrophysiol.* 2005;16:611–17.

78. Henrikson CA, Spragg DD, Cheng A, Capps M, Devaughn K, Marine JE, Calkins H, Tomaselli GF, Berger RD. Evidence for electrical remodeling of the native conduction system with cardiac resynchronization therapy. *Pacing Clin Electrophysiol.* 2007;30: 591–5.

79. Nishijima Y, Sridhar A, Viatchenko-Karpinski S, Shaw C, Bonagura JD, Abraham WT, Joshi MS, Bauer JA, Hamlin RL, Gyorke S, Feldman DS, Carnes CA. Chronic cardiac resynchronization therapy and reverse ventricular remodeling in a model of nonischemic cardiomyopathy. *Life Sci.* 2007;81:1152–9.

80. Tomaselli GF, Beuckelmann DJ, Calkins HG, Berger RD, Kessler PD, Lawrence JH, Kass D, Feldman AM, Marban E. Sudden cardiac death in heart failure. The role of abnormal repolarization. *Circulation.* 1994;90:2534–9.

Chapter 3

Electrical assessment of the failing heart

Dan Blendea and Jagmeet P. Singh

Key Points

1. Understanding the propagation of the depolarization wavefront in the failing heart is essential to the understanding of the response to cardiac resynchronization therapy.
2. Electrical activation of the ventricles, proceeds in a predominantly apex-to-base direction, sequence thought to increase ventricular pumping efficiency.
3. The short duration of ventricular activation, which is a reflection of the rapid conduction within the Purkinje fibers, facilitates synchronous activation of the heart.
4. Normal ventricular activation sequence has three important components, which include the initial trans-septal conduction, left and right ventricular endocardial activation followed by the transmural conduction to the epicardial surface.
5. The left ventricle is first activated at the endocardial level in a central area of the interventricular septum and in an area of the anterior free wall near the anterior papillary muscle. Endocardial activation of the right ventricle begins usually in the vicinity of the anterior papillary muscle. From these exits, the left and right ventricular activation travels from apex to base with small timing differences.
6. In patients with heart failure and left bundle branch block the activation wavefront spreads from the initial left ventricular breakthrough site situated most frequently along the apical septum, travels around the apex and across the inferior wall reaching the anterolateral wall, and then propagates

Pacing to Support the Failing Heart, 1st edition. Edited by K. Ellenbogen and A. Auricchio.
© 2008 American Heart Association, ISBN: 978-1-4051-7534-0

towards the basal posterior or posterolateral wall in a "U-shaped" activation pattern.

7. Ventricular epicardial activation during left bundle branch block has been demonstrated to be heterogenous, demonstrating functional lines of block, resulting in a "U-shaped" activation pattern somewhat similar to that observed at endocardial level.

8. Understanding the activation patterns and regions of slow conduction is especially important towards a better site selection for left ventricular pacing.

9. The resulting activation pattern during biventricular pacing can be influenced by several variables, inclusive of atrioventricular and interventricular pacing intervals, presence of scar, local pathologies, lead positions, and intramural delay.

10. Electrical synchrony does not necessarily imply mechanical synchrony due to the spatio-temporal heterogeneity of the relationship between electrical excitation and mechanical contraction in patients with heart failure.

Introduction

The electrical activation sequence of the heart is an important determinant of coordinated cardiac contraction and relaxation, and overall cardiac function. Abnormalities in electrical activation that cause asynchronous cardiac contraction may diminish the mechano-energetic efficiency of the heart and result in heart failure. Cardiac conduction defects can either lead to heart failure, or may occur secondarily as an integral part of the process of cardiac remodeling that accompanies advanced cardiomyopathies. Assessment of electrical activation in the failing heart has gathered renewed interest, since the emergence of cardiac resynchronization therapy (CRT) as a very effective treatment modality in patients with heart failure. The development of atrial synchronized biventricular pacing has now changed the natural history of congestive heart failure, with significant improvement in functional class and long-term clinical outcome. Understanding the propagation of the depolarization wavefront in the failing heart is essential to understand: (1) the mechanisms of heterogeneity in response to CRT, (2) the best pacing site to maximize success of CRT, and (3) the impact of optimizing the atrio-ventricular and interventricular timing on coordinating cardiac contractility.

The last decade brought to the forefront new methods for investigating the electrical activation of the heart. To the conventional catheter-based method were added the newer nonfluoroscopic, three-dimensional contact [1] and non-contact [2] mapping systems, which offer improved spatial and temporal resolution and enable in vivo overlapping of the electrical map over an anatomical reconstruction. However, these techniques are invasive and are used mainly for endocardial mapping. Contact mapping involves the use of a mapping catheter that is dragged over the endocardium. This enables the sequential acquisition of points, while the location of the electrode tip and the local electrogram in relation to the surface QRS signal is recorded. The method uses bipolar signals and facilitates the creation of a color-coded activation map, generated from regional activation timings, which can be superimposed on the three-dimensional chamber geometry. Noncontact mapping has made it possible to determine the global pattern of LV activation, through the use of a multi-electrode array mapping catheter system. This system uses unipolar signals and enables the reconstruction of the endocardial activation and ventricular chamber geometry. These catheter-based methods have been extensively validated, and despite some inherent limitations, remain the most accurate and practical techniques for delineating the electrical activation of the heart.

Electrocardiographic imaging via body surface mapping with a multi-electrode vest covering the anterior and posterior portion of the chest is another novel noninvasive imaging modality for determining cardiac excitation [3]. This technique involves the recording of ventricular activation time using isochronous maps, generated via epicardial imaging over a single beat [3]. This method can be used to generate maps of cardiac activation and repolarization during normal sinus rhythm, conduction disturbances, and ventricular pacing including in patients undergoing CRT (Figure 3.1) [4,5].

Electrical activation of the normal heart

To understand the impact of the electrical activation sequence on the failing heart and vice versa, the next section will review the basic features of the components of the conduction system involved in the electrical activation of the normal heart.

Sinus node

The sinus node (SN) was described in 1907 by Keith [6] as "a remarkable remnant of primitive fibres persisting at the sino-auricular junction," "in close connection with the vagus and sympathetic nerves," where "dominating rhythm of the heart is believed to normally arise." The SN is a spindle-like [7] or crescent-like [8] structure, approximately 10–20 mm in length, located 0.1–1 mm subepicardially in the right atrium (RA) at the junction with the superior vena cava, in the immediate vicinity of crista terminalis (Figures 3.2a and 3.2b) [8]. The nodal cells are imbedded in a matrix of fibrous tissue, with a relatively discrete boundary seen between the margins of the node and the adjacent atrial tissues [8,9]. The SN has, in most cases, radiations extend toward the superior caval vein, the subepicardium, the terminal crest, the intercaval region and toward the right atrial appendage [8,10]. These anatomical features can facilitate the communication between the SN and the right atrial myocardium, with subsequent conduction to the rest of the heart [8].

In addition to the structural variances, the SN is functionally quite heterogeneous, in regards to pacemaker activity, action potential, densities of ionic currents and expression of gap-junction proteins [11,12]. The site of the leading

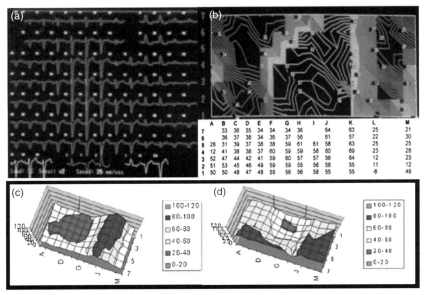

Fig. 3.1 PQRST electrodes recorded from 87 body-surface potential mapping leads (a), with the derived isochronous map of cardiac electrical activation (b). The isochronous map can be divided into three distinct regions: (1) the right ventricular (RV) region, (2) the anteroseptal (AS) region, and (3) left ventricular (LV) region. Three-dimensional graphic presentation of the horizontal plane of the matrixes of mean electrical activation times in the RV, anteroseptal region, and the LV. The isochronous maps are constructed from the values gathered during the native left bundle branch block pattern (c) and with atrio-biventricular pacing (d). (Adapted from Pastore et al. [5].) (See color plate section).

pacemaker within the SN can originate from a variable area, and can change location inside the SN depending on the milieu and fluctuations in sympathetic and parasympathetic stimulation. Shifts in the site of the leading pacemaker inside the SN shows a relationship to changes in rate (the more the superior the location the faster the heart rate), and can also translate into P wave morphology changes on the surface electrocardiogram [9,11–13]. Moreover, the initiation of the electrical impulse within the SN can be multicentric, with more than one focus initiating a single beat [12]. Regarding ionic currents, the pacemaker cells from the SN exhibit typical electrophysiological characteristics like the presence the hyperpolarization-activated current, I_f ("funny" current), and the absence of the inwardly rectifying potassium current, I_{K1} [14]. There are regional differences in the role of calcium and sodium currents toward the pacemaker activity of the SN. In the center of the node, where the calcium current is predominantly the inward current, the action potential is slow and small compared with the action potential in the periphery where the sodium current predominates [9,11]. Connexin 45, which forms low-conductance gap-junction channels, is

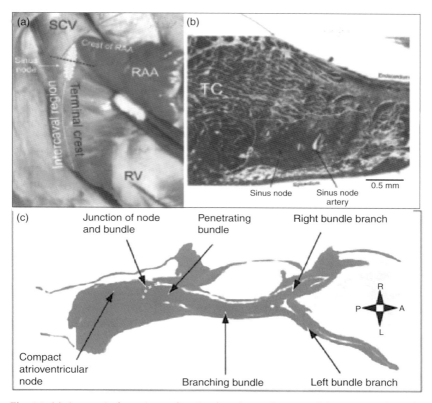

Fig. 3.2 (a) Anatomical specimen showing location and extent of the sinus node at the right atrial superior vena cava junction. (b) Histopathological section showing the sinus node and its relation to the sins node artery and to the crista terminalis (Adapted from Dobrzynski et al. [9].) (c) This illustration is scanned from Tawara's monograph of 1906, and re-oriented to attitudinally correct position. It shows the axis of conduction tissue, in orange, extending from the atrial myocardium in yellow, penetrating the insulating plane, shown in red, and branching on the crest of the muscular ventricular septum, also shown in yellow. Anatomy of the human atrioventricular junctions revisited (Adapted from Anderson et al. [10].) (See color plate section).

well-represented at the SN level. This may be responsible for the high intercellular resistance and low conductance inside the SN. The conduction velocity in the SN (0.03–0.05 m/s) is much slower than in the surrounding atrial myocardium, which is approximately 1m/s [11]. Nearly one-third of the patients with heart failure have some degree of sinus node dysfunction, resulting in impaired generation and/or propagation of the native sino-atrial electrical impulse.

Atrial conduction system

In 1916, Jean George Bachmann reported the presence of a special structure, described as a band of muscle tissue extending from the right atrium to the base of the left atrial appendage [15]. This band of tissue, which was thought to enhance inter-atrial conduction, became known afterward as Bachmann's bundle. Several subsequent anatomical and physiological reports described the existence of connections between the right and left atrial myocardium that bridge the septal raphe at three levels: anteriorly (Bachmann's bundle), centrally or superiorly, and posteriorly [16–21]. The presence of specialized conduction fibers between the SN and atrio-ventricular node (AVN) is a matter of controversy [8,17,18,22]. It is thought that internodal conduction is modulated by the geometry and arrangement of the myocardial fibers rather than conduction via the specialized conduction fibers. In the internodal areas, as elsewhere in the heart, the propagation in a direction parallel to the length of the myocardial fiber is faster than that in a perpendicular direction. [23] In failing hearts with the remodeling process involving the atrium as well, both the inter-atrial and intra-atrial activation sequences are affected.

Atrio-ventricular node

The AVN, first described in 1906 [24], is a histologically distinct bundle of fibers that provides the only electrical connection between the atria and the ventricles. The AVN has been divided in three zones: (i) atrial transitional cells, (ii) the compact AVN (or "knoten"), and (iii) the penetrating part of the AV bundle (the portion that penetrates the central fibrous body of the heart). The electrical impulse is conducted very slowly through the AVN, allowing coordination between the contraction of the atria and the ventricles. During propagation of a normal sinus beat, activation of the transitional zone accounts for at least 25% of conduction time from atrium to His bundle, with the small compact zone constituting the main source of AV nodal delay. Cycle length-dependent conduction delay is localized mainly in the compact zone [25]. Although the AVN conduction is strongly influenced by sympathetic and vagal stimulation, ion channels and gap junction channels appear very important in explaining the AVN physiology. Predominance of calcium channels (both L-type and T-type) and the paucity of sodium channels contribute to the prolonged conduction time through the AVN [26]. The gap junction channel proteins (connexins) expressed in the triangle of Koch, also play a role in the AVN conduction. Connexin-45, which forms gap junction channels with low conductivity, is well-represented at this level [26,27]. On the other hand, the more ubiquitous Connexin-43, which forms high conductance gap junction channels throughout most of the myocardium has a low expression in the compact AVN [26]. The AVN, through these innate conducting properties, protects the ventricles by blocking premature or very rapid atrial impulses. Additionally, it is important to recognize the ability of the AVN to serve as a pacemaker to the ventricles when the sinoatrial pacemaker fails or when conduction block between atria and AV node develops [25]. The site of origin of junctional rhythm seems to be most of the times at the posterior extension of the AV node, where the pacemaking channel HCN4 (responsible for the I_f current) is highly expressed [26]. The velocity of conduction at the AVN is very slow, approximately 0.04–0.05 m/s, which accounts for an AVN delay of approximately 80 ms.

His–Purkinje system

Electrical activation of the ventricles is facilitated by the rapidly conducting His–Purkinje system, with activation sequence being determined by the branching pattern of the His bundle.

The His–Purkinje system (Figure 3.2b), described for the first time in the late 1800s [28,29] is a structure that connects with the distal part of the compact AV node via the His bundle. This bundle perforates the central fibrous body and continues through the annulus fibrosus, penetrating the membranous septum, bifurcating at its superior margin into the right bundle branch and the left bundle branch. At this level, the muscular interventricular septum is vascularized by branches from both the anterior and posterior descending arteries making the His bundle and its bifurcation relatively resistant to ischemic insults. The right bundle branch is a cord-like structure that courses along the right side of the interventricular septum. It is because of the relatively superficial course that it is prone to injury during catheter movement on the right side of the heart. Closer to the right ventricular (RV) apex at the base of the anterior papillary muscle of the tricuspid valve, the right bundle terminates into the Purkinje network.

The left bundle branch, described as a broad fenestrated sheet of conduction fibers, has a short subendocardial course along the interventricular septum before bifurcating into anterior and posterior fascicles, which travel toward the left ventricular apex and both papillary muscle groups. In some cases the left bundle gives rise also to a group of central fibers, and in other cases the left bundle system appears more as a fan-like structure without a fascicular division [30]. When there is a bifascicular division, the anterior fascicle of the left bundle branch is thinner and longer that the posterior fascicle, and is therefore more susceptible to different types of insults, thereby explaining the greater preponderance of anterior fascicular defects as compared to the posterior ones. The Purkinje network is better represented at the apex than in the basal segments of the ventricles and is more resistant to ischemia than the surrounding myocardium [31]. The Purkinje fibers extensively innervate the endocardial surface of both ventricles [32], penetrating only the inner third of the endocardium, where these are electrically coupled with the working myocardial cells. The Purkinje cells are larger than working cardiac myocytes, contain more glycogen and fewer myofibrils and an abundance of lateral and end-to-end gap junctions made up primarily of Connexin-40 and Connexin-43 (which form gap junction channels of high conductance) [27] and are aligned to form multicellular bundles in longitudinal strands separated by collagen, being uniquely suited for functioning like a cable [33]. As a consequence the conduction velocity in the His–Purkinje system is approximately 3 m/s, much faster than normal myocardium ($\approx$0.5 m/s).

Normal electrical activation sequence

The normal activation wavefront starts in the SN, with the electrical impulse propagating to the atria and then to the AVN. The impulse exits from the AVN and is spread rapidly into the LV and RV through the His bundle, its branches and the network of Purkinje fibers. The His bundle and bundle branches are electrically insulated from surrounding muscle as they course toward the ventricular apex [34]. The insulation breaks down within the peripheral networks of Purkinje fibers, enabling direct impulse transmission to the working myocardium at the Purkinje–myocyte junctions. As a consequence of their disposition, activation and contraction of the ventricles proceed in a predominantly apex-to-base direction. This sequence of excitation and contraction is thought to increase ventricular pumping efficiency [35]. Although even in the normal heart there can be variability in the activation sequence, the total duration of this activation is less than 80 ms. This short duration, which is a reflection of the rapid conduction within the Purkinje fibers, facilitates synchronous activation of the heart.

The LV myocardial wall is first activated at the endocardial level in a central area of the of the interventricular septum and in an area of the anterior free wall near the anterior papillary muscle and extending toward the apex (Figure 3.3) [36]. Endocardial activation of the RV starts 5–10 ms after the beginning of LV activation in the vicinity of the anterior papillary muscle [36]. From

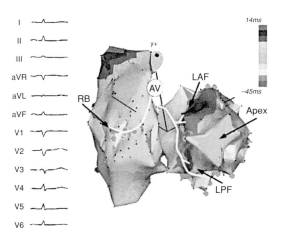

Fig. 3.3 Normal electrical activation sequence using contact mapping (CARTO system). This is a left anterior oblique view and the activation times are color coded where purple is the last and red the earliest portion of the heart to be activated. The activation of both the ventricles is near simultaneous and synchronous. The left ventricular activation precedes the right ventricle by 10 ms. The pink tags depict regions of the heart with fascicular potentials. The yellow lines are schematic representations of the right and left bundles. (Adapted Peichl et al. [86].) (See color plate section).

these exits of the Purkinje system, the LV and RV activation sequence travels from apex to base with small timing differences in activation between the septum and LV free wall [37]. The activation patterns of the LV and RV are near mirror images with the latest activated regions of the RV along the lateral wall and the basal area near the AV sulcus, while that of the LV occurring in the postero-lateral/basal area. The intramural conduction from the endo-to-epicardium is less well-understood and is considered to spread in a centrifugal manner [36]. Interestingly, the earliest ventricular epicardial activation site does not coincide with the first endocardial site to be activated. The first epicardial breakthrough occurs in the area pretrabecularis of the right ventricle 20–25 ms after the onset of ventricular endocardial activation [36]. Once, the ventricular activation breaks through epicardially, its subsequent spread occurs in a radial fashion toward the apical and basal regions [36].

Mechanical activation: The importance of a normal atrio-ventricular and ventricular activation sequence

The electrical activation of the heart determines the mechanical activation via excitation-contraction coupling. This process is mediated at the intracellular level by the entry into the cell of Ca^{2+} through L-type Ca^{2+} channels, which, in turn, triggers the release of a large amount of Ca^{2+} from the sarcoplasmic reticulum (by the mechanism known as Ca^{2+}-induced Ca^{2+} release), which, in turn, facilitates the interaction between actin and myosin filaments leading to contraction [38,39]. The delay between depolarization and the onset of myocardial contraction (electromechanical delay), which is approximately 30 ms [40], is mainly determined by the delay between intracellular Ca^{2+} increase and the development of force.

Due to this tight coupling, the electrical activation of the heart is closely followed by mechanical contraction at atrial level and, after a delay required for impulse conduction through the AVN, at the ventricular level. Because of this sequence of events, atrial contraction precedes ventricular contraction responsible for approximately 10–40% to the ventricular filling in a normal heart [41]. The relative contribution of atrial contraction to ventricular filling is affected by several variables inclusive of age, and heart rate, and is inconsistent among individuals. An optimal atrio-ventricular (AV) interval optimizes the booster pump function of the atria and consequently optimizes the volume and function of the ventricles, helps atrioventricular valve closure and prevents diastolic regurgitation [34]. The importance of an optimal AV delay becomes evident in pathologic situations. If the electrical activation and the subsequent contraction of the atria occurs too early as in a prolonged PR interval (first–degree AV block) or in dual chamber pacing with a long AV interval the mitral valve closes early thereby limiting ventricular diastolic filling time and also promotes diastolic mitral regurgitation. If the atrial contraction occurs too late, for example, in patients with dual chamber pacing and short AV intervals, the atrial contraction can get overtly truncated by the next ventricular systole resulting in impaired ventricular filling.

In a normal heart, the synchronous electrical activation of the ventricles is followed by an equally closely timed contraction. In order for the ventricles to function efficiently as pumping chambers, there needs to be a close coordination between the two ventricles and between the walls of the same ventricle (i.e. inter-ventricular and intraventricular synchrony). This electromechanical activation sequence is disrupted due to variety of circumstances, such as extrasystoles and ventricular pacing [42,43], and most importantly due to conduction system defects accompanying remodeling in the failing heart [44].

Pathophysiological changes in the conduction system of the failing heart

Studies in experimental congestive heart failure in animals have shown that ventricular failure is accompanied by atrial remodeling consisting of extensive interstitial fibrosis accompanied by cell loss, degenerative changes, and hyper-trophy. These studies have shown that the myofibril bundles are packed less tightly than in control animals and are separated by thick layers of fibrous tissue along with increased intercellular connective tissue deposition [45]. The connective tissue is composed of increased numbers of fibroblasts, large amounts of collagen, ground substance, and occasionally fat cells [45]. Although histological changes are similar in both atria, they are more extensive in the left atrium (LA), promoting the potential induction of atrial fibrillation. This remodeling itself may impact the inter-atrial and intra-atrial conduction, which may significantly affect ventricular preload and consequently the cardiac output.

Ventricular remodeling in heart failure is a progressive process that encom-passes degenerative and maladaptive changes occurring at tissue, cellular, and subcellular level. including myocyte hypertrophy, necrosis, increased apoptosis, inflammation, and fibrosis. The remodeling process affects also the ventricular conduction system. Heart failure causes remodeling of important K^+ and Ca^{2+} currents in cardiac Purkinje cells, which decreases the repolarization reserve with potential implications regarding ventricular arrhythmogenesis [46]. Heart failure is associated with marked ventricular conduction abnormalities that can be at least in part explained by disturbances of gap junction organiza-tion. The most consistently observed is the down-regulation of Connexin-43 in patients with end-stage heart failure due to idiopathic dilated cardiomyopathy or ischemic heart disease [47]. Down-regulation of Connexin-43 is accompa-nied by significant reduction in intercellular coupling and conduction velocity in association with an enhancement of transmural dispersion of action poten-tial duration.[48] Animal studies have confirmed this reduction of Connexin-43 protein expression associated with a redistribution of Connexin-43 from the intercalated disk region to lateral cell borders [48]. The changes in Connexin-43 expression in the failing myocardium contribute to both intraventricular conduction disturbances and arrhythmia substrate formation.

Conduction abnormalities in the failing heart

Sino-atrial dysfunction

Bradyarrhythmias account for almost half of the sudden in-hospital deaths in patients with congestive heart failure [49,50]. Heart failure is associated with significant remodeling of the SN [50,51], which results in a decrease in the intrinsic heart rate [50, 52–54], as well as an increase in the corrected SN recovery time, a caudal shift of the leading pacemaker site, fractionated electrograms or double potentials along the terminal crest, a decrease in the amplitude of the electrograms along the terminal crest, and abnormal propagation of the action potential from the SN [9,50]. Changes in SN sensitivity to acetylcholine and vagal stimulation have been observed in heart failure in rabbit and dog [9,51,53]. An explanation for the increase in intrinsic cycle length of the SN was provided by Verkerk et al. [55], who demonstrated, in a heart failure model in rabbits, that the increased intrinsic cycle length is caused by a decrease in diastolic depolarization rate rather than changes in action potential duration. SN hyperpolarization-activated pacemaker current (I_f – the "funny" current) was found to be reduced, and the hyperpolarization-activated cyclic nucleotide-gated (HCN) subunits 4 and 2 that encode I_f at SN level were found to be down-regulated [55,56]. Down-regulation of HCN_4 and HCN_2 expression contribute to heart failure-induced SN dysfunction. HCN_4 was found to be however up-regulated in the rest of RA myocardium [56]. It appears that the intrinsic SN cycle length is prolonged in heart failure, but that in vivo the enhanced sympathetic activity can override this and can actually decrease sinus cycle length [57].

Significant electroanatomic remodeling was demonstrated not only in the SN but also in the rest of the atria in heart failure patients. Beside the tendency for atrial enlargement. There is also evidence of loss of functioning atrial myocardium, with regions of low-voltage amplitude and spontaneous scarring that are associated with significantly impaired atrial conduction observed throughout the RA, the LA, and the level of Bachmann's bundle [58]. Patients with heart failure were also shown to have an increase in effective refractory period at the atrial level when compared with controls [58]. Experimental heart failure was found to change the atrial cellular electrophysiologic substrate, via selectively increasing the Na^+/Ca^{2+} exchanger current [59], and up-regulation of the atrial HCN_4 that underlies the depolarizing "pacemaker" current, I_f [56]. As a consequence of structural and functional alterations at the atrial level, heart failure patients demonstrate increased inducibility and duration of atrial fibrillation, which may be a consequence of the demonstrated electrophysiological abnormalities [58]. However, it is important to note the difficulty in separating heart failure-induced ionic abnormalities in patients from those caused by underlying heart disease or concomitant drug therapy, or atrial fibrillation itself [59]. Consequent to the remodeling process accompanying heart failure, there can be significant changes in the intra-atrial, inter-atrial, and inter-nodal conduction.

Ventricular activation sequence in the failing heart

The structural and functional changes accompanying heart failure can have a significant impact on impulse generation and propagation. Despite, changes in the conduction pattern, the extent of asynchrony can be significantly affected by the alteration of myocardial characteristics. The resulting myocardial conduction is not only slower but more variable depending on the underlying myopathy. The slow conduction through the myocardial wall is often unpredictable, with the presence of scar, fibrosis, and ischemia adding to the complexity of the conduction pattern.

The normal ventricular activation sequence has three important components, which include the initial trans-septal conduction, LV and RV endocardial activation followed by the transmural conduction to the epicardial surface. To understand the variability in activation sequence among different patients, it is important to first understand some of the basic terminologies derived from electroanatomic mapping: (i) Earliest LV breakthrough site, which is defined as the location from which the propogation wavefront first breaks through to spread to the rest of the LV; (ii) Transeptal activation time, which is the time difference from the onset of the QRS complex on the surface ECG to the earliest LV breakthrough site. The latter point is recognized as the largest rapid deflection of the bipolar electrogram crossing the baseline; and (iii) Transmural activation time, is the time taken from the last activated site to the end of the QRS complex. Regions of slow conduction are defined by the presence of low voltage (<0.5 mV) or fragmented signals (>50 ms).

Left bundle branch block

The most frequent intraventricular conduction abnormality that occurs in approximately 25–30% of patients with heart failure is left bundle branch block (LBBB) [60–62]. By inducing regional delays in electrical activation it leads to dyssynchronous mechanical activity having a detrimental effect on overall LV function, which ultimately translates into negative impact on prognosis in heart failure patients [61,62].

Ventricular activation pattern in LBBB has been evaluated in animal studies [63–65] (by direct interruption of the proximal left bundle branch) or in studies in humans using noninvasive electrocardiographic imaging that maps epicardial ventricular activation [66], or using intraoperative epicardial [67], or catheter-based endocardial mapping [68,69]. More recently, Auricchio et al. [44], using catheter-based high-resolution three-dimensional endocardial mapping offered more detailed assessment of the sequence of ventricular activation in patients with heart failure who have LBBB pattern on the surface ECG. LBBB can occur in patients with dilated cardiomyopathy of ischemic or nonischemic etiology and is a heterogeneous entity [44,70–72]. It can result from conduction delay located at several anatomic levels in the conduction system from the distal His bundle to the left bundle branch and further distally to the arborization of the left bundle branch system. Different degrees of conduction delays in the right bundle branch system and in the diseased myocardium outside the conduction system can be also associated, which increases the complexity of this heterogeneous entity [44,70,73]. Because the conduction defect in a LBBB may be mixed and involve other parts of the ventricular His–Purkinje system, the pattern of ventricular activation is variable and unpredictable [44,66]. Also, the variance of the centrifugal conduction from the endocardium to epicardium, due to altered conductive properties of the different myocardial layers may partly explain this variability [44].

RV activation
Studies using three-dimensional electroanatomic mapping showed that in patients with heart failure and LBBB the first endocardial ventricular activa-tion occurs in the RV free wall, immediately before [70] or after [73] the Q wave on the surface ECG. From the RV endocardial breakthrough in the free wall, the activation spreads over the right septum to the posterobasal region, that is, the RV site with the latest activation (Figure 3.4) [70].

LV breakthrough
The LV endocardial breakthrough sites can be variable in their location and number. Although, most often the earliest portion of the LV to be activated is along the apical septum, it may occur in the septobasal or midseptal region or anterior in a minority of the patients [44]. In the majority of cases LV break-through is located at a single site but some patients can have two sites of early activation (Figure 3.5a) [70]. Although in a majority of patients with heart fail-ure and LBBB, the myopathic process prolongs the transseptal conduction time, in approximately one-third of patients the transseptal conduction time may be normal [44]. The site of LV breakthrough is dictated by the conductive pattern within the heart-the midseptal or apicoseptal breakthrough sites are often due to the slow cell-to-cell transseptal conduction, while patients with septobasal or anterior breakthrough sites have faster transseptal conduction likely via septal branches of the His–Purkinje system [44].

   In patients with nonischemic cardiomyopathy, the prolongation of the LV activation is more homogeneous in comparison to coronary artery disease. In patients with coronary artery disease, despite a classic LBBB on ECG, there may be early septal activation due to preserved conduction down the anterior or

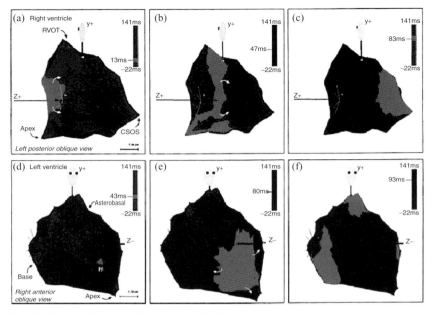

Fig. 3.4 Propagation map showing septal activation. Contact mapping (CARTO system) demonstrates the pattern of septal activation in a patient with left bundle branch block and heart failure. Right ventricular septal activation is shown in Panels (a)–(c), in the left posterior oblique view. The right side of the septum is activated from apex to base. Panels (d)–(f) show left ventricular activation in the right anterior oblique view. Earliest left ventricular activation occurs in the mid-septal region as a result of slow conduction through the left posterior fascicle (d), followed by activation, which spreads toward the apex and high septum (e,f). (Adapted from Rodriguez et al. [70].) (See color plate section).

posterior fascicle. Additionally, the presence of scar can significantly alter the activation process.

LV activation wavefront

Auricchio and colleagues demonstrated that the activation wavefront spreads from the initial LV breakthrough site both superiorly and inferiorly [44]. In most patients the activation cannot cross directly from the anterior to the lateral wall and instead travels inferiorly around the apex and across the inferior wall in a "U-shaped" pattern, reaches the anterolateral wall of the LV, and then propagates toward the basal posterior or posterolateral wall near the mitral valve annulus, which is the last LV segment to be depolarized [44]. This "U-shaped" activation pattern is thought to be generated by a functional line of block that is oriented from the base toward the apex of the LV (Figures 3.5b and 3.6). The turning point of the U-shaped activation front is located in the vicinity of the

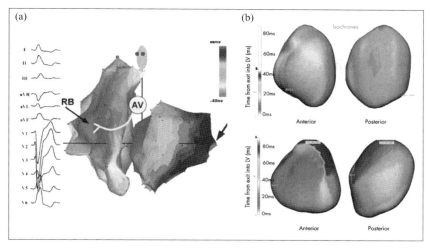

Fig. 3.5 (a) Color-coded electroanatomic isochronal maps of right ventricular and left ventricular activation in a heart failure patient with left bundle branch block, generated via contact mapping. The activation sequence is color-coded with red depicting the region with earliest activation and bluish-purple depicting the region of the heart with most delayed activation. Adapted from Peichl et al. [86].) (b) Isochronal maps comparing left ventricular activation on the anterior and posterior endocardial surfaces in a patient with idiopathic dilated cardiomyopathy (DCM) without a slow conduction zone, where there is homogeneous activation and in a patient with DCM and a slow conduction zone. In this subject, the activation wavefront arcs around the zone of slow conduction (see arrows) and reaches the region of latest activation. Times are referenced from exit of the activation wavefront into the left ventricle with earliest activation shown in red and latest in blue-white, as depicted by the reference scale. (Adapted from Lambiase et al. [100].) (See color plate section).

LV apex [44]. The LV endocardial activation time in patients with heart failure and LBBB is on average significantly longer than in subjects with normal hearts [70]. That a proportion of the heart failure patients with LBBB may also have normal or near-normal LV endocardial activation times is noteworthy [70]. It is possible that that in this subgroup of patients the LBBB morphology is consequent to a prolonged intramural activation time, accompanying the myopathic process. Simplistically, the endocardial activation time comprises about 75% of the surface QRS complex [70], while the rest of the activation delay is a consequence of mid-myocardial or epicardial activation (intramural) delay. However, there does appear to be a relationship between QRS duration, transseptal activation, and the pattern of LV activation. Patients with LBBB and a longer QRS duration (>150 ms) generally demonstrate prolonged (>40 ms) transseptal time, have a midseptal or septoapical LV breakthrough, with a more closely situated (more anterior) functional line of block as opposed to patients with LBBB but with a shorter QRS duration. LBBB with a narrower QRS duration is usually

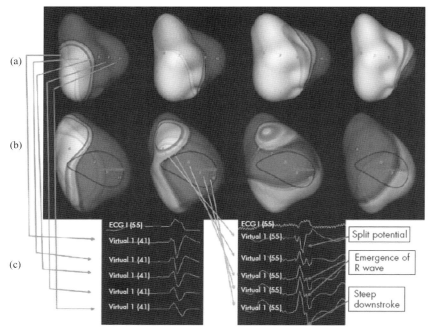

Fig. 3.6 Noncontact left ventricular mapping showing two different activation patterns. The sequence of endocardial activation using isopotential maps are shown with reference to onset of the QRS complex. In (a), the activation wavefront starting in the septum spreads across the anterior wall, with no obvious region of slow conduction (type I pattern). (b) shows the depolarization wavefront, as depicted by the isopotential map progressing from the septum along the inferior border to the postero-lateral wall of the left ventricle. An area of conduction block is noted over the anterior wall of the left ventricle, where the propagating wavefront breaks up and proceeds inferiorly. Panel (c) shows the electrogram characteristics (right side), such as the split potential, an emergence of the R wave, and a steep down stroke, as the wavefront progresses around the anterior wall. This is in contrast to the electrograms ((c), left) from depolarization wavefront in (a), where there is no area of slow conduction. (Adapted from Fung et al. [108].) (See color plate section).

characterized by a shorter transseptal time (<20 ms), an anterior or septobasal LV breakthrough, and a more distantly situated line of functional block, on the lateral wall [44].

Line of functional block

It is important to recognize that the line of conduction block is representative of a region prone to anisotropy (Figure 3.5b). This line of functional block can be altered and shifted in its location and length depending on the site of ventricular pacing. This reinforces the concept that the site of RV pacing-induced LBBB can have varied activation sequences and lines of blocks, depending on the location of the RV pacing electrode. Recent work has shown that by altering the RV pacing site, once can alter the electrical distance of the RV lead from the LV lead [74], suggesting that this may be consequence of a change in the activation wavefront. Ventricular epicardial activation during LBBB assessed non-invasively with electrocardiographic imaging has been demonstrated to be heterogenous, demonstrating functional lines of block, resulting in a "U-shaped" activation pattern somewhat similar to that observed at endocardial level. The epicardial functional lines of block generate complex barriers that may interfere with paced wave fronts [66]. Understanding the activation patterns and regions of slow conduction is especially important toward better site selection for LV and RV pacing. Different activation sequences can a have variable global and regional impact on the overall hemodynamic picture as well as on synchronicity of the papillary muscle contraction and resultant mitral regurgitation. Also important to note is that for the same QRS width and morphology, the segment of LV wall activation and consequent mechanical asynchrony pattern can differ substantially [75–77].

Right bundle branch block

Although right bundle branch block (RBBB) may be commonly observed in the community, its prevalence is greater in subjects of older age, male sex, prior myocardial infarction, and chronic lung disease [78]. Although, in subjects without overt heart disease, RBBB does not appear to have significant impact on cardiovascular mortality [79,80], in patients with coexistent cardiac disease (especially in acute coronary syndromes), the presence of RBBB and the degree of intraventricular conduction delay are associated with worse prognosis including increased all-cause mortality [78,81]. Approximately 10% of patients with heart failure who present as candidates for CRT have RBBB [82]. Experimental models have shown that cardiac dyssynchrony in failing hearts with RBBB is less than what is seen in the clinical situation. A pure RBBB is associated with less dyssynchrony between lateral and septal walls. It is important to note that these models do not account for scar, comorbidities, pulmonary hypertension, and the concomitant involvement of left-sided fascicles. As we alluded to earlier, the right bundle is fairly superficial and prone to injury secondary to right-sided pathologies or catheter manipulation. Consequently, right bundle branch block can result from interruption or delay in the conduction at any level of the right-sided intraventricular conduction system inclusive of the right bundle branch or its arborization.

RV Activation

Using a three-dimensional, high-resolution nonfluoroscopic electroanatomic mapping system, Fantoni and colleagues were the first to describe the ventricular activation sequence in patients with heart failure and RBBB [73]. They have shown that the earliest ventricular activation site is situated at the endocardial surface of the LV septum and after a significant delay the activation proceeds via transseptal conduction and breaksthrough in a single site at the RV septum. This occurred in their study group 59±16 ms after the beginning of the earliest surface QRS complex. Transseptal time was significally longer in patients with RBBB compared to LBBB patients. From the RV septal break through site the activation proceeds slowly likely as a result of cell-to-cell conduction to the anterior region and from there to the lateral wall and the RV outflow tract (Figure 3.7a). Total RV activation time is significantly longer in RBBB group as compared to LBBB group [73].

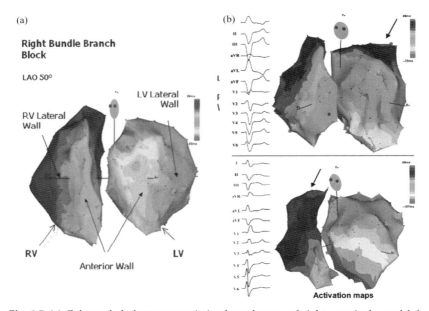

Fig. 3.7 (a) Color-coded electroanatomic isochronal maps of right ventricular and left ventricular activation in a heart failure patient with right bundle branch block, generated via contact mapping. The activation sequence is color-coded with red reflecting the region with earliest activation and bluish-purple depicting the region of the heart with most delayed activation. Two breakthrough sites can be seen on the left ventricular septum (the antero-basal region and apico-septal region). Right ventricular activation is delayed and the most-delayed portions of the heart to be activated are the postero-lateral walls of the left and right ventricles. (Adapted from Fantoni C, et al. [73].) (b) Activation maps in 2 patients with dilated cardiomyopathy and bifascicular. The intraventricular conduction delay (QRS width) is comparable between the two patients, but the conduction pattern (morphology in lead V1) is different. In both cases, the activation spreads from the posterior fascicle and is then conducted to the right ventricle via the interventricular septum. In the top panel, the last portion of the heart to be activated is the anterior wall along the mitral annulus, and in the bottom panel, the last portion of the heart to be activated is the right ventricle. (Adapted from Peichl et al. [86].) (See color plate section).

In contrast to patients with RBBB, in those with LBBB there are one or two RV breakthrough sites in the interventricular septum that occur quickly after the onset of the earliest QRS, with RV endocardial activation proceeding rapidly to the apex, lateral wall, outflow tract, and the basal region around the tricuspid ring [73].

LV Activation

The LV activation pattern is usually affected by either the presence of the under-lying cardiovascular disease or coexiting conduction defects. In normal hearts with an isolated RBBB, the LV activation is normal, and the RV activation time exceeds that of the LV. The LV endocardial activation time in patients with RBBB and cardiomyopathy is prolonged and may even be longer (135 ± 24 ms) than in patients with LBBB (109 ± 19 ms), suggesting that CHF patients with RBBB may have a diffuse disease of the conduction system beyond only right-sided involvement [73]. This hypothesis is consistent with prior pathologic findings [83]. The LV activation in patients with RBBB usually occurs from a LV septal or anterior breakthrough site, with the activation wavefront spreading to the apical and lateral regions, with the postero-lateral and basal regions around the mitral valve being activated last of all. This pattern of LV activation was similar to that observed in the LBBB group of patients further supporting the hypothesis that patients with heart failure and RBBB morphology of the ECG have in fact a diffuse disease of the conduction system that extends to the LV. Features suggestive of delayed LV activation accompanying a RBBB have also been observed found on surface ECG leads. Fantoni et al. [73] noted that the majority of heart failure patients with RBBB had a broad R wave on leads I and aVL with leftward axis, as usually seen in LBBB. An ECG pattern of delayed LV activation (i.e. LBBB) masked by RBBB had been previously described in the literature [84]. Given all these data it is not surprising that the heart failure patients with RBBB were found to have a severe underlying cardiomyopathy with lower LV ejection fraction, higher resting mean heart rate, higher NYHA class, and increased all-cause mortality [73,85].

RBBB with a left anterior hemiblock is a common pattern seen in many car-diomyopathic patients. The activation wavefront in these patients usually starts in the left inferior wall, with subsequent conduction to the RV septal endo-cardium, after approximately 50 ms [86]. The wavefront then proceeds to prop-agate along the RV lateral wall and the outflow. The LV activation time in these patients is prolonged and usually the last portion to be activated is in the anterior region close to the mitral annulus. It is noteworthy that patients with bifascicular block have longer LV activation times than patients with LBBB. This prolonged activation time is a result of the fact that the activation wavefront starts in a region (LV inferior wall), where there is a paucity of conduction tissue (Figure 3.7b).

Although, only a small fraction of patients with heart failure eligible for CRT have a RBBB, it nevertheless remains a sizable population. As described above, it is evident that a number of these patients have coexisting left-sided conduction disease, with delayed lateral wall activation and could benefit form CRT. This is substantiated from several studies that have shown possible benefit from CRT in this group of patients [87,88].

Cardiac resynchronization therapy and electromechanical consequences

Cardiac resynchronization therapy by using LV or biventricular pacing and altering the sequence of electrical activation in patients with heart failure and intraventricular conduction abnormalities improves LV efficiency and over-all hemodynamic function (Figure 3.8) [89]. Although the way in which CRT improves the synchrony of contraction has been well-studied, little informa-tion is available on the relationship between changes in electrical synchrony and the resulting changes in the contractile or mechanical synchrony with CRT. Although biventricular pacing has been shown to be beneficial, several studies

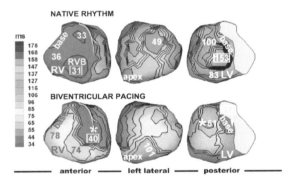

Fig. 3.8 Epicardial isochrone maps reflective of activation of the right and left ventricles during native rhythm and biventricular pacing. The epicardial surfaces of both ventricles are displayed in anterior, left lateral, and posterior views, with some overlap between adjacent views. The valve area is shaded in grey. The thick black mark in the top panel indicates the line of block, which is no longer appreciable with biventricular pacing. The native rhythm panel shows sequential activation of the right ventricle followed by a much-delayed left ventricular activation, which is suggestive of a left bundle branch–like pattern. Activation times (in milliseconds) of selected regions are shown. Earliest and latest ventricular activation times are indicated by framed numbers and are in relation to the onset of the QRS. (Adapted from Jia et al. [4].) (See color plate section).

have shown that acute hemodynamic effects of LV pacing are comparable to BiV pacing [75,90–92].

An important point to consider is that electrical synchrony does not necessarily imply mechanical synchrony because of the spatiotemporal heterogeneity of the relationship between electrical excitation and mechanical contraction in patients with heart failure. The variable response to CRT is determined by the inconsistent activation patterns between patients and the consequent variance in the electromechanical relationship. Even within the same patient, for the same LV and RV pacing lead positions, a wide range of isovolumic contraction times can exist from varying the atrio-ventricular and interventricular timing.

The LV and RV lead location during the delivery of biventricular pacing is vital [74,93]. Defining an optimal lead position is still unclear and the choice between an optimal anatomical position, targeting either the segment with maximal mechanical dyssynchrony [94] or a region with maximal electrical delay is still up for debate. There is evidence to suggest that maximal electrical separation between the right and left ventricular leads [74] and positioning the LV lead as far out into the electrical activation sequence may have a beneficial impact on clinical outcomes [93]. Modulating the AV delay, over and above this, has a significant impact on the depolarization wavefront and consequently on the extent of RV and LV pre-excitation, and ventricular contractility. Also, noteworthy is that changes in the AV delay can influence the location and size of the line-of-conduction block.

Electromechanical effect of left ventricular pacing

Data on electrical activation sequence during LV pacing is considerably limited. If atrial synchronous epicardial pacing is delivered at the lateral or posterolateral LV wall using a short AV delay, the activation starts at the level of the LV pacing lead and spreads epicardially to the lateral wall, then the anterior wall, and then around the apex, which is the latest activation occurring in the RV [4,95,96]. From the epicardial pacing site the activation also proceeds transmurally and after a short delay reaches the endocardial surface and spreads from this level in a pattern that follows in general the epicardial activation [96]. However, the highly ordered temporospatial pattern of transmural activation during sinus rhythm is replaced during LV pacing with a more heterogeneous activation [97].

Faris and colleagues [96] mapped simultaneously both endocardial and epicardial electrical activation during atrial synchronous LV free-wall pacing at varying AV delays (AV delay 0–150 ms) with the use of a 64-electrode LV endocardial basket and a 128-electrode epicardial sock in an animal model. The study offered information about ventricular electrical synchrony during CRT delivered by LV pacing alone in normal hearts with special focus on transition from dyssynchronous LV-paced activation to synchronous RA-paced activation at endocardial and epicardial level with progressive changes in AV delay.

At short AV delays during epicardial LV pacing, the LV activation pattern, as assessed using the electrical activation delay magnitude, showed a high degree of dyssynchrony equal on both endocardial and epicardial surfaces [96]. Moreover, the degree of electrical dyssynchrony was consistent over a range of short AV delays, indicating that activation did not involve fusion with the atrial stimulus via the intrinsic conduction system [96]. As the AV delay was increased, the activation became progressively more synchronous, because an increasingly larger portion of the ventricular myocardium was being activated via intrinsic conduction. Over a certain value of the AV delay, the activation wavefront did not change, indicating that the heart was primarily activated from the intrinsic conduction system rather than from the LV stimulus. It is important to note that the transition from dyssynchronous to synchronous pattern occurred approximately at the same AV delays for both epicardial and endocardial activation [96].

The same pattern of progressive fusion between the two activation wavefronts, the one generated by LV pacing and the one coming from the intrinsic activation system was observed in a study on heart failure patients who received CRT devices in whom epicardial activation was assessed noninvasively by using electrocardiographic imaging (Figure 3.9) [4]. With an optimal AV delay, patients in whom the device was programmed for LV pacing alone showed fusion between intrinsic excitation and the LV paced beat. Depending on the relative length of the PR interval and optimal AV delay, the degree of fusion varied. Fusion significantly influenced the degree of electrical synchrony during LV pacing, with synchrony improving as fusion increases [4].

Adjusting the AV delay, impacts the depolarization wavefronts, facilitating a hemodynamically beneficial fusion of the LV paced wavefront with the intrinsic conduction, minimizing the line of functional block and the synchronization of the mechanically dyssynchronous segments.

Given the fact that electrical fusion between LV pacing and spontaneous RV activation is considered the key to resynchronization in sinus rhythm patients treated with single-site left ventricular pacing there were efforts to provide simple ways define the range of AV delays that provide optimal benefit from CRT. Gianfranchi et al. [98] used QRS morphology from the surface ECG to optimize device programming in patients with CHF, sinus rhythm, and LBBB treated with single-site LV pacing. They defined the "fusion band" as the range of AV intervals within which surface the ECG showed an intermediate morphology between the native LBBB pattern and the fully paced RBBB pattern. Echo-derived parameters were collected in the fusion band and compared with the basal LBBB condition. They noted that in the fusion band diastolic filling time, LV ejection fraction and myocardial performance index showed a statistically significant improvement, and interventricular delay and mitral regurgitation progressively and significantly decreased as AV delay shortened [98].

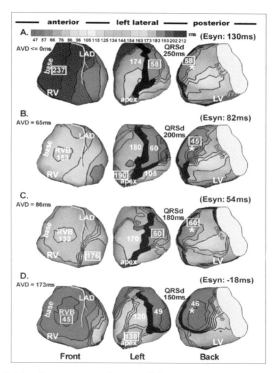

Fig. 3.9 Epicardial isochrone maps reflective of the extent of fusion of intrinsic activation with left ventricular (LV) pacing with alteration of the atrioventricular delay (AVD). The epicardial surfaces of both ventricles are displayed in anterior, left lateral and posterior views. There is a progressive increase in the AV delay from (a) to (d), with the most optimal fusion occuring at AV delay of 173 ms ((d), where the breakthrough in the right ventricular (RV) septum occurs at 45 ms, with the best electrical synchrony index (Esyn), that is, the least difference between RV and LV activation time (Esyn:-18 ms). Thick black markings are indicative of the region of conduction block. Earliest and latest ventricular activation times are indicated by framed numbers. All activation times are given with respect to the onset of the QRS. (*LAD; left anterior descending coronary artery.) (Adapted from Jia et al. [4].) (See color plate section).

LV lead location in relation to the region of slow conduction can often be affected by the underlying coronary venous anatomy, the absence of phrenic nerve capture, and an acceptable pacing threshold. The global LV depolarization from LV pacing can be unduly prolonged, especially if the pacing site is located over an area of local scarring or fibrosis, which may retard the progression of the depolarizing wavefront. Hence, optimal LV lead location is needed to facilitate optimal propagation with reduction of LV activation time results in reduced septal dyskinesis and early papillary muscle contraction, which translates into beneficial hemodynamic effects.

Electromechanical effect of biventricular pacing: The effect of AV and VV timing

Biventricular pacing is based on the premise that modifications in the pattern of electrical activation of both ventricles can lead to an increase in intraventricular as well as interventricular synchrony and ultimately to an improvement in the hemodynamic efficiency of the failing heart. The method most frequently used is atrio-biventricular pacing with a right atrial lead, a LV lead positioned epicardially in a tributary of the coronary sinus, and a RV lead implanted endocardially.

Although there is significant interpatient variability, ventricular activation during simultaneous biventricular pacing with a short AV delay follows a general pattern that can be summarized as follows. The spatial disposition of the pacing leads allows generation of two ventricular activation wavefronts, which are initiated at the LV and RV pacing sites and move in opposite directions toward each other (Figure 3.10). If pacing is delivered with a sufficently short AV delay, the left and right ventricular wavefronts generated by pacing merge, even before the instrinstic activation generated in the atria could reach the ventricles via the AVN. The RV activation wavefront breaks into the LV after a 50–60 ms delay. The RV is depolarized entirely or almost entirely by the wavefront generated by the RV lead. The initially dyssynchronous LV (because of LBBB or other preexistent intraventricular conduction abnormality) is now activated from two sites: one is situated in the interventricular septum where it breaks through at the wavefront initiated by the RV lead, and the other one is situated on the epicardial surface of the lateral LV wall where the LV lead is located. Both endocardial and epicardial mapping have demonstrated that LV activation wavefronts have to circumvent functional lines of block with variable disposition (anterior, lateral, inferior) resembling the lines of block that occur during native rhythm in heart failure patients with LBBB [4,44].

It is important to note that the resulting activation pattern can be influenced by several variables, including (i) AV and VV pacing intervals (ii) presence of scar, (iii) local pathologies, (iv) alternativelead positions, (v) variable lead positions, and (vi) variable intramural delay.

The AV interval significantly influences the pattern of activation not only during LV pacing alone but also during biventricular pacing. If atrio-biventricular pacing is delivered with very long AV interval in a heart failure patient with LBBB, the depolarization initiated in the atria descends via the AVN and right bundle branch and propagates from the RV to the LV. With intermediate AV delays, ventricular depolarization occurs with different degrees of fusion between the wavefronts generated by the right bundle branch (intrinsic conduction) and by the RV and LV leads. At short AV delays, ventricular depolarization

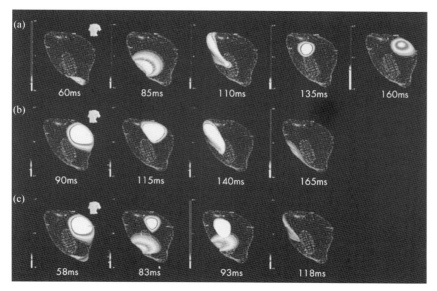

Fig. 3.10 Noncontact mapping showing the activation sequence with (a) right ventricular pacing, (b) left ventricular pacing, and (c) biventricular pacing. Timings are referenced from first pacing stimulus. (a) Activation due to the right ventricle emerges on the lower septum 60 ms postpacing, and reaches the most delayed segment in the lateral region 160 ms after initiation of the pacing stimulus. (b) Left ventricular activation breaks out from the left ventricular pacing site and takes 90 ms to exit the surrounding slow conduction zone into normally activating myocardium, with up to 165 ms to reach the septum. Hence, to facilitate optimal merging of the RV and LV wavefronts, biventricular pacing requires left ventricular stimulation to precede right ventricle activation by 32 ms, to enable maximal reduction of the left ventricular activation time to 118 ms. (Adapted from: Lambiase et al. [100].) (See color plate section).

can be due exclusively to the two activation wavefronts generated by LV and RV pacing leads leading to ventricular resynchronization.

There is considerable data to suggest that adjusting and optimizing the AV interval can result in hemodyanmic benefits [89,101–105], however, there is a paucity of information on the impact of this optimization on the electrical activation pattern. The highest improvement in systolic function is achieved with short AV interval that allows complete capture of the ventricles by the two pacing induced activation wavefronts. The exact value of this AV delay that improves synchrony is variable because it is patient-specific [89].

Another factor that influences ventricular activation during biventricular pacing is the interventricular (VV) timing (Figure 3.11). The modern CRT devices have the possibility of programming the VV pacing interval, allowing LV–RV simultaneous or sequential pacing with different degrees of LV or RV

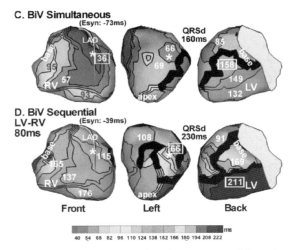

Fig. 3.11 Epicardial isochrone maps that reflect the activation of the right and left ventricles during biventricular pacing. The epicardial surfaces of both ventricles are displayed in anterior, left lateral and posterior, with some overlap between adjacent views. The valve area is shaded in grey. The thick black mark in the top panel indicates the line of block, which is no longer appreciable with biventricular pacing. The native rhythm panel shows sequential activation of the right ventricle followed by a much delayed left ventricular activation, suggestive of a left bundle branch–like pattern. Activation times (in milliseconds) of selected regions are shown. Earliest and latest ventricular activation times are indicated by framed numbers, and are in relation to the onset of the QRS. (Adapted from Jia et al. [4].) (See color plate section).

pre-excitation. These adjustments, together with AV interval adjustments can produce a multitude of patterns of ventricular depolarization by offering, in patients with LBBB and intact AV conduction, a certain degree of control over the three fronts of activation originating from the right bundle branch, the RV, and the LV pacing leads. Although in most patients simultaneous RV–LV pacing produces good hemodynamic results, pre-exciting the LV before RV pacing seem to further optimize synchrony and increase LV systolic function. Perego et al. demonstrated an increase in LV dP/dt with sequential LV–RV biventricular pacing as compared to simultaneous biventricular pacing. The highest LV dP/dt was achieved when LV was stimulated before by 25±21 ms in VDD mode and by 25±26 ms in DDD mode [106]. The clinical significance of this hemodynamic benefit remains to be proven.

Another factor that has an impact on electromechanical activation is lead position. The optimal lead positions are those that offer the greatest reduction in total activation time by producing two activation wavefronts that start from opposite positions [34]. Given that in LBBB the last LV wall to be activated during sinus rhythm is the basal posterolateral wall, placing the pacing lead in the vicinity of this area should theoretically produce maximum benefit in terms of electrical synchrony. This is not always possible with transvenous lead placement because of constraints imposed by the coronary venous anatomy, which is highly variable [107].

Response to pacing from the RV and LV site is often unpredictable, due to the pacing site-dependent changes in the line of functional block. Overall, electromechanical synchrony is dependent on the lead location, local pathology, as well as local activation and responsiveness. Minimal variation in lead positioning and/or orientation may have a large impact on the ventricular activation pattern. This highlights the fact that the variability in clinical response to CRT is driven by the heterogeneity of the LV substrate and their electrical response.

Lambiase and colleagues [100] demonstrated using noncontact endocardial mapping that electrical activation in patients with heart failure and ventricular conduction delays depends on LV lead placement. They identified areas of slow conduction within the LV, present mainly in patients with ischemic cardiomyopathy probably related to the underlying process of myocardial hibernation or fibrosis. When the LV lead was found to be positioned in such an area, the electrograms at the pacing site were of low amplitude and the conduction velocity was on average 27% of that in free wall regions with normal amplitude electrograms. Depolarization generated by an LV lead situated in a slow conduction zone was delayed an average of 70 ms while leaving the area. In order to achieve simultaneous activation of the LV with biventricular pacing in such patients, the LV had to be paced 30–40 ms before RV to allow time for depolarization to leave the slow conduction zone. Endocardial pacing outside regions of slow conduction using a roving catheter decreased LV activation time and significantly increased LV systolic performance as assessed by cardiac output and dP/dt_{max}, and was accompanied by a reduction in QRS width. There was no significant relationship noted in this study between the degree of decrease in LV activation time and the reduction in QRS width. The phenomenon was also identified in sinus rhythm when depolarization circumvented the areas of slow conduction, which only depolarized in the final phases of ventricular activation. This pattern of activation however did not occur in patients with nonischemic cardiomyopathy who had a more homogenous LV activation.

The impact of the RV pacing site on the activation sequence or fusion of the depolarization wavefront is underestimated. Recent work has demonstrated that by changing the RV pacing site, the electrical distance from the LV lead can be varied and also the dyssynchrony patterns of the LV can be altered [74]. This is again patient specific and affected by the intrinsic conduction, as well as the myopathy, which may influence local cell-to-cell conduction and recruitment of the native conduction system. Adjusting the AV interval, as alluded to above enables a variable extent of the activation wavefront originating from each of the pacing leads and intrinsic conduction.

Conclusion

The electrical activation sequence in the failing heart can vary depending on the type of the conduction defect, as well as the severity and type of cardiomyopathy (i.e. ischemic and nonischemic). The impact of LV and biventricular pacing on the activation wavefront is influenced by several factors inclusive of substrate differences, lead location, local pathology, presence of intrinsic conduction disease and recruitment of the Purkinje network, areas of slow conduction, and so forth. Interplay between the native activation sequence and the pacing induced alterations dictate the benefit derived from CRT. Adjusting the AV and V–V intervals can alter the propagation of the depolarization wavefront and in turn the response to CRT.

References

1. Gepstein L, Hayam G, Ben-Haim SA. A novel method for nonfluoroscopic catheter-based electroanatomical mapping of the heart. In vitro and in vivo accuracy results. *Circulation*. 1997;95(6):1611–22.
2. Schilling RJ, Peters NS, Davies DW. Simultaneous endocardial mapping in the human left ventricle using a noncontact catheter: comparison of contact and reconstructed electrograms during sinus rhythm. *Circulation*. 1998;98(9):887–98.
3. Ramanathan C, Ghanem RN, Jia P, Ryu K, Rudy Y. Noninvasive electrocardiographic imaging for cardiac electrophysiology and arrhythmia. *Nat Med*. 2004;10(4):422–8.
4. Jia P, Ramanathan C, Ghanem RN, Ryu K, Varma N, Rudy Y. Electrocardiographic imaging of cardiac resynchronization therapy in heart failure: observation of variable electrophysiologic responses. *Heart Rhythm*. 2006;3(3):296–310.
5. Pastore CA, Tobias N, Samesima N, Martinelli Filho M, Pedrosa A, Nishioka S, Douglas RA, Moreira LF, Ramires JF. Ventricular electrical activation in cardiac resynchronization as characterized by body surface potential mapping. *Arq Bras Cardiol*. 2007;88(3):251–7.
6. Keith A, Flack M. The Form and Nature of the Muscular Connections between the Primary Divisions of the Vertebrate Heart. *J Anat Physiol*. 1907; 41(Pt 3):172–89.
7. De PR, Ho SY, Salerno-Uriarte JA, Tritto M, Spadacini G. Electroanatomic analysis of sinus impulse propagation in normal human atria. *J Cardiovasc Electrophysiol*. 2002;13(1):1–10.
8. Sanchez-Quintana D, Cabrera JA, Farre J, Climent V, Anderson RH, Ho SY. Sinus node revisited in the era of electroanatomical mapping and catheter ablation. *Heart*. 2005;91(2):189–94.
9. Dobrzynski H, Boyett MR, Anderson RH. New insights into pacemaker activity: promoting understanding of sick sinus syndrome. *Circulation*. 2007;115(14):1921–32.
10. Anderson KR, Ho SY, Anderson RH. Location and vascular supply of sinus node in human heart. *Br Heart J*. 1979;41(1):28–32.
11. Boyett MR, Honjo H, Kodama I. The sinoatrial node, a heterogeneous pacemaker structure. *Cardiovasc Res*. 2000;47(4):658–87.
12. Schuessler RB, Boineau JP, Bromberg BI. Origin of the sinus impulse. *J Cardiovasc Electrophysiol*. 1996;7(3):263–74.

13. Boineau JP, Canavan TE, Schuessler RB, Cain ME, Corr PB, Cox JL. Demonstration of a widely distributed atrial pacemaker complex in the human heart. *Circulation.* 1988;77(6):21–37.

14. Altomare C, Terragni B, Brioschi C, Milanesi R, Pagliuca C, Viscomi C, Moroni A, Baruscotti M, DiFrancesco D. Heteromeric HCN1-HCN4 channels: a comparison with native pacemaker channels from the rabbit sinoatrial node. *J Physiol.* 2003;549(Pt 2):347–59.

15. Bachmann JG. The interauricular time interval. *Am J Physiol.* 1916;41:309–20.

16. Lemery R, Guiraudon G, Veinot JP. Anatomic description of Bachmann's bundle and its relation to the atrial septum. *Am J Cardiol.* 2003;91(12):1482–85, A1488.

17. James TN. The connecting pathways between the sinus node and a-V node and between the right and the left atrium in the human heart. *Am Heart J.* 1963;66:498–508.

18. Sherf L, James TN. Fine structure of cells and their histologic organization within internodal pathways of the heart: clinical and electrocardiographic implications. *Am J Cardiol.* 1979;44(2):345–69.

19. Ho SY, Sanchez-Quintana D, Cabrera JA, Anderson RH. Anatomy of the left atrium: implications for radiofrequency ablation of atrial fibrillation. *J Cardiovasc Electrophysiol.* 1999;10(11):1525–33.

20. Ho SY, Anderson RH, Sanchez-Quintana D. Gross structure of the atriums: more than an anatomic curiosity? *Pacing Clin Electrophysiol.* 2002;25(3):342–50.

21. Chauvin M, Shah DC, Haissaguerre M, Marcellin L, Brechenmacher C. The anatomic basis of connections between the coronary sinus musculature and the left atrium in humans. *Circulation.* 2000;101(6):647–52.

22. Anderson RH, Ho SY, Smith A, Becker AE. The internodal atrial myocardium. *Anat Rec.* 1981;201(1):75–82.

23. Ho SY, Anderson RH, Sanchez-Quintana D. Atrial structure and fibres: morphologic bases of atrial conduction. *Cardiovasc Res.* 2002;54(2):325–36.

24. Tawara S. Das Reizleitungssystem des Saugetierherzens: Eine anatomisch-histologische Studie uber das Atrioventrikularbundel und die Purkinjeschen Faden. *Jena, Germany: Gustav Fischer.* 1906:114–56.

25. Meijler FL, Janse MJ. Morphology and electrophysiology of the mammalian atrioventricular node. *Physiol Rev.* 1988;68(2):608–47.

26. Efimov IR, Nikolski VP, Rothenberg F, Greener ID, Li J, Dobrzynski H, Boyett M. Structure-function relationship in the AV junction. *Anat Rec A Discov Mol Cell Evol Biol.* 2004;280(2):952–65.

27. Kreuzberg MM, Willecke K, Bukauskas FF. Connexin-mediated cardiac impulse propagation: connexin 30.2 slows atrioventricular conduction in mouse heart. *Trends Cardiovasc Med.* 2006;16(8):266–72.

28. Schweitzer P. Jan Evangelista Purkinje (Purkine). *Clin Cardiol.* 1991;14(1):85–6.

29. His WJ. Die Tatigkeit des embryonalen Herzens und deren Bedeutung fur die Lehre von der Herzbewegung beim Erwachsenen. *Arbeiten aus der Medizinischen Klinik zu Leipzig.* 1893;1:14–49.

30. Kulbertus HE, Demoulin JC. The left hemiblocks: significance, prognosis and treatment. *Schweiz Med Wochenschr.* 1982;112(45):1579–84.

31. Friedman PL, Stewart JR, Fenoglio JJ, Jr., Wit AL. Survival of subendocardial Purkinje fibers after extensive myocardial infarction in dogs. *Circ Res.* 1973;33(5):597–611.

32. Myerburg RJ, Nilsson K, Gelband H. Physiology of canine intraventricular conduction and endocardial excitation. *Circ Res.* 1972;30(2):217–43.

33. Coghlan HC, Coghlan AR, Buckberg GD, Cox JL. "The electrical spiral of the heart": its role in the helical continuum. The hypothesis of the anisotropic conducting matrix. *Eur J Cardiothorac Surg.* 2006;29 Suppl 1:S178–S187.

34. Prinzen FW, Spinelli JC, Auricchio A. Basic physiology and hemodynamics of cardiac pacing. In: Ellenbogen KA, Kay GN, Lau CP, Wilkoff BL, eds. *Clinical cardiac pacing, defibrillation, and resynchronization therapy.* Saunders, 2007:291–335.

35. Reckova M, Rosengarten C, deAlmeida A, Stanley CP, Wessels A, Gourdie RG, Thompson RP, Sedmera D. Hemodynamics is a key epigenetic factor in development of the cardiac conduction system. *Circ Res.* 2003;93(1):77–85.

36. Durrer D, van Dam RT, Freud GE, Janse MJ, Meijler FL, Arzbaecher RC. Total excitation of the isolated human heart. *Circulation.* 1970;41(6):899–912.

37. Scher AM. Studies of the electrical activity of the ventricles and the origin of the QRS complex. *Acta Cardiol.* 1995;50(6):429–65.

38. Fabiato A. Simulated calcium current can both cause calcium loading in and trigger calcium release from the sarcoplasmic reticulum of a skinned canine cardiac Purkinje cell. *J Gen Physiol.* 1985;85(2):291–320.

39. Cheng H, Lederer MR, Xiao RP, Gomez AM, Zhou YY, Ziman B, Spurgeon H, Lakatta EG, Lederer WJ. Excitation-contraction coupling in heart: new insights from Ca2+ sparks. *Cell Calcium.* 1996;20(2):129–40.

40. Prinzen FW, Augustijn CH, Allessie MA, Arts T, Delhaas T, Reneman RS. The time sequence of electrical and mechanical activation during spontaneous beating and ectopic stimulation. *Eur Heart J.* 1992;13(4):535–43.

41. Kuo LC, Quinones MA, Rokey R, Sartori M, Abinader EG, Zoghbi WA. Quantification of atrial contribution to left ventricular filling by pulsed Doppler echocardiography and the effect of age in normal and diseased hearts. *Am J Cardiol.* 1987;59(12):1174–8.

42. Karpawich PP, Mital S. Comparative left ventricular function following atrial, septal, and apical single chamber heart pacing in the young. *Pacing Clin Electrophysiol.* 1997;20(8 Pt 1):1983–8.

43. Vassallo JA, Cassidy DM, Miller JM, Buxton AE, Marchlinski FE, Josephson ME. Left ventricular endocardial activation during right ventricular pacing: effect of underlying heart disease. *J Am Coll Cardiol.* 1986;7(6):1228–33.

44. Auricchio A, Fantoni C, Regoli F, Carbucicchio C, Goette A, Geller C, Kloss M, Klein H. Characterization of left ventricular activation in patients with heart failure and left bundle-branch block. *Circulation.* 2004;109(9):1133–9.

45. Li D, Fareh S, Leung TK, Nattel S. Promotion of atrial fibrillation by heart failure in dogs: atrial remodeling of a different sort. *Circulation.* 1999;100(1):87–95.

46. Han W, Chartier D, Li D, Nattel S. Ionic remodeling of cardiac Purkinje cells by congestive heart failure. *Circulation.* 2001;104(17):2095–2100.

47. Severs NJ, Coppen SR, Dupont E, Yeh HI, Ko YS, Matsushita T. Gap junction alterations in human cardiac disease. *Cardiovasc Res.* 2004;62(2):368–77.

48. Poelzing S, Rosenbaum DS. Altered connexin-43 expression produces arrhythmia substrate in heart failure. *Am J Physiol Heart Circ Physiol.* 2004;287(4):H1762–H1770.

49. Faggiano P, d'Aloia A, Gualeni A, Gardini A, Giordano A. Mechanisms and

immediate outcome of in-hospital cardiac arrest in patients with advanced heart failure secondary to ischemic or idiopathic dilated cardiomyopathy. *Am J Cardiol.* 2001; 87(5):655–7, A610–A651.

50. Sanders P, Kistler PM, Morton JB, Spence SJ, Kalman JM. Remodeling of sinus node function in patients with congestive heart failure: reduction in sinus node reserve. *Circulation.* 2004;110(8):897–903.

51. Opthof T, Coronel R, Rademaker HM, Vermeulen JT, Wilms-Schopman FJ, Janse MJ. Changes in sinus node function in a rabbit model of heart failure with ventricular arrhythmias and sudden death. *Circulation.* 2000;101(25):2975–80.

52. Jose AD, Taylor RR. Autonomic blockade by propranolol and atropine to study intrinsic myocardial function in man. *J Clin Invest.* 1969;48(11):2019–31.

53. Vatner SF, Higgins CB, Braunwald E. Sympathetic and parasympathetic components of reflex tachycardia induced by hypotension in conscious dogs with and without heart failure. *Cardiovasc Res.* 1974;8(2):153–61.

54. Jose AD, Collison D. The normal range and determinants of the intrinsic heart rate in man. *Cardiovasc Res.* 1970;4(2):160–7.

55. Verkerk AO, Wilders R, Coronel R, Ravesloot JH, Verheijck EE. Ionic remodeling of sinoatrial node cells by heart failure. *Circulation.* 2003;108(6):760–6.

56. Zicha S, Fernandez-Velasco M, Lonardo G, L'Heureux N, Nattel S. Sinus node dysfunction and hyperpolarization-activated (HCN) channel subunit remodeling in a canine heart failure model. *Cardiovasc Res.* 2005;66(3):472–81.

57. Janse MJ. Electrophysiological changes in heart failure and their relationship to arrhythmogenesis. *Cardiovasc Res.* 2004;61(2):208–17.

58. Sanders P, Morton JB, Davidson NC, Spence SJ, Vohra JK, Sparks PB, Kalman JM. Electrical remodeling of the atria in congestive heart failure: electrophysiological and electroanatomic mapping in humans. *Circulation.* 2003;108(12):1461–8.

59. Li D, Melnyk P, Feng J, Wang Z, Petrecca K, Shrier A, Nattel S. Effects of experimental heart failure on atrial cellular and ionic electrophysiology. *Circulation.* 2000; 101(22):2631–8.

60. Shamim W, Francis DP, Yousufuddin M, Varney S, Pieopli MF, Anker SD, Coats AJ. Intraventricular conduction delay: a prognostic marker in chronic heart failure. *Int J Cardiol.* 1999;70(2):171–8.

61. Baldasseroni S, Opasich C, Gorini M, Lucci D, Marchionni N, Marini M, Campana C, Perini G, Deorsola A, Masotti G, Tavazzi L, Maggioni AP. Left bundle-branch block is associated with increased 1-year sudden and total mortality rate in 5517 outpatients with congestive heart failure: a report from the Italian network on congestive heart failure. *Am Heart J.* 2002;143(3):398–405.

62. Hawkins NM, Wang D, McMurray JJ, Pfeffer MA, Swedberg K, Granger CB, Yusuf S, Pocock SJ, Ostergren J, Michelson EL, Dunn FG. Prevalence and prognostic impact of bundle branch block in patients with heart failure: evidence from the CHARM programme. *Eur J Heart Fail.* 2007;9(5):510–17.

63. Rodriguez MI, Sodi-Pallares D. The mechanism of complete and incomplete bundle branch block. *Am Heart J.* 1952;44(5):715–46.

64. Verbeek XA, Vernooy K, Peschar M, Van Der Nagel T, Van Hunnik A, Prinzen FW. Quantification of interventricular asynchrony during LBBB and ventricular pacing. *Am J Physiol Heart Circ Physiol.* 2002;283(4):H1370–H1378.

65. Liu L, Tockman B, Girouard S, Pastore J, Walcott G, Ken-Knight B, Spinelli J. Left ventricular resynchronization therapy in a canine model of left bundle branch block. *Am J Physiol Heart Circ Physiol.* 2002;282(6):H2238–H2244.

66. Varma N, Jia P, Rudy Y. Electrocardiographic imaging of patients with heart failure with left bundle branch block and response to cardiac resynchronization therapy. *J Electrocardiol.* 2007;40(6) Suppl:S174–S178.

67. Wyndham CR, Smith T, Meeran MK, Mammana R, Levitsky S, Rosen KM. Epicardial activation in patients with left bundle branch block. *Circulation.* 1980;61(4):696–703.

68. Cannom DS, Wyman MG, Goldreyer BN. Initial ventricular activation in left-sided intraventricular conduction defects. *Circulation.* 1980;62(3):621–31.

69. Vassallo JA, Cassidy DM, Marchlinski FE, Buxton AE, Waxman HL, Doherty JU, Josephson ME. Endocardial activation of left bundle branch block. *Circulation.* 1984;69(5):914–23.

70. Rodriguez LM, Timmermans C, Nabar A, Beatty G, Wellens HJ. Variable patterns of septal activation in patients with left bundle branch block and heart failure. *J Cardiovasc Electrophysiol.* 2003;14(2):135–41.

71. Fung JW, Yu CM, Yip G, Zhang Y, Chan H, Kum CC, Sanderson JE. Variable left ventricular activation pattern in patients with heart failure and left bundle branch block. *Heart.* 2004;90(1):17–19.

72. Xiao HB, Brecker SJ, Gibson DG. Effects of abnormal activation on the time course of the left ventricular pressure pulse in dilated cardiomyopathy. *Br Heart J.* 1992; 68(4):403–7.

73. Fantoni C, Kawabata M, Massaro R, Regoli F, Raffa S, Arora V, Salerno-Uriarte JA, Klein HU, Auricchio A. Right and left ventricular activation sequence in patients with heart failure and right bundle branch block: a detailed analysis using three-dimensional non-fluoroscopic electroanatomic mapping system. *J Cardiovasc Electrophysiol.* 2005;16(2):112–19; discussion 120–121.

74. Singh JP, Heist EK, Ruskin JN, Harthorne JW. "Dialing-in" cardiac resynchronization therapy: overcoming constraints of the coronary venous anatomy. *J Interv Card Electrophysiol.* 2006;17(1):51–8.

75. Leclercq C, Faris O, Tunin R, Johnson J, Kato R, Evans F, Spinelli J, Halperin H, McVeigh E, Kass DA. Systolic improvement and mechanical resynchronization does not require electrical synchrony in the dilated failing heart with left bundle-branch block. *Circulation.* 2002;106(14):1760–3.

76. Kass DA, Chen CH, Curry C, Talbot M, Berger R, Fetics B, Nevo E. Improved left ventricular mechanics from acute VDD pacing in patients with dilated cardiomyopathy and ventricular conduction delay. *Circulation.* 1999;99(12):1567–73.

77. Prinzen FW, Hunter WC, Wyman BT, McVeigh ER. Mapping of regional myocardial strain and work during ventricular pacing: experimental study using magnetic resonance imaging tagging. *J Am Coll Cardiol.* 1999;33(6):1735–42.

78. Hesse B, Diaz LA, Snader CE, Blackstone EH, Lauer MS. Complete bundle branch block as an independent predictor of all-cause mortality: report of 7,073 patients referred for nuclear exercise testing. *Am J Med.* 2001;110(4):253–9.

79. Fleg JL, Das DN, Lakatta EG. Right bundle branch block: long-term prognosis in apparently healthy men. *J Am Coll Cardiol.* 1983;1(3):887–92.

80. Eriksson P, Wilhelmsen L, Rosengren A. Bundle-branch block in middle-aged men: risk of complications and death over 28 years. The Primary Prevention Study in Goteborg, Sweden. *Eur Heart J*. 2005;26(21):2300–6.

81. Wong CK, Gao W, Stewart RA, van Pelt N, French JK, Aylward PE, White HD. Risk stratification of patients with acute anterior myocardial infarction and right bundle-branch block: importance of QRS duration and early ST-segment resolution after fibrinolytic therapy. *Circulation*. 2006;114(8):783–9.

82. Bristow MR, Saxon LA, Boehmer J, Krueger S, Kass DA, De Marco T, Carson P, DiCarlo L, DeMets D, White BG, DeVries DW, Feldman AM. Cardiac-resynchronization therapy with or without an implantable defibrillator in advanced chronic heart failure. *N Engl J Med*. 2004;350(21):2140–50.

83. Unger PN, Lesser ME, Kugel VH, Lev M. The concept of masquerading bundle-branch block; an electro-cardiographic-pathologic correlation. *Circulation*. 1958;17(3):397–409.

84. Richman JL, Wolff L. Left bundle branch block masquerading as right bundle branch block. *Am Heart J*. 1954;47(3):383–93.

85. McCullough PA, Hassan SA, Pallekonda V, Sandberg KR, Nori DB, Soman SS, Bhatt S, Hudson MP, Weaver WD. Bundle branch block patterns, age, renal dysfunction, and heart failure mortality. *Int J Cardiol*. 2005;102(2):303–8.

86. Peichl P, Kautzner J, Cihak R, Bytesnik J. The spectrum of inter- and intraventricular conduction abnormalities in patients eligible for cardiac resynchronization therapy. *Pacing Clin Electrophysiol*. 2004;27(8):1105–12.

87. Garrigue S, Reuter S, Labeque JN, Jais P, Hocini M, Shah DC, Haissaguerre M, Clementy J. Usefulness of biventricular pacing in patients with congestive heart failure and right bundle branch block. *Am J Cardiol*. 2001;88(12):1436–41, A1438.

88. Aranda JM, Jr., Conti JB, Johnson JW, Petersen-Stejskal S, Curtis AB. Cardiac resynchronization therapy in patients with heart failure and conduction abnormalities other than left bundle-branch block: analysis of the Multicenter InSync Randomized Clinical Evaluation (MIRACLE). *Clin Cardiol*. 2004;27(12):678–82.

89. Auricchio A, Stellbrink C, Block M, Sack S, Vogt J, Bakker P, Klein H, Kramer A, Ding J, Salo R, Tockman B, Pochet T, Spinelli J. Effect of pacing chamber and atrioventricular delay on acute systolic function of paced patients with congestive heart failure. The Pacing Therapies for Congestive Heart Failure Study Group. The Guidant Congestive Heart Failure Research Group. *Circulation*. 1999;99(23):2993–3001.

90. Riedlbauchova L, Fridl P, Kautzner J, Peichl P. Performance of left ventricular versus biventricular pacing in chronic heart failure assessed by stress echocardiography. *Pacing Clin Electrophysiol*. 2004;27(5):626–31.

91. Touiza A, Etienne Y, Gilard M, Fatemi M, Mansourati J, Blanc JJ. Long-term left ventricular pacing: assessment and comparison with biventricular pacing in patients with severe congestive heart failure. *J Am Coll Cardiol*. 2001;38(7):1966–70.

92. Blanc JJ, Bertault-Valls V, Fatemi M, Gilard M, Pennec PY, Etienne Y. Midterm benefits of left univentricular pacing in patients with congestive heart failure. *Circulation*. 2004;109(14):1741–4.

93. Singh JP, Fan D, Heist EK, Alabiad CR, Taub C, Reddy V, Mansour M, Picard MH, Ruskin JN, Mela T. Left ventricular lead electrical delay predicts response to cardiac resynchronization therapy. *Heart Rhythm*. 2006;3(11):1285–92.

94. Murphy RT, Sigurdsson G, Mulamalla S, Agler D, Popovic ZB, Starling RC, Wilkoff BL, Thomas JD, Grimm RA. Tissue synchronization imaging and optimal left ventricular pacing site in cardiac resynchronization therapy. *Am J Cardiol*. 2006;97(11):1615–21.

95. McClelland AJ, Owens CG, Navarro C, Smith B, Roberts MJ, Anderson J, Adgey AA. Usefulness of body surface maps to demonstrate ventricular activation patterns during left ventricular pacing and reentrant activation during ventricular tachycardia in men with coronary heart disease and left ventricular dysfunction. *Am J Cardiol*. 2006;98(5):591–6.

96. Faris OP, Evans FJ, Dick AJ, Raman VK, Ennis DB, Kass DA, McVeigh ER. Endocardial versus epicardial electrical synchrony during LV free-wall pacing. *Am J Physiol Heart Circ Physiol*. 2003;285(5):H1864–H1870.

97. Kavanagh KM, Belenkie I, Duff HJ. Transmural temporospatial left ventricular activation during pacing from different sites: potential implications for optimal pacing. *Cardiovasc Res*. 2008;77(1):81–8.

98. Gianfranchi L, Bettiol K, Sassone B, Verlato R, Corbucci G, Alboni P. Fusion beat in patients with heart failure treated with left ventricular pacing: may ECG morphology relate to mechanical synchrony? A pilot study. *Cardiovasc Ultrasound*. 2008; 6(1):1.

99. Verbeek XA, Vernooy K, Peschar M, Cornelussen RN, Prinzen FW. Intra-ventricular resynchronization for optimal left ventricular function during pacing in experimental left bundle branch block. *J Am Coll Cardiol*. 2003;42(3):558–67.

100. Lambiase PD, Rinaldi A, Hauck J, Mobb M, Elliott D, Mohammad S, Gill JS, Bucknall CA. Non-contact left ventricular endocardial mapping in cardiac resynchronisation therapy. *Heart*. 2004 90(1):44–51.

101. Auricchio A, Ding J, Spinelli JC, Kramer AP, Salo RW, Hoersch W, KenKnight BH, Klein HU. Cardiac resynchronization therapy restores optimal atrioventricular mechanical timing in heart failure patients with ventricular conduction delay. *J Am Coll Cardiol*. 2002;39(7):1163–9.

102. Verbeek XA, Auricchio A, Yu Y, Ding J, Pochet T, Vernooy K, Kramer A, Spinelli J, Prinzen FW. Tailoring cardiac resynchronization therapy using interventricular asynchrony. Validation of a simple model. *Am J Physiol Heart Circ Physiol*. 2006;290(3):H968–H977.

103. Zuber M, Toggweiler S, Roos M, Kobza R, Jamshidi P, Erne P. Comparison of different approaches for optimization of atrioventricular and interventricular delay in biventricular pacing. *Europace*. 2008.

104. Toggweiler S, Zuber M, Kobza R, Roos M, Jamshidi P, Meier R, Erne P. Improved response to cardiac resynchronization therapy through optimization of atrioventricular and interventricular delays using acoustic cardiography: a pilot study. *J Card Fail*. 2007;13(8):637–42.

105. Vernooy K, Verbeek XA, Cornelussen RN, Dijkman B, Crijns HJ, Arts T, Prinzen FW. Calculation of effective VV interval facilitates optimization of AV delay and VV interval in cardiac resynchronization therapy. *Heart Rhythm*. 2007;4(1):75–82.

106. Perego GB, Chianca R, Facchini M, Frattola A, Balla E, Zucchi S, Cavaglia S, Vicini I, Negretto M, Osculati G. Simultaneous vs. sequential biventricular pacing in dilated cardiomyopathy: an acute hemodynamic study. *Eur J Heart Fail*. 2003;5(3):305–13.

107. Blendea D, Shah RV, Auricchio A, Nandigam V, Orencole M, Heist EK, Reddy VY, McPherson CA, Ruskin JN, Singh JP. Variability of coronary venous anatomy in patients undergoing cardiac resynchronization therapy: a high-speed rotational venography study. *Heart Rhythm.* 2007;4(9):1155–62.

108. Fung JW, Chan JY, Yip GW, Chan HC, Chan WW, Zhang Q, Yu CM. Effect of ventricular enocardial activation pattern on echocardiographic and clinical response to cardiac resynchronization therapy. *Heart.* 2007;93:432–7.

Chapter 4

Mechanical assessment of the failing heart

Przemyslaw P. Borek and Richard A. Grimm

Key Points

1. Its versatility and cost-effectiveness make echocardiography the most widely utilized modality (clinically and experimentally) for assessing cardiac performance in heart failure patients.
2. Information obtained from cardiac imaging is highly useful in tailoring heart failure management and in determining prognosis.
3. Cardiac systolic dysfunction is the most common etiology of heart failure and can be assessed with echocardiography by visual estimation or formal calculation of left ventricular volumes and ejection fraction.
4. The most commonly used method for assessing left ventricular ejection fraction is via the biplane method of discs also known as the modified Simpson's rule.
5. Cardiac diastolic dysfunction, also a common cause of heart failure, is usually assessed by Doppler evaluation of blood flow or myocardial tissue kinetics.
6. No single echocardiographic measurement of diastolic function is sufficient to accurately diagnose diastolic dysfunction.
7. Dyssynchronous left ventricular contraction leads to inefficient systole, abnormal chamber filling, increased mitral regurgitation and higher susceptibility to cardiac arrhythmias.
8. Despite its angle-dependency and other technical limitations, evaluation of longitudinal myocardial velocities with TDI is the most studied and most commonly used modality in the clinical evaluation for cardiac dyssynchrony.

Pacing to Support the Failing Heart, 1st edition. Edited by K. Ellenbogen and A. Auricchio.
© 2008 American Heart Association, ISBN: 978-1-4051-7534-0

9. Speckle tracking imaging is a novel echocardiographic modality which allows for angle independent evaluation of LV dyssynchrony via quantification of regional myocardial strain.

10. Echocardiographic evidence of reverse left ventricular remodeling has been associated with improved symptoms and increased longevity in patients treated with cardiac resynchronization therapy.

Introduction

Prior to the advent of echocardiography, systolic heart function was quantifiable by two-dimensional cine imaging, and diastolic heart function was evaluated by catheter measurement of intracardiac pressures. Both were performed during cardiac catheterization, which involved arterial instrumentation, contrast, and radiation exposure. Interestingly, sonography was first incorporated into cardiac assessment around the 1950s, when W. D. Keidel, a German investigator, used ultrasound to determine cardiac volumes [1]. Drs. Helmut Herts and Inge Edler of Sweden first began to use an ultrasonoscope to examine the heart and were credited with pioneering the field of cardiac echocardiography [2]. From the time echocardiography was begun, its diagnostic capabilities have grown tremendously as a result of growing knowledge and expanding technology. The field rapidly progressed from simple M-Mode imaging to two-dimensional echocardiography with incorporation of Doppler, and more recently, to sophisticated three-dimensional imaging. Its versatility and cost-effectiveness make echocardiography the most frequently clinically and experimentally used modality to assess cardiac performance. In fact, echocardiography is "the single most useful diagnostic test in the evaluation of heart failure patients" according to the American College of Cardiology/American Heart Association [3]. Other diagnostic modalities, such as nuclear imaging, tomography (CT), or magnetic resonance imaging (MRI), are also useful for heart-function assessment; however, due to various technical and/or fiscal limitations these modalities are far less used in clinical practice.

Cardiac systolic dysfunction is the most common etiology of heart failure [4]. It is usually assessed via echocardiography by visual estimation of ejection fraction (EF) by an experienced echocardiographer or through formal calculation of left ventricular ejection fraction (LVEF), and more recently via more sophisticated techniques, such as Tissue Doppler Imaging (TDI), speckle tracking (STI), or three-dimensional echocardiography. Stress echocardiography testing using exercise or dobutamine can be used to evaluate for cardiac ischemia, and in the case of dobutamine, to also evaluate for myocardial viability.

Diastolic heart dysfunction, also a common cause of heart failure [5], especially in the elderly, is usually assessed by Doppler evaluation of blood flow or myocardial tissue kinetics. These widely studied modalities are sensitive enough to classify various stages of diastolic dysfunction and provide excellent prognostic information.

Therefore, it is not surprising that echocardiography is also used for dyssynchrony assessment. Doppler imaging is the most studied and widely applied technique for quantification of the degree of interventricular or intraventricular dyssynchrony. Newer, less studied, three-dimensional echocardiography and two-dimensional speckle tracking methods are on the horizon and expected to overcome many of the shortcomings of Doppler imaging.

Cardiac imaging is also used in the management and follow-up of heart failure patients. Even though, the success of medical or surgical therapy is frequently assessed by patient's symptoms and longevity, additional information obtained from cardiac imaging is highly useful in tailoring further heart failure management and in determining a patients' prognosis. For instance, heart attack survivors with low ejection fraction carry a worse cardiovascular prognosis and have a higher risk of sudden cardiac death when compared to similar patients with normal ejection fraction [6]. Those patients also tend to benefit most from defibrillator (ICD) or biventricular pacing (BiV) therapy [7]. As a result, the current ICD and/or BiV therapy guidelines use some echocardiographic indices of LV systolic performance. Furthermore, it has been suggested that echocardiography (TDI) is useful for selecting potential candidates for BiV therapy by detecting mechanical dyssynchrony particularly when conventional selection criteria (i.e. QRS duration) are borderline. Finally, echocardiography has been used to assess response to BiV pacing and for pacing optimization in responders and nonresponders alike, to cardiac resynchronization therapy (CRT).

This chapter will focus on echocardiographic assessment of the failing heart. We will first discuss various echocardiographic modalities used to assess cardiac function and dysfunction, both, systolic and diastolic; and then focus on echocardiographic evaluation of mechanical dyssynchrony and ventricular remodeling.

Systolic myocardial dysfunction

In the early days of echocardiography left ventricular (LV) systolic function was assessed by linear measurements (M-Mode) of systolic and diastolic LV dimensions in the minor axis from which fractional shortening and other indexes could be assessed. M-Mode imaging was superseded by two-dimensional echocardiography, which allows far greater spatial resolution and, therefore, more precise evaluation of LVEE. It estimates LVEF from various views of the LV taking into account some of the regional abnormalities not necessarily assessed by the linear measurements. The emergence of three-dimensional echocardiography allows for even more precise evaluation of systolic performance by more precisely quantifying volumes, thereby, eliminating the shortcomings of geometric assumption used in two-dimensional echocardiography. In addition, the improved regional assessment by three-dimensional echocardiography allows for evaluation of mechanical dyssynchrony. TDI can also be used to evaluate LV systolic performance by computing mitral annular systolic velocities that have been shown to be more prognostic than the two-dimensional EF measurements [8]. Furthermore, TDI and a newer technique of two-dimensional speckle tracking can be used to estimate regional myocardial strain for evaluation of regional systolic function and mechanical dyssynchrony.

Linear measurements of LV function

M-Mode was the earliest technique used to assess LV performance. It uses single beam (linear) interrogation of a desired LV segment, perpendicular to the long axis of the LV, from which systolic and diastolic dimensions can be measured directly and then incorporated into calculation of LV function. Indexes of LV performance such as fractional shortening or velocity of circumferential shortening could be assessed via this modality and have been shown to be reproducible with low intra-observer and inter-observer variability [9–13]. The major advantage of this technique is the high temporal resolution of M-Mode imaging allowing for precise identification of even the finest movement throughout the cardiac cycle. One of the limitations of linear measurement is that it only provides information regarding myocardial performance along a single line of interrogation. In conditions, such as ischemic heart disease, where regional abnormalities are prevalent, this techniques can both, underestimate LV performance by sampling in the diseased area only, or overestimate LV performance by solely interrogating the healthy segments. Another major limitation of the linear measurement is its poor accuracy as often times the true short axis view of the ventricle is difficult to obtain leading to overestimation of LV dimensions. For those and other reasons, linear measurements of LV performance are not recommended in clinical practice [14].

Two and three-dimensional measurements of LV function

Two-dimensional assessment of LV performance relies on the measurement of LV area or volume in both systole and diastole and subsequent calculation of indexes such as fractional area change, stroke volume, or EF. These indices have also been validated and have a low intra-observer and inter-observer variability [9–13]. The most commonly used method for assessing LV EF is the biplane method of discs known as the modified Simpson's rule. This technique takes advantage of the elliptical contour of the LV in the apical views and, by dividing it into equal height short axis disks, calculates LV dimensions by summation of volumes from a stack of disks. End-systolic and end-diastolic dimensions are derived from apical two-chamber and/or four-chamber views, and these measurements then yield stroke volume and EF (Figure 4.1). Unfortunately, as with linear assessment of LV performance, accuracy is also of considerable concern with two-dimensional EF assessment due to geometric assumptions or interpellations used in this technique. In clinical practice, true two-chamber view

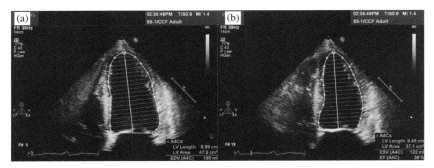

Fig. 4.1 The modified Simpson's rule for assessment of LV EF. (a) End-diastolic LV dimension in the apical four-chamber view. (b) End-systolic LV dimension in the apical four-chamber view. Note the disks used to extrapolate LV volume. The difference between the two volume measurement represents SV.

may be difficult to obtain or interpret as a result of poor image quality due to poor acoustic windows. This often precludes endocardial border visualization playing a major role in limiting the accuracy of LV volume and EF assessment. Fortunately, tissue harmonic imaging and the use of echocardiographic contrast have improved image quality allowing for more accurate results [15–19]. Furthermore, off-axis two-dimensional LV chamber views may be inadvertently used in volume calculation leading to erroneous EF assessment. Ensuring proper bean alignment with true LV center helps mitigate this problem. In addition, the LV apex is often times foreshortened in the apical view that may result in inaccurate LV volume measurements, as well. Fortunately, the true apex can be easily identified as it is the thinnest area of the myocardium and typically does not move much during systole and diastole. Finally, even though, large territory wall motion abnormalities are less likely to be omitted during two-dimensional LV function assessment, small territory abnormalities could be missed.

Three-dimensional echocardiography, which is not subject to geometric assumptions or plane positioning errors, was recently introduced in an attempt to alleviate the above mentioned problems with the two-dimensional assessment [20]. Initially, three-dimensional imaging was performed via laborious off-line reconstruction from a set of two-dimensional images followed by systolic and diastolic volumes and EF calculations [21]. More recently, on-line three-dimensional data acquisition was made possible by real time three-dimensional echocardiographic imaging using a matrix array transducer [22]. The acquired data, still require further processing using manual tracing or semi-automatic algorithms, which ultimately yield chamber size and function. Numerous studies have proven improved three-dimensional versus two-dimensional imaging accuracy for determining LV volumes and global or regional performance when echocardiographic standardized to magnetic resonance imaging (MRI) [23–26], however the cumbersome postprocessing required for three-dimensional volume determination does not compensate for the small, clinically less significant, differences between the two techniques. Real-time three-dimensional volume acquisition and automated volume and EF calculations, have enabled the three-dimensional modality to become more practical and, thereby, more applicable to common clinical practice.

Regional left ventricular function

Global LV function assessment provides information regarding the overall performance of the ventricle. It provides valuable prognosis and serves an important role in establishing guidelines for management of various cardiac conditions. However, in situations where regional LV wall motion assessment is sought out, as in the case ischemic heart disease, additional tools have been developed to assist in that evaluation process.

The most common method for assessing LV regional wall motion abnormalities uses operator based assessment of prespecified myocardial segments. By dividing the entire myocardium into known segments, regional wall motion abnormalities can be assessed and assigned along a progressive gradation of myocardial tissue kinetics ranging from normal (1) to hypokinesis, (2) akinesis, (3) dyskinesis (4), and aneurysmal (5). A wall motion score index (WMSI) can be calculated as the sum of individual scores divided by the number of visualized segments. A WMSI of 1 is normal. Currently, the 17-segment model (supported by the American Heart Association Writing Group on Myocardial Segmentation for Cardiac Imaging) is widely proposed for most accurate and reproducible regional LV assessment via most imaging modalities including nuclear, CAT scan (CT), MRI, and echocardiography (Figure 4.2) [27]. This model was recently developed to replace the 16-segment model (supported by the American Society of Electrocardiography) that had been faulted for poor characterization of the apical segment [28]. Despite the current AHA recommendations, the 16-segment model remains in use among cardiologists for echocardiographic assessment of regional LV function. This is substantiated by the argument that the true apex is normally akinetic, therefore, should not be taken into consideration when assessing for regional wall motion abnormalities. In the authors' opinion, either technique is more than adequate and can be used for functional assessment. When assessing myocardial tissue kinetics using either model, both the extent and the severity of an abnormality can be assessed, characterized, and frequently correlated with a coronary artery distribution. Only, the 17-segment model allows for correlation of myocardial kinetics among other modalities, such as nuclear imaging or MRI [27].

The specificity of the segmental models is negatively offset by nonischemic wall motion abnormalities caused by tethering, translocation, conduction abnormalities, pacing, or post–open-heart surgery state, which can all lead to overestimation of LV dysfunction. There are, however, certain clues that help

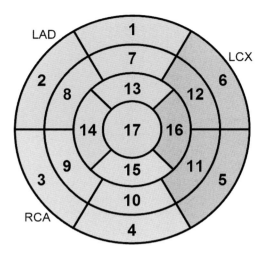

Fig. 4.2 The 17-segment model used for assessment of regional LV function. Note the correlation to coronary artery distribution. The outer segments represent the corresponding basal segments. The mid segments represent the mid ventricular myocardium and the most inner segment is the apex.

distinguish ischemic from nonischemic etiologies of wall motion abnormalities. In the left bundle branch block conduction abnormality, anterior septal activation precedes that of the rest of the LV with a characteristic early downward displacement of the anterior septal wall during M-Mode imaging. The wall thickness is preserved and contractility attenuated, which distinguishes these mechanics from abnormalities related to ischemia or infarction. In a paced ventricular rhythm where the right ventricular apex is stimulated first, the distal septum is activated the earliest as compared to the rest of the LV. Wall thickness is preserved but, again, contractility will be variably attenuated in that segment in keeping with the pacing paradox that states that the region that contracts first performs worst [29]. In the post–open-heart surgery state where the heart is no longer constrained by the pericardium there is paradoxical (outward) septal motion due to anterior systolic displacement of the ventricle. Wall thickeness and thickening are preserved. Often times, it may be difficult to assess systolic function in patients with the above mentioned conditions, even by very experienced operators. Understanding coronary artery distribution and relying on M-Mode echocardiography for the presence and timing of wall thickening are frequently useful in making a correct assessment.

Three-dimensional echocardiography can also be used to assess regional wall motion abnormalities [30]. Given that this model is more precise than its two-dimensional counterpart, regional abnormalities in even small areas of myocardium can be discerned and correlated to coronary distribution. This technique is currently in its early stages and, despite some technical limitations pertaining to image quality, appears to be quite promising in terms of its clinical utility.

Peak systolic velocity (Sm) of the myocardium as assessed by TDI has been used in region wall motion assessment, as well. The technique uses simultaneous pulsed-wave Doppler velocity measurement of multiple LV myocardial segments in apical views throughout the cardiac cycle. The segmental velocities are displayed on a graph with time as the independent variable. Duration of systole is ascertained by ECG tracing. TDI-derived peak systolic velocities have been used as an adjunct to WMSI in quantifying regional wall motion abnormalities [31,32]. Furthermore, by averaging Sm velocities from six segments around the mitral annulus one can predict overall systolic function and prognosis, such that a cut-off value of greater than 7.5 cm/sec has a sensitivity of 79% and specificity of 88% in predicting normal global LV ejection fraction, and a cut-off of less than 3 cm/sec has been associated with increased cardiac mortality in normal subjects and those with known cardiac disease [33].

Because TDI-generated myocardial velocity is subject to error due to translational movement of the heart or due to tethering of abnormal segments by normally contracting segments, myocardial deformation (strain), and strain rate were recently developed for more accurate assessment of regional myocardial performance. Lagrangian strain represents the ratio of change in dimension (length) over the original dimension (Delta L/Lo). Unfortunately, that measurement can not be obtained directly from TDI; instead, it is derived from velocity measurements in two different, yet adjacent, points in the myocardium. The difference in two adjacent velocities divided by their original distance represents strain rate, which, when integrated over time, results in an estimation of strain. The major pitfall of this modality is that in order to obtain accurate tissue velocities the pulsed Doppler beam must be aligned in parallel with the region of interest giving rise to significant angle-dependence. In addition, because the interrogation is performed in the apical views only, it is quite apparent that this modality evaluates myocardial strain mostly in the longitudinal axis of the LV, and therefore, does not take into account radial or circumferential components of myocardial contraction.

Speckle tracking imaging (STI), which uses the movement of unique speckle patterns created by reflection and scattering of echo beams throughout the myocardium, is a novel method for assessing various aspects of cardiac performance, from global LV function assessment to regional wall motion abnormalities, dyssynchrony, and potentially even diastolic function evaluation [34]. The premise and major advantage behind this modality is that the unique speckle patterns can be traced frame by frame through the cardiac cycle to yield tissue deformation in two-dimensional. Because speckles are distributed throughout the myocardium, wall motion and strain can be assessed in multiple segments independent of the angle of interrogation allowing for accurate assessment of regional function and mechanical dyssynchrony [35]. Furthermore, STI allows for assessment of shear strain and ventricular torsion, indexes that up until now were only measurable by sophisticated MRI [36,37]. This technique is in its early stages and requires a significant amount of postacquisition processing using various semi-automated software designed for tracking of designated speckles throughout the cardiac cycle.

Diastolic myocardial dysfunction

Diastolic heart failure accounts for more than 50% of all heart failure patients [5]. It tends to affect the elderly and is more prevalent among women [38,39]. Even though, once thought of as a more favorable condition when compared to systolic dysfunction, diastolic dysfunction carries similarly poor prognosis and may lead to subsequent development of systolic dysfunction [40,41]. Conditions such as hypertension, diabetes, obesity and sleep apnea, coronary artery disease, and hypertrophic or restrictive/infiltrative cardiomyopathy have all been linked with the development of diastolic heart failure irrespective of systolic LV function [42,43]. In fact, diastolic dysfunction is defined as the presence of signs or symptoms of heart failure in the absence of systolic dysfunction (EF >50% and LV end-diastolic volume index <97 ml/m2) [44]. It should, however, be noted, that often times patients with established systolic dysfunction have abnormalities of diastolic function as well. Further investigation of suspected diastolic dysfunction calls for documentation of abnormal LV relaxation and elevated diastolic pressures. Previously diagnosed only in the catheterization laboratory via documentation of elevated LV end-diastolic pressure (>16 mmHg) or elevated pulmonary capillary wedge pressure (>12 mmHg), contemporary, diagnosis of diastolic dysfunction can be established using conventional echocardiography using Doppler measurements [44]. Mitral inflow velocity, mitral annular velocity, velocity of mitral inflow propagation, and pulmonary vein inflow velocity are some of the more common Doppler methods used to assess diastolic function in clinical practice. However, no single Doppler index of diastolic function should ever be used alone; instead, it should be combined with other Doppler indexes as well as other echocardiographic data, such as LV mass or LA volume index.

Blood flow Doppler and mitral inflow velocity

Even though, transmitral inflow velocity is one of the earliest and most criticized methods for diastology evaluation, it remains an integral part of diastolic dysfunction assessment in conjunction with other methods. Its predictive value for diagnosing diastolic dysfunction has been quite variable (due to the lead-dependency for the measure); however, when combined with the pulmonary inflow velocity pattern, the two are greater than 90% predictive [45]. Mitral

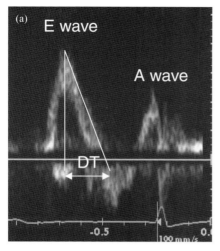
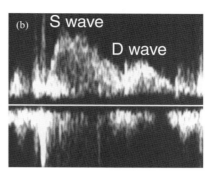

Fig. 4.3 (a) Normal pulmonary vein inflow pattern associated with normal diastolic function. Note the S wave is greater than the D wave. (b) Normal transmitral blood flow Doppler recording. Note the E velocity is greater than the A velocity. Deceleration time (DT) is normal.

inflow velocity uses pulsed-wave Doppler velocity sampling from the tips of the mitral valve leaflets in the four-chamber view. Normal transmitral blood inflow pattern consists of an early diastolic passive flow from the left atrium into the LV designated as the E wave. This measurement exceeds, both in volume and velocity, the late diastolic active blood flow due to atrial contraction, designated as the A wave. As a result the normal inflow pattern has an early to late velocity ratio that is greater than one (E/A >1) (Figure 4.3). With aging, or other conditions known to cause LV stiffening, the ventricle becomes less compliant. The decrease in chamber compliance leads to a lesser contribution from passive filling (E velocity less than 1 m/sec) and more dependence on atrial contraction as shown in Figure 4.4 (E/A ratio <1). Note the deceleration time (DT) of the E wave is longer as a result of prolonged time needed to equalize the LA pressure with the poorly compliant LV. As the disease process progresses, high filling pressure results in left atrial remodeling. Ultimately, the remodeled atrium generates higher pressure that overcomes the noncompliant LV leading to reversal of the inflow pattern to a more normal-appearing profile, often referred to as the pseudonormal pattern, as shown in Figure 4.5 (peak E velocity >1 m/sec, E/A ratio >1). This pattern can be difficult to distinguish from the normal pattern; however, clues from other Doppler indices or from chamber dimensions render the distinction more apparent. The most advanced stage of diastolic dysfunction is the restrictive filling pattern. Transmitral inflow pattern is suggestive of this stage when the E wave velocity amplitude is high, the A

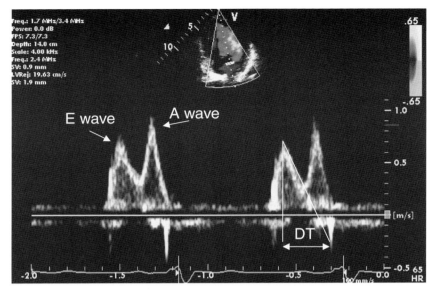

Fig. 4.4 Transmitral flow Doppler tracing consistent with stage I diastolic dysfunction. Note the E velocity is less than the A velocity, and the deceleration time (DT) is longer than the normal pattern. (See color plate section).

wave amplitude is markedly diminished (peak E velocity >> 1, E/A ration >> 1), and the E wave DT is less than 150 ms. The DT is very short because of exceedingly high left atrial pressures and rapid ventricular filling (Figure 4.6). Besides its dependence on filling pressures, ventricular relaxation, and age, one of the other major limitations of mitral inflow Doppler measurement is the difficulty of obtaining accurate measurements during elevated heart rates, such as during sinus tachycardia or atrial fibrillation. Furthermore, in the case of atrial fibrillation, which may affect up to 15% of patients with heart failure, the E/A ratio can not be calculated.

Tissue Doppler and mitral annular velocity

This index of diastolic function uses pulsed-wave Doppler velocity sampling from the medial and lateral aspects of the mitral annulus in the four-chamber view (Figure 4.7). As shown in Figure 4.7, the velocity sampling yields three distinct waves. The E' wave represents LV relaxation and because it is relatively independent of preload and unaffected by sinus tachycardia or atrial fibrillation, it is an exceptionally sensitive marker of diastolic dysfunction [46]. Peak E' velocity decreases (when diastolic dysfunction increases) from a normal value of about 10–15 cm/sec to severely abnormal values of less than 3 cm/sec in restrictive filling. It should be noted that typically, the annular velocity recorded at the

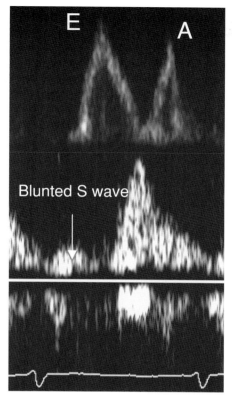

Fig. 4.5 Top tracing: Transmitral inflow with E>A suggestive of normal diastolic Function. However, the bottom tracing reveals blunted systolic pulmonary vein inflow, classifying this pattern as pseudonormal or stage II diastolic dyfunction.

medial aspect of the mitral annulus is slightly slower than that from the lateral annulus and currently there is no consensus as to which annular velocity should be used for assessment of diastolic function. The European Society of Cardiology [44] recommends averaging both velocities, other authorities recommend using either the medial or the lateral annular velocity only. The A' wave represents annular velocity as a result of atrial contraction and is not used to assess diastolic function. The previously mentioned S wave represents annular velocity due to systolic contraction and is used in assessment of LV function and dyssynchrony.

When combined with the transmitral inflow pattern, the peak E' velocity can be used to estimate the LV filling pressures. The peak E velocity from any transmitral inflow pattern is dependent on LV driving pressure, LV relaxation kinetics and age, and increases with increasing filling pressures. The E' velocity, on the other hand results from elastic recoil of the base and is mostly dependent

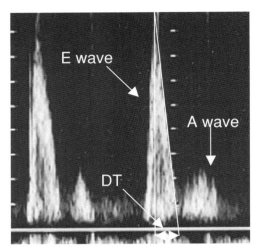

Fig. 4.6 Transmitral Doppler inflow pattern consistent with restrictive physiology (stage III/IV). Note the large E/A ratio (>>1) and very short deceleration time (DT).

on LV relaxation kinetics and age, and typically decreases with worsening diastolic function. By creating a ratio of E to E', the effects of LV relaxation kinetics and age cancel out and the LV driving/filling pressure can be estimated. Increasing E/E' ratio correlates well with high LV filling pressures, such that E/E' ratio of more than 15 indicates a PCWP of more than 20 mmHg. The same holds true for low E/E' ratio where E/E' ration less than 8–10 indicates a PCWP of less than 15 mmHg [47]. As previously mentioned, since TDI-derived tissue velocity measurements are independent of heart rate, the above mentioned

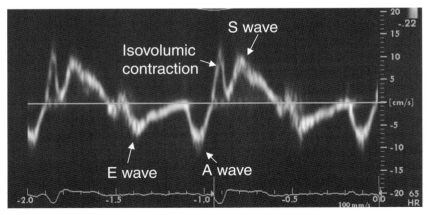

Fig. 4.7 Tissue Doppler tracing from the medial mitral annulus. Note the wave generated by the isovolumic contraction (not part of the S wave).

E/E′ index can be used to estimate filling pressures during sinus tachycardia or atrial fibrillation [48].

Mitral inflow velocity of propagation

The premise behind propagation velocity (Vp) involves the concept that blood fills the LV as result of a pressure gradient created by chamber relaxation and suctioning (negative pressure) such that flow (velocity) at the base of the LV is the highest and decreases as the blood moves toward the apex. Stated differently, the pressure gradient is highest when measured between the base and the apex and diminishes as blood moves toward the apex. Using color M-Mode sampling through the center of mitral inflow in the four-chamber view, spanning from the mitral valve annulus to the LV apex (distance of about 4 cm), the velocities along the single interrogation line are displayed in a color-coded fashion optimizing spatial and temporal flow characteristics. The slope of the highest velocity (distance down the LV cavity divided by time) represents Vp and has been correlated with LV diastolic function [49–51]. Normal Vp is about 45–50 cm/sec or greater. The major pitfall in assessing color M-mode flow propagation velocity is the low reproducibility due to misalignment of color M-mode cursor and mitral inflow. Furthermore, contrary to what was once thought, Vp is also not preload independent and this may be the reason why it has fallen out of favor in assessing diastolic function.

Blood flow Doppler and pulmonary vein inflow velocity

Pulmonary vein inflow velocity assessment is performed in a fashion very similar to the transmitral inflow velocity. Pulsed-wave Doppler is used to sample inflow velocity typically at the ostium of the right inferior pulmonary vein in the four-chamber view. Pulmonary vein inflow depends greatly on LA pressure, which, in turn, is greatly dependent on LV relaxation [52]. Under normal circumstances, the normally relaxed LV allows a majority of the volume in the LA to move down across the open mitral valve to the LV in diastole, thereby reducing LA pressure. During ventricular systole the LA begins to fill, in fact, the majority of LA filling occurs during that phase (S wave). The LA continues to fill during ventricular diastole as a result of decreased LA pressure caused by opening of the mitral valve (D wave). Atrial contraction causes some reversal in the pulmonary vein flow (A wave). Abnormally compliant LV does not allow for adequate atrial emptying during ventricular diastole leading to abnormally elevated LA pressures after the closure of the mitral valve. This prevents adequate LA filling during ventricular systole giving rise to a blunted systolic inflow (blunted S wave) and a predominant diastolic filling pattern of the LA. Because of elevated early diastolic LA pressure, atrial contraction leads to a more prominent atrial reversal. When combined with mitral inflow pattern, the pulmonary vein inflow can help distinguish between normal diastolic function (S>D) and the pseudonormal pattern (blunted S) seen in early stages of abnormal LV compliance [53] (See Figure 4.5). Furthermore, the pulmonary vein inflow pattern has also been used to assess LV loading pressure, such that a difference between the pulmonary atrial flow reversal duration (Ard) and the mitral A wave duration (Ad) of greater than 30 ms has been correlated with an LV end-diastolic pressure of greater than 18 mmHg [54,55]. The major limitation of this method is the technical difficultly of obtaining adequate sampling of the pulmonary vein inflow.

Left atrial volume

The left atrium serves as a conduit for blood flow from the pulmonary veins into the LV. In addition, left atrial contraction (LA kick) provides up to 30% of LV filling. The LA size can be estimated echocardiographically using M-Mode generated linear measurements such as the anteroposterior (AP) linear dimension obtained from the parasternal long view. Unfortunately, the true LA size in not adequately represented by a single linear measurement. For that reason, LA volume computed using the previously described Simpson's rule has emerged as the more preferred technique for LA size assessment. LA volume is further corrected for body surface area to yield the LA volume index. The LA volume index has been shown to be independent of age, unlike any of the Doppler indexes of diastolic dysfunction [56]. Because any increase in LA size is usually only associated with increased filling pressures, LA volume is a very powerful predictor of the severity and chronicity of diastolic dysfunction [57,58]. Furthermore, because LA volume increases linearly with worsening diastolic dysfunction, it has often been referred to as the "glycosylated hemoglobin of diastolic dysfunction" Increased LA volume index has been associated with the development of atrial fibrillation, a stroke, and with increased cardiovascular mortality risk of [59–62].

Clinical use of diastolic indexes

As previously stated, no single echocardiographic measurement of diastolic function is fully sufficient and it should never be used for assessment. Instead, synthesizing multiple echocardiographic diastolic parameters including chamber anatomy and combining them with clinical history and plasma markers, such a BNP is often necessary to make the appropriate diagnosis. Based on the above-mentioned Doppler indexes, diastolic dysfunction can be further classified echocardiographically into four progressive stages from abnormal relaxation (stage 1) to pseudonormal (stage 2), reversible restrictive filling (stage 3), and irreversible restrictive filling (stage 4) [63]. The main purpose of this classification scheme is to estimate filling pressures that correlate well with symptoms and prognosis, and also to assess the response to heart failure therapy. Patients with Stage 1 dysfunction have abnormal LV relaxation, but normal filling pressures and are typically asymptomatic with normal activity. Exercise induced tachycardia or atrial fibrillation, however, may make them symptomatic due to shortening of diastole. Management in this stage involves treatment of underlying conditions (HTN, diabetes, coronary artery disease, etc.) and heart rate/rhythm control. Stage 2 patients have abnormal relaxation and elevated filling pressures and may present with exertional dyspnea and lower extremity edema. They are typically managed with diuretics to decrease the filling pressures, rate/rhythm control, and RAAS modulators. Patients with stage 3 and stage 4 dysfunction have exceedingly high filling pressures and are most symptomatic. Their treatment is mostly limited to the use of diuretics and careful titration of RAAS modulators.

Measurement of mechanical dyssynchrony

LV dyssynchrony is a relatively new concept in clinical cardiology despite its description in patients with Wolf–Parkinson–White syndrome in the 1970s [64]. There are three recognized components of cardiac dyssynchrony and some or all of them may be present in individual patients. First, intraventricular or LV dyssynchrony can be best described as asynchronous, or out of phase, contraction of opposing segments of the LV as a result of abnormal electromechanical activation, most often associated with intraventricular conduction abnormalities (IVCD), left bundle branch block (LBBB), or RV apical pacing. Second, interventricular dyssynchrony refers to out of phase contraction between the right and left ventricles, also seen with ventricular conduction abnormalities. Third, atrioventricular dyssynchrony, which is associated with prolonged PR/AV interval, can be described as atrial contraction that occurs out of phase with LV contraction leading to premature termination of LV filling. Dyssynchronous LV contraction results in inefficient systole as the work generated by one region is dissipated by the opposing region leading to shifting of blood in the LV chamber rather than ejecting it. During controlled preload, afterload, and contractility, dyssynchronous contraction leads to a decrease in stoke volume in face of increased oxygen consumption making the stroke work of the heart up to 20–30% less efficient [65]. LV dyssynchrony affects diastolic function, as well, and has been shown to cause significant diastolic dysfunction. Isovolumic LV relaxation is prolonged in dyssynchrony due to high LV end-systolic pressure (LVESP) that results from late contraction of the lateral free wall well past the closure of the aortic valve and even past the opening of the mitral valve [66]. This pattern leaves less time for LV filling leading to a decrease in cardiac output and an increase in LVEDP and PCWP. Elevated LVESP has also been shown to cause diastolic mitral regurgitation (MR) that causes further decrease in preload [67]. Dyssynchronous contraction of the LV also leads to increased mitral regurgitation as a result of abnormal activation of the anterolateral papillary muscle [68]. Chronically, dyssynchronous contraction leads to electrical and structural remodeling [69–71]. Abnormal calcium handling, decreased gap junction expression, and longer conduction times result in increased arrhythmia susceptibility [72–73]. LV chamber hypertrophy, dilation, and reduced efficiency in the face of reduced coronary reserve lead to increased ischemia susceptibility, creating a vicious cycle that perpetuates this process into more advanced heart failure and higher risk of sudden cardiac death [69–74]. As a result, when comparing patients with similar degrees of LV dysfunction, those with LBBB, IVCD or RV pacing have a worse overall prognosis [75]. Fortunately, CRT has been shown to reverse this deleterious process. Synchronized pacing in patients with severe heart failure (NYHA Class III/IV) with low ejection fraction (EF <35%) and widened QRS (>120 ms) has been shown to improve patients' symptoms, decrease hospitalizations, and improve LV function and chamber dimensions [76–84]. Furthermore, more recently, large randomized trials have proven CRT with and without an ICD as a life-saving therapy [85,86].

Unfortunately, not all patients who receive BiV therapy benefit. The rate of nonresponders is as high as 30–40% in large clinical trials [87]. Patient selection based on widened QRS, an imperfect surrogate of mechanical dyssynchrony, may be partly responsible for the discrepancy in response to CRT [88]. Location of the LV pacing site and presence of infarct related scar have been shown to be important factors for optimizing the efficacy of BiV pacing, as well, and may also be responsible for the high nonresponder rates [89,90]. Furthermore, evidence from echocardiographic investigations has revealed that up to 30% of patients with severe heart failure and normal QRS duration have evidence of mechanical dyssynchrony [91]. These patients have been shown to derive favorable effect from CRT, however, are not eligible for BiV pacing according to the current QRS-based guidelines and recommendations [91,92]. These unsatisfying findings spawned the search for the modality that would directly assess mechanical dyssynchrony. MRI using strain analysis was the first technique used for that purpose. In fact, the correlation between the level of dyssynchrony and systolic improvement with synchronous pacing was first demonstrated using this technique [93–95]. Unfortunately, MRI strain analysis is quite complex, unavailable in many centers and relatively expensive. As a result, some of the previously described echocardiographic techniques used to quantify systolic and diastolic function have been used to provide similar information. Multiple echocardiographic parameters have been investigated and some of them have proven quite capable of identifying significant mechanical dyssynchrony and predicting patient response to CRT [96]. These modalities will be discussion below. In addition, two-dimensional and three-dimensional volume and EF measurements have been useful in assessing echocardiographic response to CRT, and will be discussed in the next section.

M-Mode
Septal to Posterior Wall Mechanical Delay (SPWMD) was proposed as an index of intraventricular dyssynchrony by Pitzalis et al. in 2002 [97]. This technique

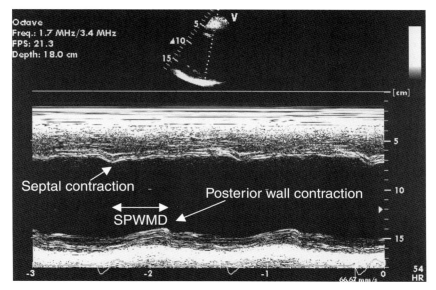

Fig. 4.8 M-mode imaging demonstrating septal to posterior wall mechanical delay (SPWMD).

uses M-Mode interrogation and computation of peak contraction delay between the septum and the posterior wall in the parasternal short- or long-axis view of the LV at the level of the papillary muscles (Figure 4.8). A delay of greater than 130 ms has been shown to be predictive of significant symptomatic and echocardiographic response to CRT and overall prognosis in small clinical trials [97,98]. The major advantages of this technique are the widespread availability of the modality, the relative ease of data acquisition, and low processing cost. The major pitfall, however, is that this technique evaluates dyssynchrony between only two segments of the ventricle. Furthermore, in up to 40% of patients, this index is unobtainable due to septal wall akinesis in the setting of previous infrac-tion or RV volume overload, or due to suboptimal imaging quality. Subsequent studies using this technique proved its low feasibility in predicting response to CRT in HF patients [99].

A relatively new M-Mode LV dyssynchrony index, lateral wall postsystolic displacement (LWPSD), is defined as the difference between the interval from QRS onset to maximal systolic displacement of the basal posterolateral wall of the LV and the interval from QRS onset to the beginning of transmitral E wave velocity. A positive value implies significant postsystolic contraction of the posterolateral wall and, despite single segment interrogation, has been shown to be predictive of CRT response in a small population of HF patients with LBBB

[100]. Its value in assessing mechanical dyssynchrony in patients with severe HF and narrow QRS has not yet been established.

Pulsed-wave Doppler

Pulsed-wave Doppler blood flow measurements have been used to identify interventricular dyssynchrony. RV and LV pre-ejection periods (PEP) can be measured from the onset of the QRS to the initiation of RVOT and LVOT Doppler-measured systolic flow, respectively; and interventricular mechanical delay can be calculated as the difference between the two measurements. An IVMD of greater than 40 ms, or a baseline aortic PEP greater than 160 ms, are associated with significant interventricular dyssynchrony and have been shown to be predictive of response to CRT in a small trial [101]. Moreover, the recently published CARE-HF trial showed a trend toward better clinical outcomes in patients with a baseline interventricular delay of greater than 49 ms [86]. The presence of severe pulmonary hypertension or RV dysfunction can impair the diagnostic accuracy of this technique as a result of RV PEP prolongation.

Tissue Doppler imaging

Interventricular dyssynchrony can also be assessed by tissue Doppler imaging (TDI). As previously described is the section on diastology, TDI uses pulsed-wave Doppler sampling of myocardial tissue velocities. Interventricular mechanical delay can be computed is a fashion very similar to the blood flow Doppler measurement by comparing the time difference between the interval from QRS onset to RV free wall systolic velocity versus the interval from QRS onset to LV lateral wall systolic velocity in the four-chamber view. Similarly, a difference of greater than 40 ms implies interventricular dyssynchrony.

However, TDI-assessed systolic myocardial velocities have in actuality emerged as an index of intraventricular dyssynchrony. Despite some of its limitations, evaluation of longitudinal myocardial velocities is by far the most studied and the most commonly used modality in clinical evaluation for cardiac dyssynchrony.

One of the earlier described indices of LV dyssynchrony using TDI was the difference in time between the intervals from QRS onset to medial versus lateral basal wall onset (Sm_0) or peak (Sm peak) velocity measured in the four-chamber view (Figure 4.9) [102]. A value greater than or equal to 65 ms was shown to be predictive of symptomatic and echocardiographic improvements from CRT in a small population of patients with severe heart failure and LBBB [103]. This technique was later modified to interrogate basal and mid-ventricular segments (up to 12) in two-chamber, three-chamber and four-chamber views with similarly high predictive accuracy of CRT response in HF patients with prolonged QRS [101,104,105]. The major disadvantage of the pulsed-wave Doppler method is that each individual segment interrogation must be performed on line making the process time-consuming and susceptible to influences of heart rate

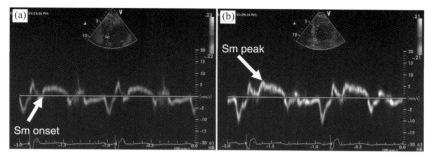

Fig. 4.9 Tissue Doppler imaging. Time from QRS onset to onset (a) or peak (b) of systolic movement (Sm) from the basal septal wall is measured and compared to the timing from the basal lateral wall. (See color plate section).

variability, breathing and patient movement. Furthermore, the Sm peak may be difficult to identify in some patients.

Due to these technical limitations, pulsed-wave Doppler has been largely replaced by color-coded TDI, which allows for simpler and more practical data acquisition and processing. With this technique time-velocity data can be analyzed off line such that opposing segments can be evaluated simultaneously limiting, but not eliminating, errors related to heart rate variability, breathing, or patient movement (Figure 4.10). The first color-coded TDI method consisted of a comparison of velocity tracings between the basal septum and the basal lateral wall from the four-chamber view (two-site method). Subsequent improvements incorporated interrogation of additional segments, initially by adding information from the base of the anterior and inferior walls from the two-chamber view (four-site method), and later, by analyzing all three apical views and combining data from the basal and mid ventricular segments from the septum and lateral wall, the anteroseptum, and the posterior wall and the anterior and inferior walls (12-site method). A delay of greater than 65 ms between any opposing walls has been shown to be predictive of symptomatic and echocardiographic improvements from CRT and better prognosis after CRT [106]. A 12-segment standard deviation of the time to Sm peak model that integrates information from the three apical views and computes a mechanical dyssynchrony index (Ts-SD) was developed and tested by Yu et al. [107]. A Ts-SD cutoff value greater than 33 ms, when applied to patients with severe heart failure and widened QRS, has been shown to be highly predictive of CRT-derived LV reverse remodeling defined as greater than 15% decrease in LV end-systolic volume [107]. In another study, Ts-SD greater than 34.4 ms was the most powerful predictor of reverse remodeling after CRT when compared to eight different echocardiographic parameters of dyssynchrony including TDI strain rate imaging [108]. To further refine this model, Yu et al. applied Tissue Synchronization Imaging (TSI) to better identify the regions of greatest delay. TSI adds a color-coded

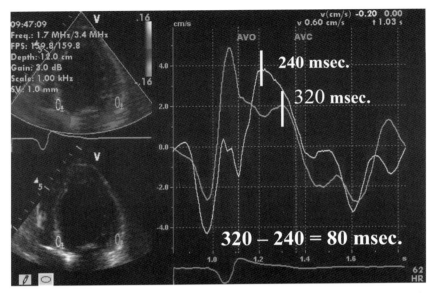

Fig. 4.10 Color-coded Tissue Doppler Imaging. Areas of interest can be selected simultaneously during off line processing. Myocardial velocities are displayed simultaneously allowing for precise calculation of mechanical delay (here between the basal septum and the basal lateral wall). (See color plate section).

overlay onto two-dimensional images. Using the 12-site model, the segments with the most delayed mechanical activation can be easily visually identified and included in the Ts-SD computation, thereby, theoretically, adding to the simplicity and ease of computation of the delay [109].

As previously stated, evidence from small clinical trials supports the use of CRT is HF patient with narrow QRS but with echocardiographic evidence of mechanical dyssynchrony. In their work with 33 severe heart failure patients with narrow QRS (<120 ms) Bleeker et al. [110] used septal to lateral wall time to peak systolic velocity delay and showed that a cutoff value of 65 ms was predictive of CRT-derived improvement in HF class and in echocardiographic LV reverse remodeling. Yu et al. [92] reported similar results in this population of patients ($n = 51$) using their Ts-SD index of greater than 34 ms.

Despite their wide clinical use for the assessment LV dyssynchrony, TDI measurements of longitudinal velocity have some concerning limitations. First, depending on the method used, only basal or basal and mid-segments are analyzed. Second, TDI parameters, as assessed in the apical views, reflect longitudinal motion of cardiac contraction only. Magnetic resonance imaging (MRI) in normal subjects and in heart failure patients has consistently revealed that the heart contracts predominantly in the circumferential axis [111], thereby, questioning the reliability of sole longitudinal assessment. On that same note, accurate measurements of even the longitudinal velocities may be difficult to perform due to significant angle dependency with TDI, especially in patients with severe LV dysfunction and LV ballooning. Third, TDI does not assess true tissue contraction; instead it measures tissue velocity based on motion that is highly affected by tethering and translocation. For example, the basal segments may display normal longitudinal velocity after myocardial infarction if the mid-ventricular segments contract in a normal fashion. All these concerns are especially valid after the recent European Society of Cardiology Congress 2007 where the PROSPECT trial was presented and raised concerned about the utility of the TDI-derived indexes of dyssynchrony assessment in severe HF patients with widened QRS [112]. Furthermore, the recently published RethinQ trial showed rather discouraging results for TDI in predicting response to CRT in patients with severe heart failure, narrow QRS, and echocardiographic (M-Mode or TDI velocity) evidence of mechanical dyssynchrony. The study enrolled 172 ICD eligible HF patients with evidence of mechanical dyssynchrony by TDI and randomized them to ICD-CRT versus ICD alone. After a 6-month follow up period there was no benefit from CRT in patients with narrow QRS (<120 ms) suggesting that TDI was not predictive of response to CRT in that population of patients when an endpoint of peak VO_2 consumption was analyzed [113]. In favor of the TDI method was the finding of a favorable result from CRT in patients with a QRS duration between 120 ms and 130 ms.

In order to address some of the shortcomings of TDI velocity measurements of dyssynchrony, strain and strain rate imaging was recently introduced. Unlike the velocity measurements, strain and strain rate measurements have a theoretical advantage of differentiating between active contraction and passive motion due to translocation or tethering.

As previously mentioned in the section on systolic function assessment, TDI-derived strain rate is defined as the difference in velocity between two adjacent myocardial regions divided by the original distance and represents rate of deformation. Strain is the magnitude of deformation and can be computed by integrating strain rate over time (using TDI) or calculated directly (not by TDI) by dividing the change in distance between two points by their original distance. Negative strain rate represents contraction whereas positive values reflect relaxation. Normal values for strain and strain rate in the apical views range from 15% to 25% and 1 to 1.5 sec, respectively [114]. TDI-derived longitudinal strain is still limited by its angle dependence, time consuming post processing and low signal-noise ratio. Never the less, the technique has been shown to be useful in assessing dyssynchrony and identifying echocardiographic responders to CRT [115–118]. However, as previously mentioned, Yu et al. demonstrated superiority of TDI longitudinal velocity Ts-SD over TDI longitudinal strain rate for predicting reverse LV remodeling [108]. Dohi et al. [119] investigated the use of TDI strain rate imaging in assessing radial mechanical dyssynchrony in 38

CRT patients [119]. Radial strain was computed using TDI strain rate calculation from the anteroseptum and posterior wall in the short axis view of LV. A peak strain delay value greater than 130 ms combined with favorable lead positioning was shown to be highly predictive (95% sensitivity, 88% specificity) of immediate improvement in stroke volume regardless of QRS duration. Unfortunately, limitations due angle dependence and low signal-to-noise ratio plague this technique, as well.

Speckle tracking imaging

Speckle tracking imaging (STI) is a novel non-Doppler two-dimensional strain technique used to assess LV dyssynchrony. Through the use of semi-automated, postprocessing software, myocardial motion can be analyzed by tracking natural acoustic markers (speckles) over several frames in a manner very similar to tagged MRI strain analysis (Figures 4.11 and 4.12). LV rotation or torsion (twisting), previously only assessable by MRI, can be reliably estimated and used to compute global and regional LV function [36,120]. This technique, using similar methodology, also allows for angle independent evaluation of LV dyssynchrony via estimation of regional strain. Suffoletto et al, [120] applied this technique

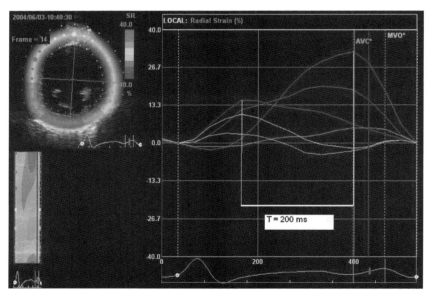

Fig. 4.11 Speckle Tracking Imaging. Regional radial strain is displayed over time. The timing in the areas of normal contraction [anteroseptum (red), anterior wall (yellow) and lateral wall (light blue)] may be compared to the timing in the delayed contracting segments [here the inferoseptum (dark blue), inferior wall (purple) and posterolateral wall (green)]. A difference of greater than 130 ms is consistent with significant LV dyssynchorny. (See color plate section).

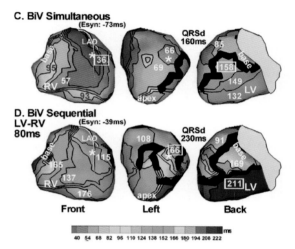

C. BiV Simultaneous
(Esyn: -73ms)

D. BiV Sequential LV-RV 80ms
(Esyn: -39ms)

QRSd 160ms

QRSd 230ms

Front Left Back

40 54 68 82 96 110 124 138 152 166 180 194 208 222 ms

Color Plate 3.11 Epicardial isochrone maps that reflect the activation of the right and left ventricles during biventricular pacing. The epicardial surfaces of both ventricles are displayed in anterior, left lateral and posterior, with some overlap between adjacent views. The valve area is shaded in grey. The thick black mark in the top panel indicates the line of block, which is no longer appreciable with biventricular pacing. The native rhythm panel shows sequential activation of the right ventricle followed by a much delayed left ventricular activation, suggestive of a left bundle branch–like pattern. Activation times (in milliseconds) of selected regions are shown. Earliest and latest ventricular activation times are indicated by framed numbers, and are in relation to the onset of the QRS. (Adapted from Jia et al. [4].)

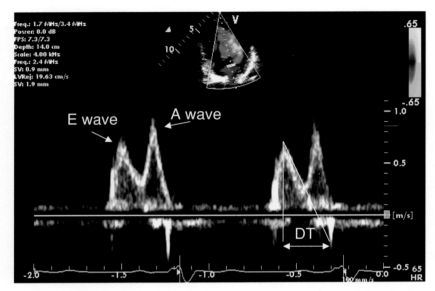

Color Plate 4.4 Transmitral flow Doppler tracing consistent with stage I diastolic dysfunction. Note the E velocity is less than the A velocity, and the deceleration time (DT) is longer than the normal pattern.

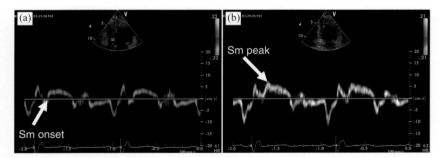

Color Plate 4.9 Tissue Doppler imaging. Time from QRS onset to onset (a) or peak (b) of systolic movement (Sm) from the basal septal wall is measured and compared to the timing from the basal lateral wall.

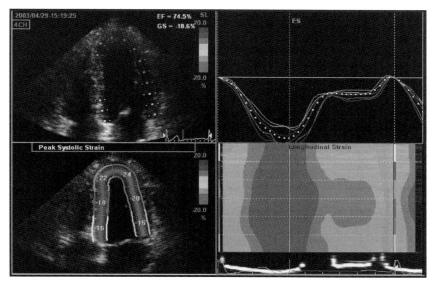

Fig. 4.12 Longitudinal strain assessment using the speckle tracking technique. Right: the speckle tracking algorithm is applied to the apical four-chamber view. The strain analysis displayed on the left reveals synchronous contraction is all segments. (See color plate section).

in 64 patients undergoing CRT to assess radial strain in 6 standard segments in the mid-ventricular short axis view. A time difference between septal peak strain and posterior wall peak strain greater than 130 ms was highly predictive of significant increase in LV EF after close to 9 months of follow up [121]. By combining non-Doppler two-dimensional radial strain from STI with TDI longitudinal velocity assessment (two-site in all patients, Ts-SD in a subgroup of 67 patients), Gorcsan et al, [122] were able to predict echocardiographic response to CRT in 190 HF patients (mean EF 23%, mean QRS 169 ms) with 88% sensitivity and 80% specificity, which was significantly better than either technique alone. However, strain measurements may not be applicable to all patients with conduction abnormalities and some measurements may be more accurate then others. Donal et al. [123] attempted to correlate radial and longitudinal strain from STI with QRS duration in 95 HF patients (EF <40%) with ischemic (ICM) and nonischemic (NICM) etiologies of LV dysfunction. They concluded that "correlation between electrical and mechanical indexes [of dyssynchrony] in patients with ICM versus NICM was dissimilar," such that both longitudinal and radial strain correlated well with QRS duration in NICM patients, however, only radial strain correlated with QRS duration in ICM patients. This finding supports the use of radial strain in assessment of dyssynchrony and further questions the utility of longitudinal strain assessment (TDI or STI-rendered) for this purpose. However, in a recently submitted work by Lim et al. [134], the authors used STI-derived longitudinal strain delay index, a measure of the component of impaired contractility related to mechanical dyssynchrony, to identify responders to CRT (unpublished data). The longitudinal strain delay index was defined as the sum of the difference between peak and end-systolic strain across 16 segments and is a combination and relative weighing of contractility and time delay. As a result, this index has a unique ability to identify potentially CRT-recruitable viable myocardium; hence, it predicts response to CRT in ischemic and nonischemic patients. Longitudinal strain delay index cut-off of 25% identified 82% of responders and 92% of nonresponders in a population of 35 ischemic and nonischemic HF patients (EF <35%, QRS >120 ms). Interestingly, as reported by Helle and Valle [36] in their original description of STI, during radial strain assessment, the longitudinal displacement of the heart during contraction precludes tracking of the same speckles as they move in and out of the imaging plane. This is especially problematic at the base of the LV where the longitudinal displacement is most pronounced [36]. The aforementioned phenomenon may further support the use of the above mentioned longitudinal strain delay index.

The need for adequate image quality and laborious post processing are limitations to this technique. However, overall, STI-derived strain indexes are quite promising for the assessment of regional LV function and LV dyssynchrony across all 17 myocardial segments. Larger clinical trials are needed to further validate this technique.

Three-dimensional echocardiography

Previously described in the section on systolic LV assessment, three-dimensional imaging has also found its applicability in the assessment of LV dyssynchrony. The major advantage of this technique is that it allows for dyssynchrony assessment across all elements of contraction (radial, circumferential, and longitudinal) in 16 LV segments in the same cardiac cycle (Figure 4.13). Semi-automated tracing algorithms allow for regional wall motion assessment and calculation of a systolic dyssynchrony index (SDI) that corresponds to the standard deviation of the average time interval needed to reach minimal end-systolic volume in 16 LV segments [124]. Marsan et al. [125] reported their experience with real-time, three-dimensional echo (RT3DE) in 56 patients with CRT in whom an SDI cutoff of 5.6% yielded a sensitivity of 88% and a specificity of 87% (AUC 0.96) for predicting acute echocardiographic response (>15% reduction in LV end-systolic volume). Furthermore, CRT responders demonstrated a significant reduction in SDI immediately after initiation of pacing, as opposed to the nonresponders in whom SDI did not change . Van de Veire et al. [126] recently published their experience with 49 CRT patients with another three-dimensional index of dyssynchrony, which is synonymous to two-dimensional Ts-SD (Yu index) and similarly computes standard deviation of time delay in 12 LV segments (Triplane

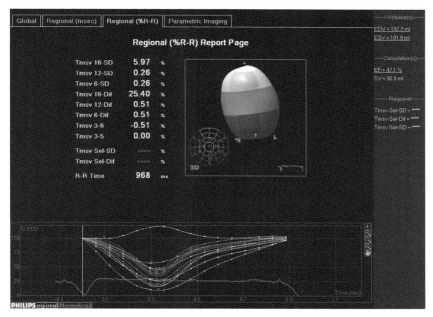

Fig. 4.13 Three-Dimensional Echocardiography. Volumes across all 17 segments are displayed graphically as shown. Minimal volumes imply peak contraction, and their timing may be used to compute regional dyssynchrony. (See color plate section).

Ts-SD). A triplane Ts-SD index greater than 35.8 ms was shown to predict acute reverse LV remodeling (>15% decrease in LV end-systolic volume) 48 hours after CRT [126]. Low spatial and temporal resolution, low feasibility (~80% [127]), and inability to distinguish between active and passive contraction are the major disadvantages of all three-dimensional imaging techniques. Nonetheless, as with STI, three-dimensional strain is very promising and requires further validation in large clinical trials.

MRI

As previously mentioned, MRI was one of the first techniques used in the assessment of LV dyssynchrony. Previously mostly used in research settings, currently, this modality is gaining considerable popularity clinically due to the improved acquisition and processing techniques. Initially, tagged MRI-based regional strain analysis provided highly accurate and reproducible. Tag lines are noninvasively applied tissue labels created by the spatial modulation of magnetization technique (SPAMM). These tags move along with the tissue throughout the cardiac cycle allowing for computation of regional contraction via strain data analysis. The major advantage of tagged-MRI is that it is window and angle independent, and provides full assessment of ventricular contraction in three-dimensional reconstructions and provides high spatial resolution. However, even though, the circumferential, radial and longitudinal strain measurements could be computed from the rich MRI data allowing for subsequent dyssynchrony assessment, this process is quite time consuming and not practical for clinical use. Furthermore, MRI is contraindicated in patients with an existing cardiac device. A more recently introduced harmonic phase (HARP) analysis of tagged MRI significantly shortens the processing time making this technique more attractive for clinical application. Simply put, this technique measures local strain by analyzing pre-specified frequency components (harmonic peaks) of the tag lines in a given tissue over time. When the tissue contracts, the tag lines become closer together increasing their frequency, and when the tissue is stretched, the opposite occurs. Strain-encoded MRI (SENC) analysis is potentially even more clinically applicable due to its instantaneous real-time quantitative strain measurements with virtually no need for postprocessing. Once strain data is obtained, a dyssynchrony index can be computed using various aspect of regional strain variance. Although, large clinical trials using this technique are lacking, there is some animal and human data validating this technique for evaluating local myocardial performance. Given the recent advancements in MRI, it is likely that it will become more frequently incorporated into clinical practice, however, its use in dyssynchrony assessment will likely be limited due to its limited availability, relatively high complexity, and expense.

Ventricular remodeling

Pathologic LV remodeling is the final common pathway to the development of heart failure. LV remodeling is classified as concentric hypertrophy when it results from conditions that cause chronic pressure overload (HTN, aortic stenosis), or eccentric hypertrophy when it is caused by chronic volume overload (mitral regurgitation, aortic insufficiency) or complications of ischemic heart disease. In conditions that result in chronic volume overload, the transition to heart failure may be protracted, sometimes occurring up to a decade later. This is in contrast to LV remodeling that result from sudden loss of myocyte mass as a result of a myocardial infarction (MI). Post-MI LV remodeling is associated with early LV dilation and its extent is dependent on the size and location of the infarction, activation of the sympathetic nervous system and up-regulation of the RAAS [128]. Regardless of the etiology, LV remodeling leads to progressive chamber dilation, distortion of the cavity, disruption of mitral valve geometry and deterioration of contractile function of the ventricle [6]. The American Society of Echocardiography recommends evaluating LV remodeling via estimation of LV volumes and EF by the previously described methods in the systolic dysfunction section of this chapter (see the modified Simpson's rule). These parameters have been shown to be predictive of death, recurrent MI, heart failure and arrhythmic complications in large clinical trials [128].

Reverse remodeling is a relatively new concept that in part stemmed from the findings of partial recovery of LV size and function in patients with heart failure who were subjected to CRT. As previously discussed, large CRT trials have documented improved symptoms and increased longevity in their patient population [85,86]. These improvements have been mirrored by echocardiographic demonstration of decreased LV size (>15% decrease in LV end-systolic volume), increased LV function (>5% increase in EF) and decreased mitral regurgitation with CRT [129]. These findings persist for up to 3 months after cessation of pacing, suggesting that they are related to actual structural LV remodeling [130]. These findings also suggest that evidence of reverse LV remodeling on post-CRT surveillance could serve a prognostic value. Yu et al. [131] compared hard clinical outcomes in echocardiographic responders to CRT (>10% reduction in LV end-diastolic volume at 3–6 months) versus echocardiographic nonresponders, and found that regardless of the improvement in symptoms, echocardiographic responders carried a statistically lower all-cause mortality, cardiovascular mortality, and incidence of HF. Not surprisingly, sustained reverse LV remodeling with continuous CRT is a function of etiology of LV dysfunction as presented by St. John Sutton et al. [132]. By analyzing data from the MIRACLE trial the authors concluded that, despite sustained universal symptomatic improvement with CRT at 6-months and 12-months follow up after implantation, sustained LV remodeling occurred to a lesser extent in patients with ischemic versus nonischemic cardiomyopathy. Presence of myocardial scar or progression of the ischemic disease may partially explain this phenomenon [133]. For the former, further research evaluating the utility of imaging-guided LV lead placement is warranted.

Conclusion

The field of cardiac imaging has emerged as a powerful tool in the diagnosis, management, and prognostic evaluation of heart failure patients. Echocardiography leads this field due to its versatility, real-time capability, and cost-effectiveness. Systolic and diastolic functions can easily, accurately, and reproducibly be assessed by a myriad of echocardiographic techniques. Conventional two-dimensional imaging is most commonly used to assess the LV systolic performance; however, the newer three-dimensional echocardiographic techniques appear to be quite promising for more precise evaluation. Diastolic function is best assessed by pulsed-wave blood flow and tissue Doppler imaging.

Similarly, echocardiography has emerged as the preferred modality for assessing cardiac dyssynchrony pre-CRT and ventricular remodeling after CRT in HF patients with severe LV dysfunction and widened QRS. Despite its angle dependency and other technical limitations, two-dimensional TDI longitudinal velocity assessment of dyssynchrony is the most studied technique and has been shown to be predictive of response to CRT in cohort studies, however, has been less impressive in controlled and randomized clinical trials. More predictive of response to CRT are the newer strain imaging techniques, especially those using the recently developed angle-independent, speckle-tracking imaging technique.

References

1. Keidel WD. Uber eine Methode zur Registrierung der Volumanderungern des Herzens am Menschen. *Z Kreislaufforsch.* 1950;39:257.
2. Edler I, Hertz CH. Use of ultrasonic reflectoscope for the continuous recording of movements of heart walls. *Kungl Fysiogr Sallsk Lung Forth.* 1954;24:40.
3. Hunt SA; American College of Cardiology; American Heart Association Task Force on Practice Guidelines (Writing Committee to Update the 2001 Guidelines for the Evaluation and Management of Heart Failure). *J Am Coll Cardiol.* 2005; Sep 20;46(6):1–82.
4. Lloyd-Jones DM, Larson MG, Leip EP, et al. Lifetime risk for developing congestive heart failure: the Framingham Heart Study. *Circulation.* 2002;106:3068.
5. Zile M, Brutsaert D. New concepts in diastolic dysfunction and diastolic heart failure: Part I. Diagnosis, prognosis and measurement of diastolic function. *Circulation.* 2002;105:1387.
6. St. John Sutton M, Pfeffer MA, Plappert T, et al. Quantitative two-dimensional echocardiographic measurements are major predictors of adverse cardiovascular events after acute myocardial infarction. The protective effects of Captopril. *Circulation.* 1994;89:68–75.
7. Goldberger Z, Lampert R. Implantable Cardioverter-Defibrillators: Expanding Indications and Technologies. *JAMA.* February 15, 2006–Vol 295, No. 7.
8. Sanderson JE. Heart failure with a normal ejection fraction. *Heart.* 2007;93:155–8.
9. Ilercil A, O'Grady MJ, Roman MJ, et al. Reference values for echocardiographic measurements in urban and rural populations of differing ethnicity: the Strong Heart Study. *J Am Soc Echocardiogr.* 2001;14:601–11.
10. Devereux RB, de Simone G, Pickering TG, et al. Relation of left ventricular midwall function to cardiovascular risk factors and arterial structure and function. *Hypertension.* 1998;31:929–36.
11. Palmieri V, Dahlof B, DeQuattro V, et al. Reliability of echocardiographic assessment of left ventricular structure and function: the PRESERVE study: Prospective Randomized Study Evaluating Regression of Ventricular Enlargement. *J Am Coll Cardiol.* 1999;34:1625–32.
12. Nidorf SM, Picard MH, Triulzi MO, et al. New perspectives in the assessment of cardiac chamber dimensions during development and adulthood. *J Am Coll Cardiol.* 1992;19:983–8.
13. Pearlman JD, Triulzi MO, King ME, Newell J, Weyman AE. Limits of normal left ventricular dimensions in growth and development: analysis of dimensions and variance in the two-dimensional echocardiograms of 268 normal healthy subjects. *J Am Coll Cardiol.* 1988;12:1432–41.

14. Lang RM, Bierig M, Devereux RB, et al. Recommendations for chamber quantification. *Eur J Echocardiogr.* 2006;7;79–108
15. Malm S, Frigstad S, Sagberg E, Larsson H, Skjaerpe T. Accurate and reproducible measurement of left ventricular volume and ejection fraction by contrast echocardiography: a comparison with magnetic resonance imaging. *J Am Coll Cardiol.* 2004;44: 1030–5.
16. Hundley WG, Kizilbash AM, Afridi I, Franco F, Peshock RM, Grayburn PA. Administration of intravenous perfluorocarbon contrast agent improves echocardiographic determination of left ventricular volumes and ejection fraction: comparison with cine magnetic resonance imaging. *J Am Coll Cardiol.* 1998;32:1426–32.
17. Yu EHC, Sloggett CE, Iwanochko RM, Rakowski H, Siu SC. Feasibility and accuracy of left ventricular volumes and ejection fraction determination by fundamental, tissue harmonic, and intravenous contrast imaging in difficult-to-image patients. *J Am Soc Echocardiogr.* 2000;13:216–24.
18. Spencer KT, Bednarz J, Rafter PG, Korcarz C, Lang RM. Use of harmonic imaging without echocardiographic contrast to improve two-dimensional image quality. *Am J Cardiol.* 1998;82:794–99.
19. Lang RM, Mor-Avi V, Zoghbi WA, Senior R, Klein AL, Pearlman AS. The role of contrast enhancement in the echocardiographic assessment of the left ventricle. *Am J Cardiol.* 2002;90:28–34.
20. Jacobs LD, Salgo IS, Goonewardena S, et al. Rapid online quantification of left ventricular volume from real-time three-dimensional echocardiographic data. *Eur Heart J.* 2006;27:460–8.
21. Houck RC, Coke J, Gill EA. Three-dimensional echo: Transition from theory to real-time, a technology now ready for prime time. Current Problems in Diagnostic *Radiology.* 2005;34:85.
22. Sugeng L, Weinert L, Lang RM. Left ventricular assessment using real time three dimensional echocardiography. *Heart.* 2003;89 Suppl 3:iii29–36.
23. Jenkins C, Bricknell K, Hanekom L, Marwick TH. Reproducibility and accuracy of echocardiographic measurements of left ventricular parameters using real-time three dimensional echocardiography. *J Am Coll Cardiol.* 2004;44:878–86.
24. Sugeng L, Mor-Avi V, Weinert L, et al. Quantitative assessment of left ventricular size and function: side-by-side comparison of realtime three-dimensional echocardiography and computed tomography with magnetic resonance reference. *Circulation.* 2006;114:654–61.
25. Mor-Avi V, Sugeng L, Weinert L, et al. Fast measurement of left ventricular mass with real-time three-dimensional echocardiography: comparison with magnetic resonance imaging. *Circulation.* 2004;110:1814–8.
26. Caiani EG, Corsi G, Zamorano J. Improved semiautomated quantification of left ventricular volumes and ejection fraction using 3-dimensional echocardiography with a full matrix-array transducer. Comparison with magnetic resonance imaging. *J Am Soc Echocardiogr.* 2005;18:779.
27. Cerqueira MD, Weissman NJ, Dilsizian V, Jacobs AK, Kaul S, Laskey WK, Pennell DJ, Rumberger JA, Ryan T, Verani MS. American Heart Association Writing Group on Myocardial Segmentation and Registration for Cardiac Imaging: Standardized myocardial segmentation and nomenclature for tomographic imaging of the heart: a statement for healthcare professionals from the Cardiac Imaging Committee of the

Council on Clinical cardiology of the American Heart Association. *Circulation*. 2002, 105:539–42.

28. Schiller NB, Shah PM, Crawford M, DeMaria A, Devereux R, Feigenbaum H, Gutgesell H, Reichek N, Sahn D, Schnittger I, et al. Recommendations for quantitation of the left ventricle by two-dimensional echocardiography. American Society of Echocardiography Committee on Standards, Subcommittee on Quantitation of Two Dimensional Echocardiograms. *J Am Soc Echocardiogr.* 1989; Sep-Oct;2(5):358–67.

29. Prinzen FW, Hunter WC, Wyman BT, McVeigh ER. Mapping of regional myocardial strain and work during ventricular pacing: experimental study using magnetic resonance imaging tagging. *J Am Coll Cardiol.* 1999; May;33(6):1735–42.

30. Corsi C, Lang RM, Veronesi F, et al. Volumetric quantification of global and regional left ventricular function from real-time three dimensional echocardiographic images. *Circulation* 2005;112:1161–70.

31. Marwick TH, Case C, Leano R, et al. Use of tissue Doppler imaging to facilitate the prediction of events in patients with abnormal left ventricular function by dobutamine echocardiography. *Am J Cardiol.* 2004;93:142–6.

32. Hanekom L, Jenkins C, Jeffries L, et al. Incremental value of strain rate analysis as an adjunct to wall-motion scoring for assessment of myocardial viability by dobutamine echocardiography: a follow-up study after revascularization. *Circulation.* 2005;112:3892–900.

33. Alam M, Wardell J, Andersson E, Samad BA, Nordlander R. Effects of first myocardial infarction on left ventricular systolic and diastolic function with the use of mitral annular velocity determined by pulsed wave Doppler tissue imaging. *J Am Soc Echocardiogr.* 2000;13:343–52.

34. Amundsen BH, Helle-Valle T, Edvardsen T, et al. Noninvasive myocardial strain measurement by speckle tracking echocardiography validation against sonomicrometry and tagged magnetic resonance imaging. *J Am Coll Cardiol.* 2006;47:789–93.

35. Suffoletto MS, Dohi K, Cannesson M, Saba S, Gorcsan J 3rd. Novel speckle-tracking radial strain from routine black-and-white echocardiographic images to quantify dyssynchrony and predict response to cardiac resynchronization therapy. *Circulation.* 2006;113:960–8.

36. Helle-Valle T, Crosby J, Edvardsen T, Lyseggen E, Amundsen BH, Smith HJ, Rosen BD, Lima JA, Torp H, Ihlen H, Smiseth OA. New noninvasive method for assessment of left ventricular rotation: speckle tracking echocardiography. *Circulation.* 2005; Nov 15;112(20):3149–56.

37. Notomi Y, Lysyansky P, Setser RM, et al. Measurement of ventricular torsion by two-dimensional ultrasound speckle tracking imaging. *J Am Coll Cardiol.* 2005;45:2034–41.

38. Owan TE, Hodge DO, Herges RM, Jacobsen SJ, Roger VL, Redfield MM. Trends in prevalence and outcome of heart failure with preserved ejection fraction. *N Engl J Med.* 2006;355:251–59.

39. Abhayaratna WP, Marwick TH, Smith WT, Becker NG. Characteristics of left ventricular diastolic dysfunction in the community: an echocardiographic survey. *Heart.* 2006;92:1259–64.

40. Bhatia RS, Tu JV, Lee DS, Austin PC, Fang J, Haouzi A, Gong Y, Liu PP. Outcome of heart failure with preserved ejection fraction in a population-based study. *N Engl J Med.* 2006;355:260–69.

41. Aurigemma P. Diastolic heart failure—a common and lethal condition by any name. *N Engl J Med.* 2006;355:308–10.

42. Fischer M, Baessler A, Hense HW, Hengstenberg C, Muscholl M, Holmer S, Doring A, Broeckel U, Riegger G, Schunkert H. Prevalence of left ventricular diastolic dysfunction in the community: results from a Doppler echocardiographic-based survey of a population sample. *Eur Heart J.* 2003;24:320–28.

43. Klapholz M, Maurer M, Lowe AM, et al. New York Heart Failure Consortium. Hospitalization for heart failure in the presence of a normal left ventricular ejection fraction: results of the New York Heart Failure Registry. *J Am Coll Cardiol.* 2004;43:1432–8.

44. Paulus WJ, Tschöpe C, Sanderson JE, et al. How to diagnose diastolic heart failure: a consensus statement on the diagnosis of heart failure with normal left ventricular ejection fraction by the Heart Failure and Echocardiography Associations of the European Society of Cardiology. *Eur Heart J.* 2007; Oct; 28(20):2539.

45. Badano LP, Albanese De Biaggio P, Rozbowsky P, Miani D, Fresco C, Fioretti PM. Prevalence, clinical characteristics, quality of life, and prognosis of patients with congestive heart failure and isolated left ventricular diastolic dysfunction. *J Am Soc Echocardiogr.* 2004;17:253–61.

46. Sohn DW, Chai IH, Lee DJ, et al. Assessment of mitral annulus velocity by Doppler tissue imaging in the evaluation of left ventricular diastolic function. *J Am Coll Cardiol.* 1997;30:474–80.

47. Ommen SR, Nishimura RA, Appleton CP, et al. Clinical utility of Doppler echocardiography and tissue Doppler imaging in the estimation of left ventricular filling pressures: a comparative simultaneous Doppler catheterization study. *Circulation.* 2000;102:1788–94.

48. Nagueh SF, Mikati I, Kopelen HA, Middleton KJ, Quinones MA, Zoghbi WA. Doppler estimation of left ventricular filling pressure in sinus tachycardia. A new application of tissue Doppler imaging. *Circulation.* 1998;98:1644–50.

49. Garcia MJ, Smedira NG, Greenberg NL, et al. Color M-mode Doppler flow propagation velocity is a preload insensitive index of left ventricular relaxation: animal and human validation. *J Am Coll Cardiol.* 2000;35:201–8.

50. Garcia MJ, Ares MA, Asher C, Rodriguez L, Vandervoort P, Thomas JD. An index of early left ventricular filling that combined with pulsed Doppler peak E velocity may estimate capillary wedge pressure. *J Am Coll Cardiol.* 1997;29:448–54.

51. Brun P, Tribouilloy C, Duval AM, Iserin L, Meguira A. Left ventricular flow propagation during early filling is related to wall relaxation: a color M-mode Doppler analysis. *J Am Coll Cardiol.* 1992;20:420–32.

52. Thomas JD, Zhou J, Greenberg N, Bibawy G, McCarthy PM, Vandervoort PM. Physical and physiological determinants of pulmonary venous flow: numerical analysis. *Am J Physiol.* 1997;272:H2453–65.

53. Tabata T, Thomas JD, Klein AL. Pulmonary venous flow by Doppler echocardiography: revisited 12 years later. *J Am Coll Cardiol.* 2003;41:1243–50.

54. Rossi A, Loredana L, Cicoira M, Bonapace S, Zanolla L, Zardini P, Golia G. Additional value of pulmonary vein parameters in defining pseudonormalization of mitral inflow pattern. *Echocardiography.* 2001;18:673–9.

55. Yamamoto K, Nishimura RA, Burnett JC Jr, Redfield MM. Assessment of left ventricular end-diastolic pressure by Doppler echocardiography: contribution of duration

of pulmonary venous versus mitral flow velocity curves at atrial contraction. *J Am Soc Echocardiogr.* 1997;10:52–9.

56. Munagala VK, Jacobsen SJ, Mahoney DW, Rodeheffer RJ, Bailey KR, Redfield MM. Association of newer diastolic function parameters with age in healthy subjects: a population-based study. *J Am Soc Echocardiogr.* 2003; Oct;16(10):1049–56.

57. Douglas PS. The left atrium: a biomarker of chronic diastolic dysfunction and cardiovascular disease risk. *J Am Coll Cardiol.* 2003;42:1206–7.

58. Pritchett AM, Mahoney DW, Jacobsen SJ, Rodeheffer RJ, Karon BL, Redfield MM. Diastolic dysfunction and left atrial volume: a population-based study. *J Am Coll Cardiol.* 2005; Jan 4;45(1):87–92.

59. Tanabe K, Yamaguchi K, Tani T, Yagi T, Katayama M, Tamita K, Kinoshita M, Kaji S, Yamamuro A, Morioka S, Okada Y, Kihara Y. Left atrial volume: predictor of atrial fibrillation in patients with degenerative mitral regurgitation. *J Heart Valve Dis.* 2007; Jan;16(1):8–12.

60. Moller JE, Hillis GS, Oh JK, Seward JB, Reeder GS, Wright RS, Park SW, Bailey KR, Pellikka PA. Left atrial volume: a powerful predictor of survival after acute myocardial infarction. *Circulation.* 2003; May 6;107(17):2207–12.

61. Benjamin EJ, D'Agostino RB, Belanger AJ, Wolf PA, Levy D. Left atrial size and the risk of stroke and death. The Framingham Heart Study. *Circulation.* 1995;92:835.

62. Moller JE, Hillis GS, Oh JK, Seward JB, Reeder GS, Wright RS, Park SW, Bailey KR, Pellikka PA. Left atrial volume: a powerful predictor of survival after acute myocardial infarction. *Circulation.* 2003;107:2207–12.

63. Nishimura RA, Tajik AJ: Evaluation of diastolic filling of left ventricle in health and disease: Doppler echocardiography is the clinician's Rosetta Stone. *J Am Coll Cardiol.* 1997;30:8–18.

64. Hishida H, Sotobata I, Koike Y, Okumura M, Mizuno Y. Echocardiographic patterns of ventricular contraction in the Wolff-Parkinson-White Syndrome. *Circulation.* 1976; Oct;54(4):567–70.

65. Nelson GS, Berger RD, Fetics BJ, Talbot M, Spinelli JC, Hare JM, Kass DA. Left ventricular or biventricular pacing improves cardiac function at diminished energy cost in patients with dilated cardiomyopathy and left bundle-branch block. *Circulation.* 2000;102;3053–9.

66. Grines CL, Bashore TM, Boudoulas H, Olson S, Shafer P, Wooley CF. Functional abnormalities in isolated left bundle branch block. The effect of interventricular asynchrony. *Circulation.* 1989; Apr;79(4):845–53.

67. Xiao HB, Lee CH, Gibson DG. Effect of left bundle branch block on diastolic function in dilated cardiomyopathy. *Br Heart J.* 1991; Dec;66(6):443–7.

68. Soyama A, Kono T, Mishima T, Morita H, Ito T, Suwa M, Kitaura Y. Intraventricular dyssynchrony may play a role in the development of mitral regurgitation in dilated cardiomyopathy. *J Card Fail.* 2005; Oct;11(8):631–7.

69. van Oosterhout MF, Prinzen FW, Arts T. Asynchronous electrical activation induces asymmetrical hypertrophy of the left ventricular wall. *Circulation.* 1998;98:588–95.

70. van Oosterhout MF, Arts T, Muijtjens AM. Remodeling by ventricular pacing in hypertrophying dog hearts. *Cardiovasc Res.* 2001;49:771–8.

71. van Oosterhout MF, Arts T, Bassingthwaighte JB. Relation between local myocardial growth and blood flow during chronic ventricular pacing. *Cardiovasc Res.* 2002;53:831–40.

72. Spragg DD, Akar FG, Helm RH. Abnormal conduction and repolarization in late activated myocardium of dyssynchronously contracting hearts. *Cardiovasc Res.* 2005;67:77–86.

73. Spragg DD, Leclercq C, Loghmani M. Left ventricular mechanical dyssynchrony in heart failure induces transmural and trans-chamber protein expression gradients. *Circulation.* 2003;108:14–5.

74. Vernooy K, Verbeek XA, Peschar M, Crijns HJ, Arts T, Cornelussen RN. Left bundle branch block induces ventricular remodeling and functional septal hypoperfusion. *Eur Heart J.* 2005; Jan; 26(1):91–8.

75. Iuliano S, Fisher SG, Karasik PE, Fletcher RD, Singh SN. QRS duration and mortality in patients with congestive heart failure. *Am Heart J.* 2002; Jun;143(6):1085.

76. Abraham WT, Fisher WG, Smith AL, et al. Cardiac resynchronization in chronic heart failure. *N Engl J Med.* 2002; Jun 13;346(24):1845–53.

77. Young JB, Abraham WT, Smith AL, et al. Combined cardiac resynchronization and implantable cardioversion defibrillation in advanced chronic heart failure: the MIR-ACLE ICD Trial. *JAMA.* 2003; May 28;289(20):2685–94.

78. Higgins SL, Hummel JD, Niazi IK, et al. Cardiac resynchronization therapy for the treatment of heart failure in patients with intraventricular conduction delay and malignant ventricular tachyarrhythmias. *J Am Coll Cardiol.* 2003; Oct 15;42(8):1454–9.

79. Bradley DJ, Bradley EA, Baughman KL, Berger RD, Calkins H, Goodman SN, Kass DA, Powe NR. Cardiac resynchronization and death from progressive heart failure: a meta-analysis of randomized controlled trials. *JAMA.* 2003; Feb 12;289(6):730-40.

80. Søgaard P, Egeblad H, Kim WY, et al. Tissue Doppler imaging predicts improved systolic performance and reversed left ventricular remodeling during long-term cardiac resynchronization therapy. *J Am Coll Cardiol.* 2002; Aug 21;40(4):723–30.

81. Auricchio A, Stellbrink C, Sack S. Pacing Therapies in Congestive Heart Failure (PATH-CHF) Study Group. Long-term clinical effect of hemodynamically optimized cardiac resynchronization therapy in patients with heart failure and ventricular conduction delay. *J Am Coll Cardiol.* 2002;39:2026–33.

82. Cazeau S, Leclercq C, Lavergne T. Multisite Simulation in Cardiomyopathies (MUSTIC) Study Investigators. Effects of multisite biventricular pacing in patients with heart failure and intraventricular conduction delay. *N Engl J Med.* 2001;344:873–80.

83. Auricchio A, Stellbrink C, Butter C, et al. Pacing Therapies in Congestive Heart Failure II Study Group, Guidant Heart Failure Research Group. Clinical efficacy of cardiac resynchronization therapy using left ventricular pacing in heart failure patients stratified by severity of ventricular conduction delay. *J Am Coll Cardiol.* 2003;42: 2109.

84. Lozano I, Bocchiardo M, Achtelik M. VENTAK CHF/ CONTAK CD Investigators Study Group. Impact of biventricular pacing on mortality in a randomized crossover study of patients with heart failure and ventricular arrhythmias. *Pacing Clin Electrophysiol.* 2000;23:1711–2.

85. Bristow MR, Saxon LA, Boehmer J, et al., Comparison of Medical Therapy, Pacing and Defibrillation in Heart Failure (COMPANION) Investigators. Cardiac resynchronization therapy with or without an implantable defibrillator in advanced chronic heart failure. *N Engl J Med.* 2004;350:2140–50.

86. Cleland J, Daubert JC, Erdmann E, et al. The effect of cardiac resynchronization on morbidity and mortality in heart failure. *N Engl J Med.* 2005;352:1539–49.

87. Kass DA. Ventricular resynchronization: pathophysiology and identification of responders. *Rev Card Med.* 2003;4:S3–13.

88. Bleeker GB, Schalij MJ, Molhoek SG, et al. Relationship between QRS duration and left ventricular dyssynchrony in patients with end-stage heart failure. *J Cardiovasc Electrophysiol.* 2004;15:544–9.

89. Bleeker GB, Kaandorp TA, Lamb HJ, Boersma E, Steendijk P, de Roos A, van der Wall EE, Schalij MJ, Bax JJ. Effect of posterolateral scar tissue on clinical and echocardiographic improvement after cardiac resynchronization therapy. *Circulation.* 2006; Feb 21;113(7):969–76.

90. White JA, Yee R, Yuan X, Krahn A, Skanes A, Parker M, Klein G, Drangova M. Delayed enhancement magnetic resonance imaging predicts response to cardiac resynchronization therapy in patients with intraventricular dyssynchrony. *J Am Coll Cardiol.* 2006; Nov 21;48(10):1953–60.

91. Bleeker GB, Holman ER, Steendijk P, Boersma E, van der Wall EE, Schalij MJ, Bax JJ. Cardiac resynchronization therapy in patients with a narrow QRS complex. *J Am Coll Cardiol.* 2006; Dec 5;48(11):2243–50.

92. Yu CM, Chan YS, Zhang Q, Yip GW, Chan CK, Kum LC, Wu L, Lee AP, Lam YY, Fung JW. Benefits of cardiac resynchronization therapy for heart failure patients with narrow QRS complexes and coexisting systolic asynchrony by echocardiography. *J Am Coll Cardiol.* 2006; Dec 5;48(11):2251–7.

93. Wyman BT, Hunter WC, Prinzen FW, McVeigh ER. Mapping propagation of mechanical activation in the paced heart with MRI tagging. *Am J Physiol.* 1999; 276: H881–91.

94. Wyman BT, Hunter WC, Prinzen FW, Faris OP, McVeigh ER. Effects of single- and biventricular pacing on temporal and spatial dynamics of ventricular contraction. *Am J Physiol Heart Circ Physiol.* 2002; 282: H372–9.

95. Curry CW, Nelson GS, Wyman BT et al. Mechanical dyssynchrony in dilated cardiomyopathy with intraventricular conduction delay as depicted by 3D tagged magnetic resonance imaging. *Circulation.* 2000;10i:E2.

96. Bax JJ, Abraham T, Barold SS, et al. Cardiac resynchronization therapy: Part 1–issues before device implantation. *J Am Coll Cardiol.* 2005; Dec 20;46(12):2153–67.

97. Pitzalis MV, Iacoviello M, Romito R, Massari F, Rizzon B, Luzzi G, Guida P, Andriani A, Mastropasqua F, Rizzon P. Cardiac resynchronization therapy tailored by echocardiographic evaluation of ventricular asynchrony. *J Am Coll Cardiol.* 2002; Nov 6;40(9):1615–22.

98. Pitzalis MV, Iacoviello M, Romito R, et al. Ventricular asynchrony predicts a better outcome in patients with chronic heart failure receiving cardiac resynchronization therapy. *J Am Coll Cardiol.* 2005;45:65–9.

99. Marcus GM, Rose E, Viloria EM, Schafer J, De Marco T, Saxon LA, Foster E. Septal to posterior wall motion delay fails to predict reverse remodeling or clinical improvement in patients undergoing cardiac resynchronization therapy. *J Am Coll Cardiol.* 2005; Dec 20;46(12):2208–14.

100. Sassone B, Capecchi A, Boggian G, Gabrieli L, Saccà S, Vandelli R, Petracci E, Mele D. Value of baseline left lateral wall postsystolic displacement assessed by M-mode to predict reverse remodeling by cardiac resynchronization therapy. *Am J Cardiol.* 2007; Aug 1;100(3):470–5.

101. Penicka M, Bartunek J, De Bruyne B, Vanderheyden M, Goethals M, De Zutter M, Brugada P, Geelen P. Improvement of left ventricular function after cardiac

resynchronization therapy is predicted by tissue Doppler imaging echocardiography. *Circulation.* 2004; Mar 2;109(8):978–83.

102. Garrigue S, Reuter S, Labeque JN, et al. Usefulness of biventricular pacing in patients with congestive heart failure and right bundle branch block. *Am J Cardiol.* 2001;88:1436–41.

103. Bader H, Garrigue S, Lafitte S, Reuter S, Jaïs P, Haïssaguerre M, Bonnet J, Clementy J, Roudaut R: Intra-left ventricular electromechanical asynchrony: a new independent predictor of severe cardiac events in heart failure patients. *J Am Col Cardiol.* 2004, 43:248–56.

104. Bordachar P, Lafitte S, Reuter S, et al. Echocardiographic parameters of ventricular dyssynchrony validation in patients with heart failure using sequential biventricular pacing. *J Am Coll Cardiol.* 2004;44:2157–65.

105. 105. Ansalone G, Giannantoni P, Ricci R, et al. Doppler myocardial imaging in patients with heart failure receiving biventricular pacing treatment. *Am Heart J.* 2001;142:881–96.

106. Bax JJ, Marwick TH, Molhoek SG, et al. Left ventricular dyssynchrony predicts benefit of cardiac resynchronization therapy in patients with end-stage heart failure before pacemaker implantation. *Am J Cardiol.* 2003;92:1238–40.

107. Yu CM, Fung WH, Lin H, Zhang Q, Sanderson JE, Lau CP. Predictors of left ventricular reverse remodeling after cardiac resynchronization therapy for heart failure secondary to idiopathic dilated or ischemic cardiomyopathy. *Am J Cardiol.* 2003;91:684.

108. Yu CM, Fung JW, Zhang Q, Chan CK, Chan YS, Lin H, Kum LC, Kong SL, Zhang Y, Sanderson JE. Tissue Doppler imaging is superior to strain rate imaging and post-systolic shortening on the prediction of reverse remodeling in both ischemic and nonischemic heart failure after cardiac resynchronization therapy. *Circulation.* 2004; Jul 6;110(1):66–73.

109. Yu CM, Zhang Q, Fung JW, Chan HC, Chan YS, Yip GW, Kong SL, Lin H, Zhang Y, Sanderson JE. A novel tool to assess systolic asynchrony and identify responders of cardiac resynchronization therapy by tissue synchronization imaging. *J Am Coll Cardiol.* 2005; Mar 1;45(5):677–84.

110. Bleeker GB, Holman ER, Steendijk P, Boersma E, van der Wall EE, Schalij MJ, Bax JJ. Cardiac resynchronization therapy in patients with a narrow QRS complex. *J Am Coll Cardiol.* 2006; Dec 5;48(11):2243–50.

111. Helm RH, Leclercq C, Faris OP, Ozturk C, McVeigh E, Lardo AC, Kass DA. Cardiac dyssynchrony analysis using circumferential versus longitudinal strain: implications for assessing cardiac resynchronization. *Circulation.* 2005; May 31;111(21):2760–7.

112. Cleland JGF, Abdellah AT, Khaleva O, Colleta AP, Clark AL. Clinical trials update from the European Society of Cardiology Congress 2007: 3CPO, ALOFT, PROSPECT and statins for heart failure. *Eur J Heart Failure.* 2007;1070–3.

113. Beshai JF, Grimm RA, Nagueh SF, Baker JH 2nd, Beau SL, Greenberg SM, Pires LA, Tchou PJ. Cardiac-resynchronization therapy in heart failure with narrow QRS complexes. *N Engl J Med.* 2007; Dec 13;357(24):2461–71.

114. Sun JP, Popovic ZB, Greenberg NL, et al. Noninvasive quantification of regional myocardial function using Doppler-derived velocity, displacement, strain rate, and strain in healthy volunteers: effects of aging. *J Am Soc Echocardiogr.* 2004;17:132–8.

115. Popović ZB, Grimm RA, Perlic G, Chinchoy E, Geraci M, Sun JP, Donal E, Xu XF, Greenberg NL, Wilkoff BL, Thomas JD. Noninvasive assessment of cardiac

resynchronization therapy for congestive heart failure using myocardial strain and left ventricular peak power as parameters of myocardial synchrony and function. *J Cardiovasc Electrophysiol.* 2002; Dec;13(12):1203–8.

116. Sogaard P, Egeblad H, Kim WY, et al. Tissue Doppler imaging predicts improved systolic performance and reversed left ventricular remodeling during long-term cardiac resynchronization therapy. *J Am Coll Cardiol.* 2002;40:723–30.

117. Sogaard P, Egeblad H, Pedersen AK, et al. Sequential versus simultaneous biventricular resynchronization for severe heart failure: evaluation by tissue Doppler imaging. *Circulation.* 2002;106:2078–84.

118. Breithardt OA, Stellbrink C, Herbots L, et al. Cardiac resynchronization therapy can reverse abnormal myocardial strain distribution in patients with heart failure and left bundle branch block. *J Am Coll Cardiol.* 2003;42:486–94.

119. Dohi K, Suffoletto MS, Schwartzman D, Ganz L, Pinsky MR, Gorcsan J 3rd. Utility of echocardiographic radial strain imaging to quantify left ventricular dyssynchrony and predict acute response to cardiac resynchronization therapy. *Am J Cardiol.* 2005; Jul 1;96(1):112–6.

120. Notomi Y, Lysyansky P, Setser RM, Shiota T, Popović ZB, Martin-Miklovic MG, Weaver JA, Oryszak SJ, Greenberg NL, White RD, Thomas JD. Measurement of ventricular torsion by two-dimensional ultrasound speckle tracking imaging. *J Am Coll Cardiol.* 2005; Jun 21;45(12):2034–41.

121. Suffoletto MS, Dohi K, Cannesson M, Saba S, Gorcsan J 3rd. Novel speckle-tracking radial strain from routine black-and-white echocardiographic images to quantify dyssynchrony and predict response to cardiac resynchronization therapy. *Circulation.* 2006; Feb 21;113(7):960–8.

122. Gorcsan J 3rd, Tanabe M, Bleeker GB, Suffoletto MS, Thomas NC, Saba S, Tops LF, Schalij MJ, Bax JJ. Combined longitudinal and radial dyssynchrony predicts ventricular response after resynchronization therapy. *J Am Coll Cardiol.* 2007; Oct 9;50(15):1476–83.

123. Donal E, Tournoux F, Leclercq C, De Place C, Solnon A, Derumeaux G, Mabo P, Cohen-Solal A, Daubert JC. Assessment of longitudinal and radial ventricular dyssynchrony in ischemic and nonischemic chronic systolic heart failure: a two-dimensional echocardiographic speckle-tracking strain study. *J Am Soc Echocardiogr.* 2008; Jan;21(1):58–65.

124. Kapetanakis S, Kearney MT, Siva A, Gall N, Cooklin M, Monaghan MJ. Real-time three-dimensional echocardiography: a novel technique to quantify global left ventricular mechanical dyssynchrony. *Circulation.* 2005; Aug 16;112(7):992–1000.

125. Marsan NA, Bleeker GB, Ypenburg C, Ghio S, van de Veire NR, Holman ER, van der Wall EE, Tavazzi L, Schalij MJ, Bax JJ. Real-Time Three-Dimensional Echocardiography Permits Quantification of Left Ventricular Mechanical Dyssynchrony and Predicts Acute Response to Cardiac Resynchronization Therapy. *J Cardiovasc Electrophysiol.* 2007; Dec 20.

126. Van de Veire NR, Bleeker GB, Ypenburg C, De Sutter J, Ajmone Marsan N, Holman ER, van der Wall EE, Schalij MJ, Bax JJ. Usefulness of triplane tissue Doppler imaging to predict acute response to cardiac resynchronization therapy. *Am J Cardiol.* 2007; Aug 1;100(3):476–82.

127. Burgess MI, Jenkins C, Chan J, Marwick TH. Measurement of left ventricular dyssynchrony in patients with ischaemic cardiomyopathy: a comparison of real-time

three-dimensional and tissue Doppler echocardiography. *Heart.* 2007; Oct;93(10): 1191–6.

128. Grayburn PA, Appleton CP, DeMaria AN, Greenberg B, Lowes B, Oh J, Plehn JF, Rahko P, St John Sutton M, Eichhorn EJ. Echocardiographic predictors of morbidity and mortality in patients with advanced heart failure: the Beta-blocker Evaluation of Survival Trial (BEST). *J Am Coll Cardiol.* 2005; Apr 5;45(7):1064–71.

129. St John Sutton MG, Plappert T, Abraham WT, Smith AL, DeLurgio DB, Leon AR, Loh E, Kocovic DZ, Fisher WG, Ellestad M, Messenger J, Kruger K, Hilpisch KE, Hill MR Effect of cardiac resynchronization therapy on left ventricular size and function in chronic heart failure. *Circulation.* 2003; Apr 22;107(15):1985–90.

130. Yu CM, Chau E, Sanderson JE, Fan K, Tang MO, Fung WH, Lin H, Kong SL, Lam YM, Hill MR, Lau CP. Tissue Doppler echocardiographic evidence of reverse remodeling and improved synchronicity by simultaneously delaying regional contraction after biventricular pacing therapy in heart failure. *Circulation.* 2002; Jan 29;105(4):438.

131. Yu CM, Bleeker GB, Fung JW, Schalij MJ, Zhang Q, van der Wall EE, Chan YS, Kong SL, Bax JJ. Left ventricular reverse remodeling but not clinical improvement predicts long-term survival after cardiac resynchronization therapy. *Circulation.* 2005; Sep 13;112(11):1580–6.

132. St John Sutton M, Plappert T, Hilpisch KE. Sustained reverse left ventricular structural remodeling with cardiac resynchronization at one year is a function of etiology. *Circulation.* 2006;113:266–72.

133. Bleeker GB, Kaandorp TA, Lamb HJ, Boersma E, Steendijk P, de Roos A, van der Wall EE, Schalij MJ, Bax JJ. Effect of posterolateral scar tissue on clinical and echocardiographic improvement after cardiac resynchronization therapy. *Circulation.* 2006; Feb 21;113(7):969–76.

134. Pascal Lim, Adisai Buakhamsri, Zoran B. Popovic, Neil L. Greenberg, Dimpi Patel, James D. Thomas, Richard A. Grimm. Longitudinal Strain Delay Index by Speckle Tracking Imaging. A New Marker of Response to Cardiac Resynchronization Therapy. *Circulation.* 2008;118.

Chapter 5

Clinical trials and response to CRT

Kenneth M. Stein

Key Points

1. Based on clinical trial data, "conventional" criteria for implantation of a cardiac resynchronization therapy system include: (1) moderate to severely symptomatic congestive heart failure despite optimal medical therapy (NYHA functional Class III or Class IV); (2) severe left ventricular systolic dysfunction ejection fraction(LVEF ≤35%); (3) a wide QRS complex (QRS duration ≥120–130 ms); and (4) sinus rhythm.
2. For conventionally indicated patients, resynchronization therapy improves exercise capacity, reduces symptoms, leads to beneficial left ventricular (LV) remodeling, and improves the neurohumoral milieu.
3. For conventionally indicated patients, resynchronization therapy significantly improves survival compared to "optimal" medical therapy.
4. For conventionally indicated patients, resynchronization therapy reduces heart failure hospitalizations and is highly cost effective.
5. In contrast to patients meeting conventional indications for cardiac resynchronization therapy (CRT), patients in other groups have not been proven to derive symptomatic benefit from resynchronization.
6. Resynchronization therapy results in significant left ventricular remodeling in minimally symptomatic patients with significant left ventricular dysfunction and wide QRS complexes. Ongoing clinical trials are studying whether this will translate into improved long-term outcomes in this population.

Pacing to Support the Failing Heart, 1st edition. Edited by K. Ellenbogen and A. Auricchio.
© 2008 American Heart Association, ISBN: 978-1-4051-7534-0

7. Although atrial fibrillation is common in advanced heart failure, there is a paucity of data regarding the benefit of resynchronization therapy in this setting. If CRT is used in a patient with AF, it is critical to achieve adequate rate control to permit a high percentage of biventricular pacing.

8. Right ventricular apical pacing leads to intraventricular dyssynchrony and diminished left ventricular function. Limited observational data suggests that upgrading existing right ventricular pacing systems to biventricular systems can be performed safely with similar implantation success and similar clinical response rates as *de novo* implantation.

9. A substantial minority (generally one-quarter to one-third) of patients in clinical trials are "no-responders," whether defined in terms of symptomatic improvement or echocardiographic response.

10. Among the possible causes of "non-responsive" are selection of patients without sufficient intraventricular dyssynchrony, suboptimal device programming, and failure to place the left ventricular lead in an optimal position.

Introduction

Cardiac resynchronization therapy (CRT) for congestive heart failure represents a new paradigm in cardiology: the use of an electrical therapy (cardiac pacing) to treat a mechanical problem. Multiple randomized clinical trials have proven that resynchronization therapy improves symptoms, increases quality of life, reduces hospitalizations, and prolongs survival in appropriately selected patients. As a result, in a relatively brief time, this therapy has become a standard treatment for patients with severe left ventricular dysfunction, moderate-to-severely symptomatic congestive heart failure despite optimal medical therapy, and left bundle branch block (LBBB) [1, 2].

It is fitting to reevaluate this wealth of clinical trial data (Table 5.1). This chapter reviews the results of these trials with respect to the clinical response to resynchronization therapy (both functional and structural) and the improvement in survival associated with resynchronization therapy in appropriate patients. In addition, we will review the critical unanswered questions that these trials raise, particularly with respect to the role of resynchronization therapy in minimally symptomatic patients, the role of resynchronization therapy in patients with persistent atrial fibrillation, and the vexing issue of nonresponders to resynchronization therapy.

Clinical response to cardiac resynchronization

For appropriately selected patients, resynchronization therapy improves exercise capacity and reduces symptoms. The most commonly reported measures of functional capacity include 6-minute hall walk distance (a measure of the

Table 5.1 Randomized multicenter clinical trials of CRT.

Trial	Publication date	N	Entry criteria	Design	Primary endpoint(s)/ outcome
MUSTIC [7]	2001	48	LVEF ≤35% LVEDD >60 NYHA Class III QRS >150 NSR	Single-blind, crossover	23% increase in 6 MHWD after 3 months ($p<0.001$)
PATH-CHF [8]	2002	41	"Dilated Cardiomyopathy" NYHA Class III or Class IV QRS ≥120 PR ≥150 NSR	Single-blind, crossover comparison of optimized univentricular (LV only) vs biventricular pacing	No difference between LV only and biventricular pacing in VO$_2$max, O$_2$ uptake at anaerobic threshold or 6 MHWD. All parameters improved significantly vs. baseline after 12 months.
MIRACLE [9]	2002	453	NYHA Class III or Class IV LVEF ≤35% LVEDD ≥55 QRS ≥130 NSR 6MHWD ≤450	Double-blind, parallel	Significant improvement in 6MHWD, NYHA class and QoL after 6 months

Trial	Year	N	Inclusion criteria	Design	Results
MUSTIC AF [18]	2002	43	NYHA Class III LVEF <35% LVEDD >60 Persistent AF with bradycardia requiring permanent ventricular pacing and an RV paced QRS >200 6MHWD<450	Single-blind, crossover	No significant difference in 6 MHWD
CONTAK-CD [10]	2003	490	NYHA Class II–IV LVEF ≤35% QRS ≥120 NSR ICD indication	Single-blind, originated as a crossover trial but changed midway to a parallel design	No significant change in a composite of mortality, CHF hospitalization, and ventricular tachyarrhythmias requiring device therapy at 3–6 months
MIRACLE ICD [11]	2003	369	NYHA Class III or Class IV LVEF ≤35% LVEDD ≥55 QRS ≥130 NSR ICD indication	Double-blind, parallel	Significant improvements in quality of life and NYHA class but not 6 MHWD after 6 months

(continued)

Table 5.1 (continued)

Trial	Publication date	N	Entry criteria	Design	Primary endpoint(s)/outcome
PATH-CHF II [12]	2003	69	LVEF ≤30% NYHA Class II–IV VO_2max ≤18 QRS ≥120 NSR	Single-blind, crossover, stratified by baseline QRS	Significant improvements in VO_2max, VO_2 at anaerobic threshold, and 6 MHWD after 3 months
COMPANION [29]	2004	1,520	NYHA Class III or Class IV LVEF ≤35% QRS ≥120 PR ≥150 NSR CHF hospitalization in the preceding year	Unblinded, parallel comparison of medical therapy, CRT-pacemaker and CRT-Defibrillator (1:2:2)	Significant reduction in the composite of death or hospitalization for any cause
MIRACLE ICD II [19]	2004	186	LVEF ≤35% LVEDD ≥55 NYHA Class II QRS ≥130 NSR ICD indication	Double-blind, parallel	No significant change in VO_2max after 6 months

Trial	Year	N	Inclusion criteria	Design	Results
CARE-HF [21]	2005	813	NYHA ClassIII or Class IV LVEF ≤35% LVEDD ≥30 (indexed to height) QRS ≥120 (pts with a QRS interval of 120–149 were required to meet two of three echo criteria for dyssynchrony)	Unblinded parallel	Significant reduction in the composite of death or hospitalization for a major cardiovascular event
PAVE [39]	2005	184	Chronic AF requiring AV node ablation and pacing therapy 6MHWD <450	Single-blind, parallel comparison of CRT vs. RV-only pacing	Significantly greater increase in 6MHWD with CRT vs. RV-only pacing after 6 months
OPSITE [40]	2005	56	Chronic AF and: (1) requiring AV node ablation and pacing therapy or (2) drug-refractory CHF, depressed LV function, and/or LBBB	Single-blind, crossover comparison of biventricular, LV-only and RV-only pacing	Compared with RV pacing, BiV pacing showed a significant improvement in some measures of QoL. BiV pacing and RV-only pacing yielded similar improvements in 6MHWD
RETHINQ [20]	2007	172	NYHA Class III, LVEF ≤35% QRS duration <130 but with echo evidence of mechanical dyssynchrony (TDI or M-mode) NSR	Double-blind, parallel	No significant change in proportion of patients with an increase in VO_2max ≥1.0 ml/kg/min after 6 months

LVEF: left ventricular ejection fraction, LVEDD: left ventricular end diastolic dimension, NSR: normal sinus rhythm, 6 MHWD: 6-minute hall walk distance, QoL: quality of life, ICD: implantable cardioverter defibrillator, CHF: congestive heart failure, AF: atrial fibrillation, LBBB: left bundle branch block, TDI: tissue Doppler imaging ability to perform activities of daily living [3]), peak oxygen consumption during a cardiopulmonary stress test (VO_2max), and quality of life (usually assessed using the Minnesota Living with Heart Failure Questionnaire [4]). Diminished 6-minute hall walk distance [5] and diminished VO_2max [6] are both strong indicators of poor prognosis in advanced heart failure. The results of the major randomized clinical trials reporting outcomes for these variables are summarized in Figure 5.1.

In such trials as MUSTIC [7], PATH-CHF [8], MIRACLE [9], CONTAK CD [10], MIRACLE ICD [11], and PATH-CHF II [12], resynchronization therapy consistently improved functional capacity and reduced heart failure symptoms. Specifically, resynchronization was associated with a 1–23% improvement in 6-minute hall walk distance, a 7–10% increase in VO_2max, and an 11–31% improvement in quality of life scores. The MUSTIC trial was designed as a blinded crossover trial comparing active and inactive pacing. After the end of the crossover period, when patients were asked which phase they preferred, an overwhelming majority (85%) chose the period of active pacing [7]. In the MIRACLE trial, total exercise time during treadmill testing improved by more than 1 minute in patients receiving resynchronization therapy compared with those getting inactive pacing; this represents a 13% improvement over baseline [9].

Reflecting the overall impact of these changes, the data consistently show that resynchronization therapy results in a one NYHA functional class improvement in symptoms, corresponding (on average) to a change from moderate heart failure symptoms to mild heart failure symptoms. Thus, in the MIRACLE trial 52% of patients improved by one functional class whereas a much smaller number improved by two functional classes (16%) and the remainder failed to respond to therapy [9]. It is, however, extremely important to interpret these results in the context of the 38% response rate in the placebo arm of the trial.

The MUSTIC, PATH-CHF, MIRACLE, CONTAK CD, MIRACLE ICD, and PATH-CHF II trials enrolled patients with: (1) moderate to severely symptomatic congestive heart failure despite optimal medical therapy, (2) severe left ventricular systolic dysfunction (LVEF ≤35%), (3) a wide QRS complex (generally defined as a QRS ≥120–130 ms), and (4) sinus rhythm. As a result, these inclusion criteria have become the conventional indications for resynchronization. As seen in Figure 5.1, the effects in these "conventional indication" trials are robust—indeed, far more robust then the effects observed with conventional pharmacologic therapy of heart failure. For instance, improvement in 6-minute hall walk distance was observed in only 2 of 6 trials of ACE-inhibitors, 3 of 17 trials of beta-blockers, and 1 of 4 trials of digoxin [13]. Trials of both beta-blockers and ACE inhibitors have likewise shown inconsistent results with respect to VO_2max [14, 15] and quality of life [16, 17].

In contrast to patients meeting conventional indications for CRT, patients in other groups have not been shown to benefit from resynchronization. In the

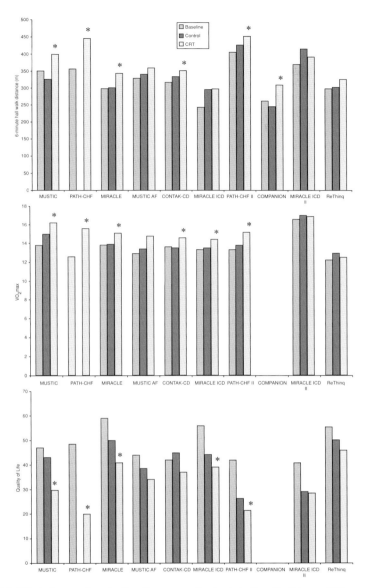

Fig. 5.1 Effect of resynchronization therapy on 6-minute hall walk distance, VO$_2$max, and Quality of Life (using the Minnesota Living with Heart Failure Questionnaire) in randomized multicenter trials. (Data were adapted from: MUSTIC [7], PATH-CHF [8], MIRACLE [9], MUSTIC AF [18], CONTAK CD [10], MIRACLE ICD [11], PATH-CHF II [12], COMPANION [29], MIRACLE ICD II [19], and RETHINQ [20]. CRT: cardiac resynchronization therapy.) (*denotes a significant improvement compared to control or baseline. Note that a decrease in quality of life score reflects an improvement in symptoms.)

MUSTIC AF trial [18], resynchronization failed to improve outcomes when used in patients with persistent atrial fibrillation and bradycardia requiring permanent pacing. In the MIRACLE ICD II trial, resynchronization did not improve 6-minute hall walk distance, VO₂max, or quality of life among patients with mildly symptomatic heart failure at the baseline [19]. The same observations were made for the subgroup of NYHA Class II patients enrolled in CONTAK CD [10]. Finally, the RETHINQ trial demonstrated that CRT did not improve exercise capacity for patients with echocardiographic evidence of intraventricular dyssynchrony but with a narrow QRS [20].

In addition to improving symptoms, randomized clinical trials have also shown that conventionally indicated patients derive objective evidence of beneficial structural changes (often referred to as "reverse remodeling") in response to CRT. Resynchronization reduces left ventricular end-systolic [10, 21–23] and end-diastolic volumes [10, 22, 23] and increases left ventricular ejection fraction [10, 21, 23]. The improvements in ejection fraction ranged from 2–7 absolute percentage points and are noteworthy given that the baseline ejection fractions in these trials were in the range of 21–25%. The data from trials reporting sufficient information to determine baseline, and treatment versus control ejection fractions are shown in Figure 5.2. A meta-analysis of randomized clinical trials of cardiac resynchronization therapy found the average absolute improvement in

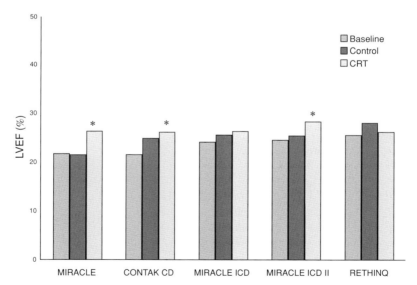

Fig. 5.2 Effect of resynchronization therapy on left ventricular ejection fraction. (Data were adapted from: MIRACLE [9], CONTAK CD [10], MIRACLE ICD [11], MIRACLE ICD II [19], and RETHINQ [20].) (*denotes a significant improvement compared to the control.)

ejection fraction to be 3 percentage points [24]. The remodeling effects of resyn-chronization therapy are progressive [22, 23] and persist for at least 18 months after the initiation of therapy [21]. Resynchronization is also associated with reduced mitral regurgitation [21–23] and with improvements in the neurohu-moral milieu as evidenced by lower plasma catecholamine levels [25], increased heart rate variability [26], and striking reductions in N-terminal pro-BNP levels (reductions of 454–567 pg/ml at 12–18 months) [25, 27].

Resynchronization and survival

In addition to improving symptoms, cardiac resynchronization therapy is also proven to improve survival in conventionally indicated populations. Although the early randomized clinical trials of CRT were not large enough to include mortality as a primary endpoint, a meta-analysis of the MUSTIC, MIRACLE, MIRACLE ICD, and CONTAK CD trials concluded that resynchronization ther-apy, with or without concomitant use of a defibrillator, reduced mortality due to progressive heart failure by 51% [28]. COMPANION was the first trial ade-quately powered to analyze total mortality as an independent endpoint [29]. In addition to significantly reducing the combined endpoint of hospitalizations and mortality, all-cause mortality was reduced by 24% ($p = 0.06$) in the group receiving CRT-pacemakers and reduced by 36% ($p = 0.003$) in the group receiv-ing CRT-defibrillators. The absolute mortality rate at 1 year was 19% in the medically treated group (a result that serves to highlight the remarkably poor prognosis for patients with advanced heart failure and left bundle branch block), 15% in the pacemaker group, and 12% in the pacemaker–defibrillator group.

The survival benefit from resynchronization therapy was confirmed in the CARE-HF trial. In this study, which almost exclusively employed CRT-pacemakers (rather than CRT-defibrillators), all-cause mortality was reduced by 36% with resynchronization therapy ($p<0.002$) [21]. The absolute mortality rate in the medical-therapy group was 13% at one year as opposed to 10% in the cardiac resynchronization group. Longer-term evaluation of the CARE-HF cohort shows that the mortality benefit increased in magnitude with longer duration follow-up: mortality at 3 years was 35% in the medical group and 24% in the CRT group [30]. Extensive subgroup analysis was performed in both the COMPANION and CARE-HF trials to attempt to identify which patient groups derive the greatest benefit from the therapy, but neither trial identified any significant heterogeneities, according to pre-implant patient characteristics [21, 29].

Although resynchronization has been proven to improve survival compared with standard medical therapy of heart failure, it should be emphasized that there is no evidence that resynchronization therapy improves survival when compared with ICD therapy alone [24]. It is also curious to note that the addition of resynchronization did not reduce ICD therapies for ventricular tachycardia/ventricular fibrillation in either the CONTAK CD or the MIRA-CLE ICD trials [10, 11]. It is possible that these observations may reflect the relatively large proportion of secondary prevention patients enrolled in these trials [31] as well as the relatively short duration of follow-up.

The improvements in functional outcome and survival associated with resynchronization therapy have translated into reduced hospitalizations for heart failure patients [7, 9, 18, 21, 29]. A meta-analysis of the trial data concluded that resynchronization reduced the risk of hospitalization for heart failure exacerbation by approximately one-third [24]. As a result, the therapy is highly cost effective. An analysis using data from COMPANION and CARE-HF calculated that an incremental cost of approximately $10,000 per quality-adjusted year of life is associated with the use of cardiac resynchronization therapy in a conventionally indicated population [32].

Unresolved questions and ongoing trials

The available clinical trials regarding cardiac resynchronization therapy provide a wealth of evidence on which to base practice. Nevertheless, numerous fundamental questions remain unanswered. Table 5.2 summarizes some of the major ongoing clinical trials of cardiac resynchronization therapy.

Minimally symptomatic patients

Perhaps foremost among the unresolved questions concerning resynchronization therapy is whether the therapy has any role for patients with severe left ventricular dysfunction but minimally symptomatic or asymptomatic heart failure. Many of these patients are candidates for prophylactic ICD implantation [33, 34]. As noted above, resynchronization therapy results in limited functional improvement for patients who are minimally symptomatic at baseline. In CONTAK CD there was no improvement in 6-minute hall walk distance, VO$_2$max, quality of life, or NYHA functional status among the NYHA Class I and Class II patients enrolled in the trial [10]. In MIRACLE ICD II trial, which only enrolled patients in NYHA Class II, there was no improvement in the primary outcome (change in VO$_2$max), and there was inconsistent improvement in secondary functional endpoints: a marginally significant improvement in NYHA functional class was observed but there was no change in quality of life score or 6-minute hall walk distance [19].

On the other hand, both the CONTAK CD and MIRACLE ICD II trials showed that resynchronization results in convincing echocardiographic evidence of reverse remodeling in minimally symptomatic patients—less than was observed in more highly symptomatic populations, but nevertheless substantial. In both trials, resynchronization led to statistically significant reductions in LV end-systolic and end-diastolic dimensions. The MIRACLE ICD II trial

Table 5.2 Selected ongoing trials.

Trial	Status	Anticipated enrollment	Entry criteria	Design	Primary endpoint
REVERSE	1-year results reported, 2-year follow-up ongoing	610	NYHA Class I–II QRS ≥120 LVEF ≤40% LVEDD ≥55 NSR	Double-blind, parallel comparison of CRT on vs. off	HF clinical composite response at 12 months
MADIT-CRT	Currently recruiting, estimated completion March 2009	1,820	NYHA Class I–II (ischemic) or OR NYHA Class II (nonischemic) LVEF ≤30% QRS ≥130 NSR	Open-label parallel comparison of CRT-D vs. ICD only	Combined endpoint of all-cause mortality and HF events
Resynchronization/ Defibrillation for Ambulatory Heart Failure	Currently recruiting, estimated completion January 2010	1,800	NYHA Class II LVEF ≤30% QRS ≥120 OR paced QRS ≥200 Conventional ICD indication NSR or chronic AT/AF with a pacing indication	Double-blind parallel comparison of CRT-D vs. ICD only	Combined endpoint of all-cause mortality and HF hospitalization

(*continued*)

Table 5.2 (continued)

Trial	Status	Anticipated enrollment	Entry criteria	Design	Primary endpoint
APAF	Currently recruiting, estimated completion May 2008	458	Permanent AF undergoing AV junction ablation and ventricular pacing for drug-refractory, severely symptomatic, uncontrolled high ventricular rate OR Permanent AF, drug-refractory heart failure, and depressed LV function	Double-blind parallel	6 months: Quality of life, New York Heart Association classification, and exercise capacity 24 months: Composite end-point of: death due to cardiovascular cause, hospitalization for worsening heart failure, worsening heart failure or failure to achieve a persistent subjective symptom improvement
AVERT-AF	Currently recruiting	180	Symptomatic permanent AF ICD indication LVEF ≤35% NYHA Class II–III	Double-blind parallel comparison of Pharmacological therapy + Single Chamber ICD vs. AVJ Ablation + CRT-D	Exercise duration at 12 months

BLOCK-HF	Currently enrolling, estimated completion December 2010	1,636	PPM indicated due to AV block NYHA Class I-III LVEF ≤50%	Double-blind parallel comparison of BiV vs. RV only pacing	Time to first event: mortality, heart failure-related urgent care, or ≥15% increase in LVESVI
PREVENT-HF	Currently enrolling	100	Class I or Class IIa indication for PPM Require ≥80% ventricular pacing NYHA Class I-II	Open label parallel comparison of RV vs. BiV pacing	LVEDV at 12 months
FREEDOM	Currently enrolling	1,500	Conventional indication for CRT	Double-blind parallel comparison of frequent electrogram-guided optimization of AV/VV delays vs. empiric or single nonelectrogram guided optimization	Clinical composite heart failure score at 12 months

(continued)

Table 5.2 (continued)

Trial	Status	Anticipated enrollment	Entry criteria	Design	Primary endpoint
SMART-AV	Currently enrolling, estimated completion Winter 2009	950	Conventional indication for CRT	Double-blind parallel comparison of fixed AV delay (120 ms) vs. echo-optimized AV delay vs. electrogram-optimized AV delay	LVESV at 6 months
PEGASUS-CRT	Currently enrolling, estimated completion February 2009	1,600	Conventional indication for CRT	Single-blind parallel comparison of DDD-70, DDDR-40 and DDD-40 modes	Clinical composite heart failure score at 12 months

Data adapted from http://www.clinicaltrials.org.

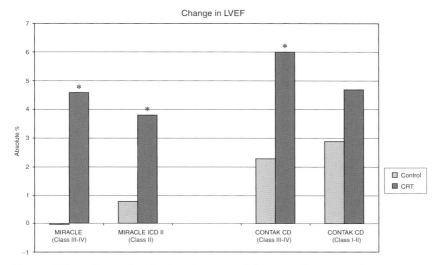

Fig. 5.3 Effect of resynchronization therapy on left ventricular ejection fraction stratified according to baseline NYHA functional status. (Data were adapted from MIRACLE [9], MIRACLE ICD II [19], and CONTAK CD [10].) (*denotes a significant improvement compared to the control.)

data showed a significant increase in ejection fraction; there was also a corresponding trend toward an increase in LVEF in the minimally symptomatic patients in CONTAK CD (Figure 5.3). The 1-year results of the REVERSE trial were recently reported (as of the time of writing, these results have been presented but not yet published, and should therefore be considered to be preliminary) [35]. The REVERSE trial evaluated 610 patients with a wide QRS and LVEF below 40% who were in NYHA functional Class I (with a prior history of symptoms) or Class II, who were randomly assigned to "CRT on" versus "CRT off" [36]. The investigators found evidence of significant reverse remodeling with CRT as well as a 53% reduction in the incidence of first hospitalization for heart failure. In addition, there was a nonsignificant trend toward a reduction in the rate of worsening CHF as assessed by a clinical composite endpoint (21% vs. 16%, $p = 0.10$). A subset of the REVERSE trial patients will continue their randomized assignments for a full 2-year follow-up.

Therefore, it is conceivable that there may be long-term hemodynamic or survival benefits to resynchronization therapy in minimally symptomatic patients. It may be that these effects were not apparent in earlier trials due to the relatively short duration of follow-up or inadequate sample size. The long-term effects of resynchronization therapy in this population are being further evaluated in the, MADIT-CRT [37], and Resynchronization/Defibrillation for Ambulatory Heart Failure [38] trials.

Atrial fibrillation

A second fundamental question concerns the role of resynchronization therapy in patients with persistent atrial fibrillation. Atrial fibrillation (AF) is common in advanced heart failure [39], but patients with persistent atrial fibrillation were excluded from the majority of randomized clinical trials of resynchronization. Three multicenter randomized trials of resynchronization therapy have enrolled patients with persistent atrial fibrillation who required permanent pacing. In the MUSTIC trial, resynchronization therapy did not result in an improvement in the primary endpoint (improvement in 6-minute hall walk distance) [18]. However, when analyzed on an efficacy basis (rather than according to the intention-to-treat principle), the resynchronization therapy group achieved borderline increases in both 6-minute hall walk distance and VO_2max. In the PAVE trial, patients receiving cardiac resynchronization therapy following atrio-ventricular (AV) node ablation experienced a greater improvement in 6-minute hall walk distance than did patients treated with RV-only pacing [40]. Furthermore, the resynchronized patients avoided the deterioration in left ventricular ejection fraction that was observed in the right ventricular (RV)-paced group. In the OPSITE trial, biventricular pacing was also associated with a modest improvement in symptoms and a greater improvement in LVEF when compared with RV-only pacing following AV node ablation for atrial fibrillation [41]. Thus, these data suggest that resynchronization therapy is a better alternative than conventional RV-only pacing for patients with moderate-to-severely symptomatic heart failure and persistent atrial fibrillation who independently require permanent pacing. This issue is being evaluated further in the ongoing APAF and AVERT-AF trials [42, 43]. The role of resynchronization in the therapy of patients with sinus rhythm who require ventricular pacing is being evaluated in the BLOCK-HF [44] and PREVENT-HF [45] studies.

The PAVE and OPSITE trials stand out among the published randomized trials of cardiac resynchronization therapy in enrolling patients irrespective of pre-implant ejection fraction. In fact, nearly half of the patients in PAVE had a left ventricular ejection fraction above 45%. Post hoc analysis of PAVE suggests that the majority of the benefit in the trial was confined to the subgroup with a pre-implant ejection fraction of less than 45% [39]. However, the opposite pattern was observed in the OPSITE trial. In that trial, the comparative benefit to biventricular pacing was greatest in those patients with normal baseline left ventricular function [40]. It is possible that these discordant results reflect the play of chance—a larger trial is necessary to resolve the issue.

Limited nonrandomized data suggest that even without undergoing AV node ablation, patients with atrial fibrillation may derive a benefit from resynchronization that can be comparable to that experienced by patients with sinus rhythm. However, there is a higher incidence of nonresponders among patients who do not undergo AV node ablation (46%) compared to those who do undergo the procedure (29%) [46]. This observation highlights the importance of achieving adequate rate control (sufficient to permit a high percentage of biventricular pacing) in these patients. Such rate control may be difficult to achieve solely with pharmacologic therapy: in one study, fully 70% of atrial fibrillation patients required AV node ablation in order to achieve adequate (>85%) biventricular pacing [47]. It should be noted that although there are numerous anecdotes of patients with persistent AF converting to sinus rhythm following the institution of CRT, this is a rare event, and there is no reduction in the incidence of new atrial fibrillation in patients receiving resynchronization for conventional indications [48].

Paced versus native left bundle branch block

Most major randomized clinical trials required that a patient's native QRS complex be wide in order to be eligible for resynchronization therapy. However, it has long been recognized that pacing from the right ventricular apex results in a wide QRS complex with a LBBB morphology. Substantial data exists showing that chronic RV apical pacing results in intraventricular dyssynchrony [49], a reduction in left ventricular function [50], and worsened outcome in patients with congestive heart failure [51, 52]. Limited observational data suggests that upgrading existing right ventricular pacing systems to biventricular systems can be performed safely with similar implantation success and similar clinical response rates as *de novo* CRT implantation [53].

"Nonresponders"

One of the most critical issues in the field of CRT concerns "nonresponders." A substantial minority of patients receiving resynchronization therapy for conventional indications derive little or no benefit, whether defined on the basis of echocardiographic response (typically a reduction in left ventricular end-systolic volume of at least 15%) or symptomatic improvement (typically improvement by at least one NYHA functional class). A closer look at the MIRACLE data is instructive: 52% of patients improved by one functional class and another 16% of patients improved by two or more functional classes. Very few patients experienced a worsening of symptoms with the therapy (2%), but fully 30% of patients were "nonresponders" [9].

Three potential explanations might explain "nonresponse" (Table 5.3). First is patient selection: Was the device implanted in a patient who never possibly could have responded? Substantial controversy exists regarding the appropriate QRS width cut-off to determine eligibility for resynchronization. Indeed, controversy exists regarding whether QRS duration should be used at all! As noted above, most resynchronization trials used a QRS duration of greater than 120–130 ms as an enrollment criterion, but this has not been uniform. In the MUSTIC trial, for example, the QRS duration cut-off was 150 ms [7]. Even in the trials with more liberal enrollment criteria, the mean QRS width for patients actually enrolled in the trial tended to be quite long: in the MIRACLE trial the mean QRS width

Table 5.3 Nonresponders to resynchronization therapy:
Potential etiologies.

Patient Selection	Patients without dyssynchrony [54, 55], including those with RBBB [53] Patients with transmural lateral myocardial infarction [58]
Device Programming	Failure to achieve adequate biventricular capture Suboptimal AV interval [63, 64] Suboptimal LV-RV timing [61]
Lead Placement	Failure to place the LV lead in an area leading to adequate resynchronization [74, 75]

in the group eventually randomized to resynchronization was 167 ms, and it is estimated that only about one-sixth of patients had a baseline QRS duration less than 145 ms [9]. Extrapolation of these results to populations with QRS durations in the 120-130 ms range is thus difficult.

The PATH-CHF II investigators prospectively stratified patients according to baseline QRS duration (QRS 120–150 vs. QRS >150 ms) and found that the benefit of resynchronization was confined to the group with a QRS duration >150 ms [12]. There was a nonsignificant tendency toward a similar result in the subgroup analysis of COMPANION [29]. The cohort of patients eligible for CRT in trials based on QRS width alone includes the group of patients with right bundle branch block (RBBB). In these patients, late activation occurs in the right ventricular free wall and there is no a priori reason to expect them to benefit from left ventricular pacing. Indeed, an analysis of pooled data from the MIRACLE and CONTAK CD trials shows that patients with right bundle branch block derive limited benefit from CRT [54].

Growing data show that patients without intraventricular dyssynchrony are unlikely to respond to resynchronization therapy, no matter how wide their QRS [55, 56]. Two randomized clinical trials have used echocardiographic measurement of dyssynchrony to aid in patient selection for resynchronization therapy. In CARE-HF patients could be enrolled on the basis of QRS duration alone, if the QRS was 150 ms or greater. Patients with a QRS of 120–149 ms were required, in addition, to demonstrate two of three echocardiographic criteria for dyssynchrony: (1) an aortic pre-ejection delay >140 ms, (2) an interventricular mechanical delay of >40 ms, and/or (3) delayed activation of the posterolateral LV wall by M-mode or tissue Doppler imaging [57]. Perhaps as a result, subgroup analysis of the CARE-HF data did not show any heterogeneity of response according to pre-implant QRS duration [21]. In the RETHINQ trial, patients with a QRS <130 ms were selected for resynchronization if they had echocardiographic evidence of intraventricular dyssynchrony, predominantly on the basis of tissue Doppler imaging. In this trial, patients with a QRS interval of less than 120 ms experienced no improvement in the primary endpoint (VO_2max), but in the prespecified subgroup of patients with a QRS interval of 120–129 ms VO_2max increased significantly with resynchronization [20]. It should be acknowledged, however, that the results of the PROSPECT trial raise concern regarding the ability of current echocardiographic techniques to reproducibly measure dyssynchrony and to distinguish clinical responders from nonresponders [58].

Data also exist to suggest that patients with transmural myocardial infarctions of the lateral wall are unlikely to improve with lateral left ventricular pacing [59]. Echocardiographic substudies of the MIRACLE [23] and MUSTIC [22] trials have shown greater reverse remodeling in patients with nonischemic as opposed to ischemic cardiomyopathies. It is, however, important to recognize that substudy analysis shows no difference in clinical outcomes between patients with ischemic versus nonischemic heart disease [10, 21, 29].

A second potential cause of "nonresponse" is suboptimal programming, particularly with respect to programming an appropriate AV delay [60, 61] but also potentially with respect to programming LV–RV timing [62]. In fact, failure to program an optimal AV delay may result in as much as a 10–15% decline in cardiac output [63]. Although many trials have shown acute hemodynamic benefits to AV optimization, limited data exist to show that systematic optimization results in a long-term improvement in clinical outcome [64, 65]. The major randomized clinical trials have used wildly different approaches to programming the AV delay: (1) in the CONTAK CD trial, a fixed, short AV delay was empirically programmed [10], (2) in the COMPANION trial, the AV delay was programmed according to a formula taking into account the baseline PR interval and baseline QRS duration [29], and (3) in the MIRACLE [9] and CARE-HF [21] trials, echocardiographic imaging of mitral valve inflow was used to determine an "optimum" AV delay. Thus far no large randomized clinical trial has been completed comparing long-term outcomes with various methods of optimizing the programmed AV delay. This issue will be addressed by the FREEDOM [66] and SMART-AV trials [67].

In addition to AV optimization, it has been proposed that programming sequential rather than simultaneous LV and RV pacing (often referred to as "VV timing") may further improve ventricular performance [68]. However, in neither of two randomized clinical trials did VV optimization following AV optimization affect the long-term clinical response to resynchronization therapy [69, 70]. The effect of other programming choices is unclear. The potential for an improvement in outcome with rate adaptive pacing is particularly interesting. Chronotropic incompetence is common in patients with advanced heart failure, [71] and may itself reduce functional capacity as well as limit the use of betablockers. Nevertheless, all of the major randomized clinical trials completed to date used (VDD) pacing or fixed-rate atrial pacing, usually with a rate deliberately programmed low to avoid atrial pacing. The potential effect of rate adaptive pacing in CRT is currently being evaluated in the PEGASUS-CRT trial [72].

A third possible cause of "nonresponse" is failure to place the left ventricular lead in an adequate position. Early data showed that the hemodynamic response to resynchronization was greatest for left ventricular leads placed on the mid-lateral wall of the left ventricle [73]. Bearing this in mind, the actual lead positions achieved in clinical trials are striking. For example, in the CONTAK CD trial, the left ventricular lead was placed on the mid-lateral wall in only 40% of all of the cases [74]. The extent to which precise lead placement affects the response to therapy is controversial. In an animal study, the area yielding 90% of the maximal response to CRT covered only 16% of the left ventricular free wall, but sites yielding 70% of the optimal dP/dt_{max} covered fully 43% of the free wall [75]. Observational data suggest that the choice of optimum lead position may need to be individualized and that leads should be placed in the region of latest left ventricular activation [76], although this has yet to be proven in a prospective manner.

Summary

In summary, CRT reduces symptoms of congestive heart failure and improves cardiac performance in patients with moderate-to-severely symptomatic heart failure, severe left ventricular systolic dysfunction, normal sinus rhythm, and a wide QRS complex. Resynchronization therapy significantly reduces hospitalizations in these patients and is highly cost-effective. Perhaps most important, resynchronization therapy for heart failure improves survival for these patients, particularly when employed in conjunction with an implantable defibrillator. However, randomized clinical trials show that a substantial minority of patients are clinical nonresponders. Therefore, critical questions remain with respect to identifying appropriate candidates for CRT, optimal device programming, and left ventricular lead placement.

References

1. Hunt SA, Abraham WT, Chin MH, Feldman AM, Francis GS, Ganiats TG, Jessup M, Konstam MA, Mancini DM, Michl K, Oates JA, Rahko PS, Silver MA, Stevenson LW, Yancy CW. ACC/AHA 2005 guideline update for the diagnosis and management of chronic heart failure in the adult: a report of the American College of Cardiology/American Heart Association Task Force on Practice Guidelines (Writing Committee to Update the 2001 Guidelines for the Evaluation and Management of Heart Failure). *J Am Coll Cardiol*. 2005; 46:1116–43.
2. The Task Force of the European Society of Cardiology. Developed in Collaboration with the European Heart Rhythm Association. Cardiac pacing and cardiac resynchronisation therapy. *Eur Heart J*. 2007;28:2256–95.
3. Guyatt GH, Sullivan MJ, Thompson PJ et al. The 6-minute walk: a new measure of exercise capacity in patients with chronic heart failure. *Can Med Assoc J*. 1985;132: 919–23.

4. Rector TS, Kubo SH, Cohn JN. Patients' Self Assessment of Their Congestive Heart Failure. Part 2: Content, reliability and validity of a new measure, The Minnesota Living With Heart Failure Questionnaire. *Heart Failure*. 1987; 3:198–209.

5. Bittner V, Weiner DH, Yusuf S, et al. Prediction of mortality and morbidity with a 6-minute walk test in patients with left ventricular dysfunction. SOLVD Investigators. *JAMA*. 1993;270:1702–7.

6. Myers J, Gullestad L, Vagelos R, Do D, Bellin D, Ross H, Fowler MB. Clinical, hemodynamic, and cardiopulmonary exercise test determinants of survival in patients referred for evaluation of heart failure. *Ann Intern Med*. 1998; 286–93.

7. Cazeau S, Leclercq C, Lavergne T, et al. Multisite Stimulation in Cardiomyopathies (MUSTIC) Study Investigators. Effects of multisite biventricular pacing in patients with heart failure and intraventricular conduction delay. *N Engl J Med*. 2001;344: 873–80.

8. Auricchio A, Stellbrink C, Sack S, et al. Pacing Therapies in Congestive Heart Failure (PATH-CHF) Study Group. Long-term clinical effect of hemodynamically optimized cardiac resynchronization therapy in patients with heart failure and ventricular conduction delay. *J Am Coll Cardiol*. 2002;39:2026–33.

9. Abraham WT, Fisher WG, Smith AL, Delurgio DB, Leon AR, Loh E, Kocovic DZ, Packer M, Clavell AL, Hayes DL, Ellestad M, Trupp RJ, Underwood J, Pickering F, Truex C, McAtee P, Messenger J; MIRACLE Study Group. Cardiac resynchronization in chronic heart failure. *N Engl J Med*. 2002;346:1845–53.

10. Higgins SL, Hummel JD, Niazi IK, Giudici MC, Worley SJ, Saxon LA, Boehmer JP, Higginbotham MB, De Marco T, Foster E, Yong PG. Cardiac resynchronization therapy for the treatment of heart failure in patients with intraventricular conduction delay and malignant ventricular tachyarrhythmias. *J Am Coll Cardiol*. 2003;42:1454–9.

11. Young JB, Abraham WT, Smith AL, et al. Combined cardiac resynchronization and implantable cardioversion defibrillation in advanced chronic heart failure: the MIRACLE ICD trial. *JAMA*. 2003;289:2685–94.

12. Auricchio A, Stellbrink C, Butter C, et al. Pacing Therapies in Congestive Heart Failure II Study Group. Clinical efficacy of cardiac resynchronization therapy using left ventricular pacing in heart failure patients stratified by severity of ventricular conduction delay. *J Am Coll Cardiol*. 2003;42:2109–16.

13. Olsson LG, Swedberg K, Clark AL, Witte KK, Cleland JGF. Six-minute corridor walk test as an outcome measure for the assessment of treatment in randomized, blinded intervention trials of chronic heart failure: a systematic review. *Eur Heart J* 2005;26: 778–93.

14. Witte KK, Thackray S, Nikitin NP, Cleland JG, Clark AL. The effects of long-term beta-blockade on the ventilatory responses to exercise in chronic heart failure. *Eur J Heart Fail*. 2005;7:612–7.

15. Williams SG, Cooke GA, Wright DJ, Tan LB. Disparate results of ACE inhibitor dosage on exercise capacity in heart failure: a Reappraisal of vasodilator therapy and study design. *Int J Cardiol*. 2001;77:239–45.

16. Reddy P, Dunn AB. The effect of beta-blockers on health-related quality of life in patients with heart failure. *Pharmacotherapy*. 2000;20:679–89.

17. Wolfel EE. Effects of ACE inhibitor therapy on quality of life in patients with heart failure. *Pharmacotherapy*. 1998;18:1323–34.

18. Leclercq C, Walker S, Linde C, et al. MUSTIC Study Group. Comparative effects of permanent biventricular and right-univentricular pacing in heart failure patients with chronic atrial fibrillation. *Eur Heart J.* 2002;23:1780–87.

19. Abraham WT, Young JB, Leon AR, et al. Multicenter InSync ICD II Study Group. Effects of cardiac resynchronization on disease progression in patients with left ventricular systolic dysfunction, an indication for an implantable cardioverter-defibrillator, and mildly symptomatic chronic heart failure. *Circulation.* 2004;110:2864–8.

20. Beshai JF, Grimm RA, Nagueh SF, et al. RethinQ Study Investigators. Cardiac-resynchronization therapy in heart failure with narrow QRS complexes. *N Engl J Med.* 2007; 357:2461–71.

21. Cleland JGF, Daubert JC, Erdmann E, Freemantle N, Gras D, Kappenberger L, Freemantle N, Gras D, Kappenberger L, Tavazzi L. Cardiac Resynchronization-Heart Failure (CARE-HF) Study Investigators. The effect of cardiac resynchronization on morbidity and mortality in heart failure. *N Engl J Med.* 2005;352:1539–49.

22. Duncan A, Wait D, Gibson D, Daubert JC; MUSTIC (Multisite Stimulation in Cardiomyopathies) trial. Left ventricular remodelling and haemodynamic effects of multisite biventricular pacing in patients with left ventricular systolic dysfunction and activation disturbances in sinus rhythm: substudy of the MUSTIC trial. *Eur Heart J.*2003;24:430–41.

23. St. John Sutton MG, Plappert T, Abraham WT, Smith AL, DeLurgio DB, Leon AR, Loh E, Kocovic DZ, Fisher WG, Ellestad M, Messenger J, Kruger K, Hilpisch KE, Hill MR. Multicenter InSync Randomized Clinical Evaluation (MIRACLE) Study Group. Effect of cardiac resynchronization therapy on left ventricular size and function in chronic heart failure. *Circulation.* 2003;107:1985–90.

24. McAlister FA, Ezekowitz J, Hooton N, Vandermeer B, Spooner C, Dryden DM, Page RL, Hlatky MA, Rowe BH. Cardiac resynchronization therapy for patients with left ventricular systolic dysfunction: a systemic review. *JAMA.* 2007;297:2502–14.

25. Braun MU, Rauwolf T, Zerm T, Schulze M, Schnabel A, Strasser RH. Long-term biventricular resynchronisation therapy in advanced heart failure: effect on neurohormones. *Heart.* 2005;91:601–5.

26. Adamson PB, Kleckner KJ, VanHout WL, Srinivasan S, Abraham WT. Cardiac resynchronization therapy improves heart rate variability in patients with symptomatic heart failure. *Circulation.* 2003;108:266–9.

27. Fruhwald FM, Fahrleitner-Pammer A, Berger R, Leyva F, Freemantle N, Erdmann E, Gras D, Kappenberger L, Tavazzi L, Daubert JC, Cleland JG. Early and sustained effects of cardiac resynchronization therapy on N-terminal pro-B-type natriuretic peptide in patients with moderate to severe heart failure and cardiac dyssynchrony. *Eur Heart J.* 2007;28:1592–7.

28. Bradley DJ, Bradley EA, Baughman KL, Berger RD, Calkins H, Goodman SN, Kass DA, Powe NR. Cardiac resynchronization and death from progressive heart failure: a meta-analysis of randomized controlled trials. *JAMA.* 2003;289:730–40.

29. Bristow MR, Saxon LA, Boehmer J, Krueger S, Kass DA, De Marco T, Carson P, DiCarlo L, DeMets D, White BG, DeVries DW, Feldman AM. Comparison of Medical Therapy, Pacing, and Defibrillation in Heart Failure (COMPANION) Investigators. Cardiac-resynchronization therapy with or without an implantable defibrillator in advanced chronic heart failure. *N Engl J Med.* 2004;350:2140–50.

30. Cleland JG, Daubert JC, Erdmann E, Freemantle N, Gras D, Kappenberger L, Tavazzi L. Longer-term effects of cardiac resynchronization therapy on mortality in heart failure [the CArdiac REsynchronization-Heart Failure (CARE-HF) trial extension phase]. *Eur Heart J.* 2006;27:1928–32.

31. Wilkoff BL, Hess M, Young J, Abraham WT. Differences in tachyarrhythmia detection and implantable cardioverter defibrillator therapy by primary or secondary prevention indication in cardiac resynchronization therapy patients. *J Cardiovasc Electrophysiol.* 2004;15:1002–9.

32. Yao G, Freemantle N, Calvert MJ, Bryan S, Daubert JC, Cleland JG. The long-term cost-effectiveness of cardiac resynchronization therapy with or without an implantable cardioverter-defibrillator. *Eur Heart J.* 2007;28:42–51.

33. Moss AJ, Zareba W, Hall WJ, Klein H, Wilber DJ, Cannom DS, et al. Multicenter Automatic Defibrillator Implantation Trial II Investigators. Prophylactic implantation of a defibrillator in patients with myocardial infarction and reduced ejection fraction. *N Engl J Med.* 2002;346:877–83.

34. Bardy GH, Lee KL, Mark DB, Poole JE, Packer DL, Boineau R, et al. Sudden Cardiac Death in Heart Failure Trial (SCD-HeFT) Investigators. Amiodarone or an implantable cardioverter-defibrillator for congestive heart failure. *N Engl J Med.* 2005;352:225–37.

35. http://www.heart.org/downloadable/heart/1207071938190 Linde%20Tuesday.pdf, accessed April 2, 2008.

36. http://www.clinicaltrials.gov/ct2/show/NCT00271154, accessed January 22, 2008.

37. http://www.clinicaltrials.gov/ct2/show/NCT00180271, accessed January 22, 2008.

38. http://www.clinicaltrials.gov/ct2/show/NCT00251251, accessed January 22, 2008.

39. Wang TJ, Larson MG, Levy D, et al. Temporal relations of atrial fibrillation and congestive heart failure and their joint influence on mortality: the Framingham Heart Study. *Circulation* 2003;107:2920–5.

40. Doshi RN, Daoud EG, Fellows C, Turk K, Duran A, Hamdan MH, Pires LA. PAVE Study Group. Left ventricular-based cardiac stimulation post AV nodal ablation evaluation (the PAVE study). *J Cardiovasc Electrophysiol.* 2005;16:1160–5.

41. Brignole M, Gammage M, Puggioni E, Alboni P, Raviele A, Sutton R, Vardas P, Bongiorni MG, Bergfeldt L, Menozzi C, Musso G. Optimal Pacing SITE (OPSITE) Study Investigators. Comparative assessment of right, left, and biventricular pacing in patients with permanent atrial fibrillation. *Eur Heart J.* 2005;26:712–22.

42. http://www.clinicaltrials.gov/ct2/show/NCT00111527, accessed January 31, 2008.

43. http://www.clinicaltrials.gov/ct2/show/NCT00547794, accessed January 31, 2008.

44. http://www.clinicaltrials.gov/ct2/show/NCT00267098, accessed January 31, 2008.

45. http://www.clinicaltrials.gov/ct2/show/NCT00170326, accessed March 5, 2008.

46. Molhoek SG, Bax JJ, Bleeker GB, Boersma E, van Erven L, Steendijk P, van der Wall EE, Schalij MJ. Comparison of response to cardiac resynchronization therapy in patients with sinus rhythm versus chronic atrial fibrillation. *Am J Cardiol.* 2004;94:1506–9.

47. Gasparini M, Auricchio A, Regoli F, et al. Four-year efficacy of cardiac resynchronization therapy on exercise tolerance and disease progression: the importance of performing atrioventricular junction ablation in patients with atrial fibrillation. *J Am Coll Cardiol.* 2006;48:734–43.

48. Hoppe UC, Casares JM, Eiskjaer H, Hagemann A, Cleland JG, Freemantle N, Erdmann E. Effect of cardiac resynchronization on the incidence of atrial fibrillation in patients with severe heart failure. *Circulation.* 2006;114:18–25.

49. Prinzen FW, Peschar M. Relation between the pacing induced sequence of activation and left ventricular pump function in animals. *Pacing Clin Electrophysiol.* 2002; 25 (pt 1):484–98.

50. Nahlawi M, Waligora M, Spies SM, Bonow RO, Kadish AH, Goldberger J. Left ventricular function during and after right ventricular pacing. *J Am Coll Cardiol.* 2004; 44:1883–8.

51. Sweeney MO, Hellkamp AS, Ellenbogen KA, Greenspon AJ, Freedman RA, Lee KL, Lamas GA. Adverse effect of ventricular pacing on heart failure and atrial fibrillation among patients with normal baseline QRSd in a clinical trial of pacemaker therapy for sinus node dysfunction. *Circulation.* 2003; 23:2932–7.

52. The DAVID Trial Investigators. Dual-chamber pacing or ventricular backup pacing in patients with an implantable defibrillator: the Dual Chamber and VVI Implantable Defibrillator (DAVID) Trial. *JAMA.* 2002; 288:3115–23.

53. Duray GZ, Israel CW, Pajitnev D, Hohnloser SH. Upgrading to biventricular pacing/defibrillation systems in right ventricular paced congestive heart failure patients: prospective assessment of procedural parameters and response rate. *Europace.* 2008;10:48–52.

54. Egoavil CA, Ho RT, Greenspon AJ, Pavri BB. Cardiac resynchronization therapy in patients with right bundle branch block: analysis of pooled data from the MIRACLE and Contak CD trials. *Heart Rhythm.* 2005;2:611–15.

55. Yu C-M, Fung J W-H, Zhang Q, Chan C-K, Chan Y-S, Lin H, Kum LCC, Kong S-L, Zhang Y, Sanderson JE. Tissue Doppler imaging is superior to strain rate imaging and postsystolic shortening on the prediction of reverse remodeling in both ischemic and nonischemic heart failure after cardiac resynchronization therapy. *Circulation.* 2004;110:66–73.

56. Bax JJ, Bleeker GB, Marwick TH, Molhoek SG, Boersma E, Steendijk P, van der Wall EE, Schalij MJ. Left ventricular dyssynchrony predicts response and prognosis after cardiac resynchronization therapy. *J Am Coll of Cardiol.* 2004; 44:1834–40.

57. Cleland JGF, Daubert JC, Erdmann E, Freemantle N, Gras D, Kappenberger L, Klein W, Tavazzi L; The CARE-HF study Steering Committee and Investigators. The CARE-HF study (CArdiac REsynchronisation in Heart Failure study): rationale, design and end-points. *Eur J Heart Fail* 2001;3:481–9.

58. S Ghio, ES Chung, AR Leon, L Tavazzi, JP Sun, P Nihoyannopoulos, J Merlino, WT Abraham, C Leclercq. Predictors of Response to CRT. *Circulation.* in press.

59. Bleeker GB, Kaandorp TAM, Lamb HJ, Boersma E, P Steendijk E, de Roos A, van der Wall EE, Schalij MJ, Bax JJ. Effect of posterolateral scar tissue on clinical and echocardiographic improvement after cardiac resynchronization therapy. *Circulation.* 2006;113:969–76.

60. Auricchio A, Stellbrink C, Block M, Sack S, Vogt J, Bakker P, Klein H. Pacing Therapies for Congestive Heart Failure Study Group; Kramer A, Ding J, Salo R, Tockman B, Pochet T, Spinelli J. Guidant congestive heart failure research group. effect of pacing chamber and atrioventricular delay on acute systolic function of paced patients with congestive heart failure. *Circulation.* 1999;99:2993–3001.

61. Auricchio A, Ding J, Spinelli JC, Kramer AP, Salo RW, Hoersch W, KenKnight BH, Klein HU; PATH-CHF Study Group. Cardiac resynchronization therapy restores optimal atrioventricular mechanical timing in heart failure patients with ventricular conduction delay. *J Am Coll Cardiol.* 2002;39:1163–9.

62. Vernooy K, Verbeek XAAM, Cornelussen RNM, Dijkman B, Crijns HJGM, Arts T, Prinzen FW. Calculation of effective VV interval facilitates optimization of AV delay and VV interval in cardiac resynchronization therapy. *Heart Rhythm.* 2007; 4:75–82.

63. Kerlan JE, Sawhney NS, Waggoner AD, Chawla MK, Garhwal S, Osborn JL, Faddis MN. Prospective comparison of echocardiographic atrioventricular delay optimization methods for cardiac resynchronization therapy. *Heart Rhythm.* 2003; 3:148–54.

64. Sawhney NS, Waggoner AD, Garhwal S, Chawla MK, Osborn J, Faddis MN. Randomized prospective trial of atrioventricular delay programming for cardiac resynchronization therapy. *Heart Rhythm.* 2004;1:562–7.

65. Morales M-A, Startari U, Panchetti L, Rossi A, Piacenti M. Atrioventricular Delay Optimization by Doppler-Derived Left Ventricular dP/dt Improves 6-Month Outcome of Resynchronized Patients. *PACE.* 2006; 29:564–8.

66. http://www.clinicaltrials.gov/ct2/show/NCT00418314, accessed January 31, 2008.

67. Personal communication, Boston Scientific.

68. Sogaard P, Egeblad H, Pedersen AK, Kim WY, Kristensen BO, Hansen PS, Mortensen PT. Sequential versus simultaneous biventricular resynchronization for severe heart failure: evaluation by tissue Doppler imaging. *Circulation.* 2002;106:2078–84.

69. RK Rao, UN Kumar, J Schafer, E Viloria, D Delurgio, E Foster. Reduced ventricular volumes and improved systolic function with cardiac resynchronization therapy: a randomized trial comparing simultaneous biventricular pacing, sequential biventricular pacing, and left ventricular pacing. *Circulation.* 2007;115:2136–44.

70. Boriani G, Müller CP, Seidl KH, Grove R, Vogt J, Danschel W, Schuchert A, Djiane P, Biffi M, Becker T, Bailleul C, Trappe HJ; Resynchronization for the Hemodynamic Treatment for Heart Failure Management II Investigators. Randomized comparison of simultaneous biventricular stimulation versus optimized interventricular delay in cardiac resynchronization therapy. The Resynchronization for the Hemodynamic Treatment for Heart Failure Management II implantable cardioverter defibrillator (RHYTHM II ICD) study. *Am Heart J.* 2006;151:1050–8.

71. Colucci WS, Ribeiro JP, Rocco MB, Quigg RJ, Creager MA, Marsh JD, Gauthier DF, Hartley LH. Impaired chronotropic response to exercise in patients with congestive heart failure. Role of postsynaptic β-adrenergic desensitization. *Circulation.* 1989;80:314–23.

72. Martin DO, Stolen KQ, Brown S, Yu Y, Christie C, Doshi SK, Smith JM, Gold MR, Day JD. Pacing Evaluation-Atrial SUpport Study in Cardiac Resynchronization Therapy (PEGASUS CRT): design and rationale. *Am Heart J.* 2007;153:7–13.

73. Auricchio A, Klein H, Tockman B, Sack S, Stellbrink C, Neuzner J, Kramer A, Ding J, Pochet T, Maarse A, Spinelli J. Transvenous biventricular pacing for heart failure: can the obstacles be overcome? *Am J Cardiol.* 1999;5S2:136–42.

74. CONTAK CD study clinical report. Data courtesy of Guidant.

75. Helm RH, Byrne M, Helm PA, Daya SK, Osman NF, Tunin R, Halperin HR, Berger RD, Kass DA, Lardo AC. Three-dimensional mapping of optimal left ventricular pacing site for cardiac resynchronization. *Circulation.* 2007; 115:953–61.

76. Ansalone G, Giannantoni P, Ricci R, Trambaiolo P, Fedele F, Santini M. Doppler myocardial imaging to evaluate the effectiveness of pacing sites in patients receiving biventricular pacing. *J Am Coll Cardiol.* 2002; 39:489–99.

Chapter 6

Implantation of a CRT device

Christian Sticherling

Key Points

1. The majority of cardiac resynchronization therapy (CRT) systems can be implanted transvenously under local anesthesia and conscious sedation.
2. The cardiac venous anatomy parallels the coronary arteries and has specific obstacles (take-off of the coronary sinus ostium, Thebesian valve, Vieussens valve).
3. The right ventricular (RV) lead should be placed first to provide back-up pacing in the case of complete atrio-ventricular (AV) block.
4. Different shapes of guiding catheters, telescopic sheath-in-sheath systems, steerable sheaths, and steerable electrophysiological (EP) catheters allow access to the coronary sinus (CS) ostium in the vast majority of cases.
5. Venography should be performed to assess the anatomy and potential target sites for LV lead placement.
6. Optimal left ventricular (LV) lead position is usually in a (postero-) lateral vein. The LV electrogram should be as late as possible in relation to the QRS complex. Avoid the anterior cardiac vein.
7. More than 90% of LV leads can be positioned transvenously in a satisfactory cardiac vein.
8. Most coronary sinus dissections are contained and do not mandate abandonment of LV lead placement.
9. Main reasons for re-operation are lead dislodgement, rise in pacing thresholds, and phrenic nerve stimulation.
10. Surgical epicardial lead placement through a variety of minithoracotomy approaches is a viable alternative approach.

Pacing to Support the Failing Heart, 1st edition. Edited by K. Ellenbogen and A. Auricchio.
© 2008 American Heart Association, ISBN: 978-1-4051-7534-0

Introduction

Cardiac resynchronization therapy has gained widespread acceptance for the treatment of patients with symptomatic congestive heart failure NYHA Class III or Class IV under optimal medical therapy, low-ejection fraction, and bundle branch block [1–9]. The number of CRT implants will continue to grow and pose new challenges to many device implanters who face the difficulty to implant a left ventricular lead through the so far neglected cardiac venous system, the coronary sinus and its tributaries.

Because the techniques to implant atrial leads and RV pacemaker or defibrillator leads as well as to place the generator subpectorally instead of subcutaneously have become common clinical practice, this chapter will focus mainly on the implantation of left ventricular pacing leads for cardiac resynchronization.

Anatomy of the coronary sinus

The venous drainage system of the heart runs for the most part parallel to the coronary artery system (Figure 6.1) [10]. The anterior cardiac vein of the left ventricle runs in the anterior interventricular groove and becomes the great cardiac vein as it enters the atrio-ventricular groove. The greater cardiac vein receives a variable number of contributing left marginal (left lateral) and posterior cardiac veins. After the Vieussens valve the greater cardiac vein becomes the coronary sinus (CS) which drains the venous blood into the posterobasal right atrium [11]. The coronary sinus also receives blood from the middle cardiac vein, which runs in the posterior interventricular groove parallel to the posterior interventricular branch of the right coronary artery. From the right heart chambers, the venous blood reaches the coronary sinus through the small cardiac vein. Although the anterior and middle cardiac veins are virtually always present, there is great

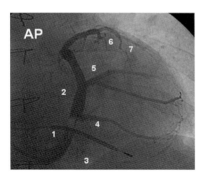
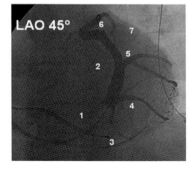

Fig. 6.1 The cardiac venous system (Fluoroscopic views in AP and LAO 45 degree angulation). An ICD lead is already positioned in the right ventricle. 1: coronary sinus; 2: greater cardiac vein; 3: middle cardiac vein; 4: posterior vein; 5: posterolateral vein; 6: anterior cardiac vein; 7: anterolateral cardiac vein.

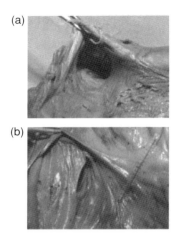

Fig. 6.2 (a) Coronary sinus ostium without Thebesian valve; (b) Cresent shaped Thebesian valve overlying the ostium. Karaca, et al., *J Interv Card Electrophysiol.* 2005;14:89.

variability in the presence and anatomy of the left marginal and posterior cardiac veins [12]. In addition to the Vieussens valve, the Thebesian valve at the ostium of the coronary sinus (Figure 6.2) can serve as an obstacle [13].

Implantation techniques

CRT implantation should preferentially be carried out in the catheterization laboratory because it is important to have high-quality fluoroscopy equipment at hand. The patient should be in a fasting state for about 6 hours, and adequate hydration should be maintained with a stable intravenous line, ideally at the side of the planned implantation. This allows the surgeon to perform a venography in the case of difficult venous access. We allow the patients to take their heart failure medication the same morning. In our experience, it is not necessary to interrupt oral anticoagulation for CRT implantation, but patients should have their (INR) reduced to about 2 [14]. Apart from rare instances, the devices can be implanted using local anesthetics and conscious sedation (e.g. midazolam and fentanyl). This has been proven to be safe and minimizes the risks of general anaesthesia in patients with severely reduced left ventricular function and common comorbidities [15]. Antibiotic prophylaxis reduces the risk for device infection [16,17]. For shock testing in defibrillator implantion, short-acting intravenous anaesthetics (e.g. propofol or etomidate) can be used.

Venous access

Left-sided venous access should be preferred because most patients will receive a CRT-defibrillator, and most guiding catheters are designed to be placed from

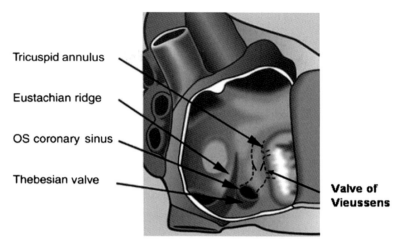

Tricuspid annulus

Eustachian ridge

OS coronary sinus

Thebesian valve

Valve of Vieussens

Fig. 6.3 Anatomy of the postero-basal right atrium and the ostium of the coronary sinus (modified from Ellenbogen).

the left side. Right-sided access will create a second right-angle turn at the junction from the subclavian vein to the superior vena cava [18]. In case of an upgrade and pre-existing intravenous leads, an intravenous line should be placed in the ipsilateral arm to visualize the venous system and to prepare oneself for a more complex implantion in the case of venous occlusion [19].

Implantation of the RV and RA leads

The right ventricular lead should be positioned first. Because the majority of patients will display a left bundle branch block (LBBB), this lead will provide back-up pacing in the case of induction of a complete AV block during catherization of the coronary sinus. Additionally, the movement of the lead body may help to visualize the level of the tricuspid valve, which may assist in localizing the ostium. The proximal portion of the Implantable Cardioverter-Defibrillator (ICD) coil is often located near the coronary sinus os. We prefer to implant the atrial lead at the end because the atrial lead is prone to dislodgement during difficult LV lead placement.

Coronary sinus cannulation

The cannulation of the coronary sinus frequently proves to be the first obstacle for the novice. One has to bear in mind, that chamber enlargement in the failing heart causes an upward shift of the long axis and a posterior shift of the short axis, which result in a lower and more posterior position of the CS ostium in the right atrium [18]. Although it is virtually always possible to succeed with a postero-anterior (PA) projection of the fluoroscopy, it may initially be helpful to briefly use an RAO 30-degree projection to look for the fat pad in the AV groove. This and possible calcifications of the right coronary artery may serve as anatomic markers for the position of the AV groove and the course of the CS. Cannulation of the CS ostium is best performed in a left anterior oblique (LAO) 30–45-degree projection. In this view, the coronary sinus runs posteriorly toward the spine. It is helpful to review the venous phase of previous coronary angiograms to get an idea of the location of the CS ostium.

Principally, the cannulation of the coronary sinus involves the following steps [18]:

1 Advancement of the guiding catheter over a 0.036 inch soft-tip J wire to the floor of the right atrium.
2 Retraction of the guidewire and upward orientation of the guiding catheter.
3 Counterclockwise torque and withdrawal of the catheter, which directs the catheter posteriorly and upward toward the ostium.

Although there are numerous shapes of guiding catheters, operators should become acquainted with "their" catheter and not change types too often. If the catheter does not engage directly by probing with the J wire one can give contrast "puffs" to visualize the ostium in the low right atrium. One has to be careful not to use too much contrast with this approach because many patients suffer from some degree of renal failure and are prone to cardiac decompensation.

We prefer to insert an "inner" sheath through the guiding catheter, thereby creating a telescopic system with gives better reach and allows for better rotational capabilities to locate the ostium. An alternative approach is the use of a deflectable electrophysiology (EP) catheter. Apart from the steerability of the catheter, this approach has the advantage of using intracardiac signals to locate the ostium. We use this approach in difficult cannulations in patients with severe impairment of their renal function. Manufacturers now also offer a steerable guiding catheter with a lumen for guidewire insertion and contrast injection.

Coronary sinus venography

Once the CS has been entered, venography should be performed to get an overview of potential target veins (Figure 6.1). Potential obstacles, like Vieussens valve, should be carefully crossed with the guide wire in order to avoid perforation [20]. Contrast injection is then carried out through a single-lumen, balloon-tip catheter after occlusion of the vessel. In order to avoid coronary sinus dissection, it is advisable to confirm that the balloon is not wedged in a side branch or underneath a valve by injecting a little contrast puff before inflating the balloon. It is helpful to store two venograms, typically in a PA or a RAO 30-degree projection and/or in a LAO 30–45-degree projection.

The use of CT angiography to delineate the CS anatomy prior to LV lead implantation has been described [21]. However, given the high radiation exposure (6–13 mSv) and the relative ease to perform a simple venography, this modality should be reserved for patients with difficult anatomies (e.g. adults

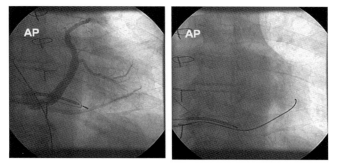

Fig. 6.4 Fluoroscopy: lateral side branch draining in the middle cardiac vein.

with certain forms of congenital heart disease). Cardiac magnetic resonance also allows visualization of the cardiac venous system without any additional radiation exposure [22].

Selection of a target vein

The target veins for cardiac resynchronization therapy should be at the left free wall (i.e. the left lateral, postero(lateral) or anterolateral (parallel to the diagonal branch of the LAD) vein). It has been shown that these positions clearly yield better results than anterior stimulation [23]. Should there be no apparent suitable vein on the venogram, this should be repeated in an occlusive position and with prolonged filming. Frequently, collateral flow then demonstrates large lateral wall drainage through a large middle cardiac vein (Figure 6.4); alternatively, one can look for anterolateral branches of the anterior cardiac vein. In the PA projection, these veins run at the anterior border of the heart silhouette parallel to the diagonal branches of the coronary artery (Figure 6.1).

LV lead placement

Depending on the anatomy of the target vein, this part of the implantation can be straightforward or develop into a tedious undertaking. Operators should have different shapes and sizes of available LV leads at hand because one size does not fit all veins [24]. Unipolar or bipolar leads in different shapes and sizes, ranging from 4 to 6 French are available. These can be used either stylet-driven or in an over-the-wire technique [18]. The anchoring mechanisms differ from small tines, over preshaped distal curves to helical fixation mechanisms (Figure 6.5). If one targets small branches of a vein, a small, flexible unipolar lead should be chosen. With this lead, one has very few options if this pacing site does not prove to be optimal because it is virtually impossible to position this lead in a greater vein in a wedge position without a high risk for dislodgment. Therefore, we often use bigger preshaped LV leads with more rigid loops at their distal segment because these give the greatest

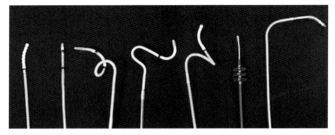

Fig. 6.5 Different anchoring mechanisms of available LV-pacing leads, showing different straight, preshaped, and helical leads.

freedom to place the lead at many locations within the venous tree. The use of bipolar leads can reduce the occurrence of phrenic nerve stimulation and may help to improve LV-pacing thresholds (e.g. by electrical repositioning, Figure 6.6) in selected cases. In case of a medium-sized vein that enters the CS at a wide angle, a preshaped bipolar lead can be readily advanced using a stylet only (Figure 6.7). If the best target vein enters the CS in an acute angle, or if a surgeon tries to manipulate the lead into a small tributary branch to ensure optimal lead stability, the over-the-wire technique should be chosen. We prefer medium to extra distal strength 0.014 inch guidewires. In the case of very acute angles, the lead might not track across the angle and dislodge the wire. In this situation,

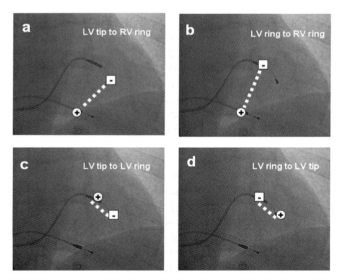

Fig. 6.6 Electrical reprogramming to avoid phrenic nerve stimulation. (a) LV tip to RV ring; extended bipolar vector; (b) LV ring to RV ring; extended bipolar pacing vector; (c) LV tip to LV ring; dedicated bipolar pacing vector; (d) LV ring to LV tip.

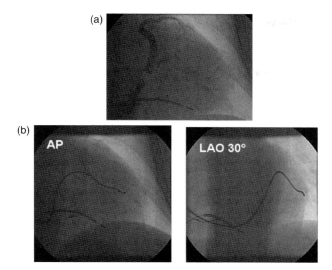

Fig. 6.7 (a) Easy access of a lateral vein (Venogram, PA projection); (b) Excellent position of a bipolar lead in a lateral vein. Note the distance between RV- and LV-pacing lead in a LAO 30-degree projection.

one can engage the vein selectively with an inner sheath and try to advance the soft-tipped guiding catheter into the side branch. Should this not be possible, we prefer to position a heavyweight 0.016 inch guidewire in the most distal position, remove the inner sheath and then advance the lead. Currently, modern lead technology allows one to advance a multipolar 4 French LV-pacing lead through the inner catheter into the subselected vein. In case of very small veins, a unipolar lead may be advantageous to ensure proper placement of the lead.

Remote robotic navigation as discussed in Chapter 12 using rare earth magnets (Niobe™, Stereotaxis, St. Louis, MO) has been used to navigate magnetic tip wires through tortuous segments. Venography or preprocedural computed tomography can be used as guides to determine the vectors and choose the target site [25,26]. Although this technology allows the placement of the wire, the problem of advancing a contemporary LV lead remains. Magnet-tipped leads, sheaths, and delivery systems are developed for future use [27].

LV lead testing
The ideal pacing site should be a position as far lateral or posterior and as far away from the right ventricular lead as possible. Visual dyssynchrony can be confirmed by fluoroscopy in a LAO projection. Several methods, such as the timing of the LV electrogram relative to the onset of the QRS complex-ideally at late as possible [28], determination of the most delayed site by electroanatomical mapping systems [29], or echocardiographic methods [30,31] have been

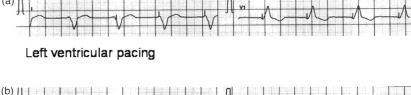

Left ventricular pacing

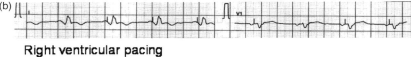

Right ventricular pacing

Fig. 6.8 Example of the QRS complexes of the surface ECG leads I (and V1) during (a) LV-pacing and (b) RV-pacing.

proposed for determination of the best left ventricular pacing site. During implantation, we always strive to achieve a negative QRS complex in lead I of the surface ECG, indicating a LV lead position on the left lateral wall (Figure 6.8) [32].

Once one has placed the lead in the desired anatomical and/or electrical position, the lead impedance and pacing threshold should be tested. One may accept higher thresholds (e.g. 3.5V @ 0.5 ms) than usual, if no other promising target veins appear to be readily accessible. Unfortunately, the intimate relation between the left lateral wall and the left phrenic nerve will frequently cause phrenic nerve stimulation resulting in diaphragmatic contraction. Even intermittent diaphragmatic stimulation is unacceptable. Therefore, one should test for phrenic nerve stimulation with 10V @ 0.5 ms during deep inspiration and maximal expiration. Generally, phrenic nerve stimulation mandates repositioning of the lead. In rare cases with a very low LV-pacing threshold and very high threshold for phrenic nerve stimulation, one gets away without repositioning. If the patient sits or stands after the implantation, the LV pacing threshold frequently rises and the diaphragmatic threshold may fall. Different programming options, like true LV bipolar pacing or change of the unipolar pacing pathway, may then solve the problem through "electrical repositioning." However, intraoperative avoidance of phrenic nerve stimulation by repositioning of the LV lead is time well spent and will reduce the risk for re-operation later. Figure 6.9 gives an example of the frequently encountered trade-off between optimal anatomical position, high LV-pacing thresholds, and phrenic nerve stimulation.

Removal of the guiding catheter

Once the LV lead is in place, the guiding catheter has to be removed without dislodging the lead. For that purpose numerous slitting tools are available. During removal of the catheter, a stylet or a stabilizing wire should be kept inside the lead up to the level of the CS. Care has to be taken as to not leave excessive slack in the lead, which may pull the tip out of the vein (Figure 6.10). Should the

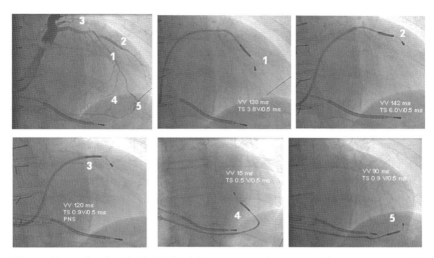

Fig. 6.9 Example of multiple LV lead locations to achieve a satisfactory position. The numbers in the first panel refer to the lead positions illustrated in the following panels. (VV: difference between activation of RV and LV lead; TS: pacing threshold; PNS: phrenic nerve stimulation).

LV lead become dislodged at this step, the LV lead placement has to start from scratch because then the lead usually cannot be maneuvered back into the CS system without the back-up of the guiding catheter.

Sheathless LV-pacing lead implantation is possible and has been described to result in a 70% implantation success [33]. This approach does not require one to perform venography. Without the knowledge of the precise anatomic details of the coronary sinus, one may fortuitously implant the lead in a lateral vein,

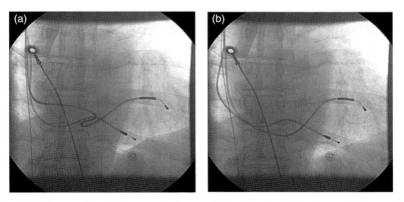

Fig. 6.10 PA projection. (a) Too much slack on LV lead in the right atrium; (b) Correct LV lead position in the right atrium.

but this may not be the best location. Furthermore, many better implant sites cannot be reached without the support of the guiding catheter.

Troubleshooting

Using the transvenous route, implantation success rate in large series of study patients are in the realm of 90% (Table 6.1) [4,6,34,35]. Single, experienced operators report much higher acute implant success rates underlining the importance of operator experience [35,36].

Reasons and strategies to overcome potential failure of LV lead implantation are summarized in Table 6.2.

Phrenic nerve stimulation

As mentioned above, one frequently encounters the problem of phrenic nerve stimulation during placement of the LV lead in a lateral vein. Phrenic nerve stimulation can also occur later and may be due to microdislodgement or a different electrical milieu with the patient standing or sitting. Even short episodes of phrenic nerve stimulation are clearly not tolerable for the patient and result in the necessity for re-operation in 3–5% of patients [7,34]. The best preventive measure for avoiding subsequent phrenic nerve stimulation is to not tolerate *any* extracardiac stimulation at 10V @ 0.5 ms intraoperatively and assure proper fixation of the LV lead to avoid dislodgement (see above). However, at times one has to compromise as to not to give up an excellent pacing site. Newer CRT-systems are capable of multiple left ventricular pacing configurations (Figure 6.6). One study found phrenic nerve stimulation (PNS) in 8% of patients during implantation and an additional 11% of patients during a 3-month follow-up, defining PNS as stimulation at twice the pacing threshold output [37]. PNS could be managed by changing the left ventricular pacing configuration in all patients equipped with a device with this function. In contrast, patients with another system had either their LV lead abandoned or underwent re-operation.

High pacing thresholds

High LV-pacing thresholds may be accepted if the position is desirable. However, one has to bear in mind that high LV-pacing thresholds in patients with ischemic heart disease are frequently due to scarred myocardium. There is evidence that the presence of a transmural scar in the posterolateral segment of the left ventricle is associated with a worse clinical outcome after CRT [38,39]. Therefore, one should consider positioning the LV lead at a different location if a transmural posterolateral scar is known.

Access problems

Particularly in CRT upgrades, one may encounter occlusion of the ipsilateral subclavian vein. Therefore, one should perform venography via an ipsilateral

Table 6.1 Comparison of implantation success rates and need for re-operation in selected large CRT series.

Authors	Studies	Success rate	Median follow-up (min)	Re-operation rate	LV lead-high threshold/ dislodgement	Extracardiac stimulation	Others	Infection
Alonso et al. 2001		102/116 (88%)	15	19/102 (19%)	15/102 (15%)	3/102 (3%)	0/102	3/102(3%)
Knight et al. 2004	VENTAK CHF CONTAK CD	443/512 (87%)	30	59/443 (13%)	32/443 (7%)	8/443 (2%)	14/443 (3%)	5/443 (1%)
Leon et al. 2005	MIRACLE, MIRACLE ICD, InSyncIII	1,903/2,078 (92%)	6	174/1,903 (9%)	108/1,903 (6%)	23/1,903 (1.2%)	30/1,903 (1.6%)	13/1,903 (0.7%)
Bristow et al. 2004 [52]	COMPANION	1,080/1,212 (89%)	15–16	NR	27/1,080 (2.5%)	104/1,080 (9.6%)	22/1,080 (2%)	11/1,080 (1%)
Cleland et al. 2005	CARE-HF	390/404 (95%)	29	NR	24/390 (6%)	NR	8/390 (2%)	3/390 (0.8%)
Overall:		3,918/4,322 (90.7%)		252/2,448 (10%)	206/3,918 (5%)	138/3,528 (4%)	72/3,918 (2%)	35/3,918 (0.9%)

Table 6.2 Causes for difficult LV lead placement and possible solution.

Problem	Solution
Difficult venous access Vein occlusion	• Perform i.v. venography on the ipsilateral arm (esp. with pre-existing leads) to assure patency of the vein. • Recanalization and percutaneous venoplasty of stenosis or occlusions of the vein. • LV lead implantation on the contralateral side and subcutaneous tunnelling to the device if pre-existing leads should be used. • Implantation of a new system on the contralateral side (and abandonment of possible pre-existing leads).
Difficulties in accessing the coronary sinus	• Check the late phase of a pre-existing coronary angiogram to assess coronary sinus anatomy. • Look for the "fat pad" in the atrio-ventricular groove in a RAO 30-degree projection (location of CS ostium). • Use telescopic sheath-in-sheath system to extend reach and gain more flexibility in maneuvering the catheter. • Use a steerable EP catheter through the guiding catheter (and record intracardiac electrocardiogram if possible). • Use steerable guiding catheter. • Perform contrast atriography. • Be very careful with repetitive contrast "puffs" (pre-existing renal failure; volume effect).
Inability to reach the target vein	Use selective "inner sheath" guiding catheters to intubate side branch. • Implant small 4Fr LV-pacing lead through the inner catheter. • Try to advance the guiding catheter into the side branch using the inner catheter as a rail. • Try to advance a heavyweight guidewire as far distally as possible, remove inner sheath and try to slide pacing-lead over the wire. • Use a different lead (e.g. unipolar instead of bipolar). • Look for possible alternative target veins. • Consider surgical epicardial lead placement.
Ramified CS system	• Look for different routes to reach the lateral wall (e.g. through the middle cardiac vein). • Use a small OTW (over the wire) LV lead and try to advance it in a very small vein. • Consider surgical epicardial lead placement.

(continued)

Table 6.2 (continued)

Problem	Solution
Phrenic nerve stimulation (PNS)	• Try to avoid any PNS intraoperatively. • Consider targeting a small side branch slightly posteriorly. • Consider using a bipolar lead. • Look for alternative pacing site. • "Electrical repositioning" may help to overcome the problem if an excellent pacing site should not be given up. • Consider surgical epicardial lead placement.
High LV-thresholds	• Accept higher pacing thresholds than usual. • Avoid pacing over scar tissue. • Consider the use of a bipolar lead and test different pacing pathways (electrical reprogramming).
V lead dislodgements	Choose appropriate lead for the given vein: • Small side branch: wedge a small flexible unipolar lead in a side branch. • Middle sized-vein: use bipolar lead, preshaped or another anchoring mechanism (no tines), assure proper wedging. • Big vein: try to access small side branch for anchoring, choose appropriate anchoring mechanism.
Barriers by Thebesian Valve and Valve of Vieussens	Thebesian valve at the CS ostium: • Use telescopic sheath-in-sheath system to extend reach and gain more flexibility in maneuvering the catheter. • Use a steerable EP catheter through the guiding catheter (and record intracardiac electrocardiogram if possible). • Use steerable guiding catheter. • Carefully probe with a 0.035″ guidewire Vieussens valve: • Carefully try to pass with a J-shaped 0.035″ guidewire or steerable EP catheter. • Do not force the guiding sheath or the balloon-tip catheter across (high risk for CS dissection).
Coronary sinus dissection	• Manipulate carefully, ideally with a J-shaped, 0.035″ guide wire, to avoid dissection. • Give a contrast puff before inflating the balloon (side branch, valve). • Most dissections are contained and have no hemodynamic consequences. • Try to position the LV lead if you are in the true lumen. • If uncertain, delay the LV lead placement for 2 weeks. • In case of hemodynamic compromise or CS perforation, perform immediate echocardiography and pericardiocentesis if necessary (call for surgery back-up).

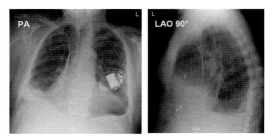

Fig. 6.11 Upgrade of a DDD-ICD system in a patient with an occluded left-sided subclavian vein. Implantation of the LV-pacing lead in the contralateral subclavian vein and subcutaneous tunneling to the device pocket.

vein before starting the operation. There are numerous options to overcome this problem. One can try to cross the occlusion with a wire and perform a venoplasty with or without stent placement [40]. Another option is to implant the LV lead on the contralateral side and tunnel the lead in front of the sternum to the device pocket (Figure 6.11). Finally, epicardial lead placement is another option. The presence of a persistent left superior vena cava, even in the absence of a patent right superior vena cava, does not preclude successful transvenous LV placement (Figure 6.12) [41].

Recognition and management of complications

In general, the risks and complication rates of implanting a CRT-system are very low. Many are comparable to the risks associated with the transvenous implantation of conventional pacemakers or defibrillators [1–5,7,35,42]. These comprise bleeding ($\sim$ 1%), infection ($\sim$1%), hematoma ($\sim$ 1%), pneumothorax ($\sim$1%), pericardial effusion with and without tamponade ($\sim$1%), and myocardial infarction, stroke, and death ($\sim$1/500) (Table 6.2).

There are certain additional risks specifically related to the transvenous placement of the LV lead: coronary sinus dissection and perforation ($\sim$1%), lead dislodgement ($\sim$5%), extracardiac stimulation ($\sim$5%), and the risks of using

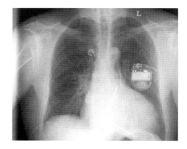

Fig. 6.12 CRT implantation through a persistent left SVC.

intravenous contrast, like renal failure (Tables 6.1 and 6.2). Also, the potential for ventricular proarrhythmia has been reported [43].

Coronary sinus dissection, perforation, and tamponade

In one early, large series of 2,078 patients, 45 (2.1%) experienced coronary sinus dissection [44]. Frequently, CS dissection occurs if the balloon-tip catheter for the venogram is advanced forcefully or inflated in the presence of an anatomic obstacle, usually the Vieussens valve or a small tributary branch (Figure 6.13a). Therefore, one should never probe with the balloon-tip catheter for the CS ostium and always inject some dye before inflating the balloon. Fortunately, coronary sinus dissection or perforation usually produces no or little clinical consequence because the CS is embedded in adipose tissue, the venous blood circulates rapidly at low pressure, and the perforation is contained by the pericardium. This is reflected by a contrast stain that is not immediately "washed out" (Figure 6.13b). One can usually proceed if the patient remains hemodynamically stable and the dissection does not occlude the CS [44]. Otherwise, the implantation should been abandoned and delayed for at least 2 weeks when the injury typically has resolved. Immediate echocardiography should be performed in the case of hemodynamic instability to assess the need for pericardiocentesis. In the case of perforation of the coronary sinus with a guiding catheter

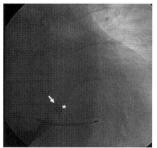

* Valve of Vieussens;   arrow: Dissection of greater cardiac vein

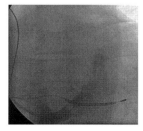

Fig. 6.13 Contained perforation of the greater cardiac vein without hemodynamic compromise.

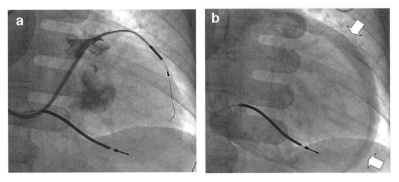

Fig. 6.14 (a) Perforation of the greater cardiac vein with the guiding catheter; the LV lead flotates freely pericardial space. (b) Contrast accumulates circumferentially in the pericardium (arrows) resulting in a hemopericardium.

or the LV lead, contrast is washed out immediately, indicating an uncontained perforation (Figures 6.14a and 6.14b). If the contrast becomes visible in the pericardium, hemodynamic deterioration becomes very likely. The hemodynamic consequences should be monitored and pericardiocentesis should be prepared and surgical back-up be sought immediately. One may consider temporarily occluding the perforation with a 4–6 mm angioplasty balloon, if a wire can be advanced to the pericardium, until a definitive solution is obtained.

Loss of capture/Lead dislodgement

Loss of LV capture can be the reason for sudden deterioration of a CRT-responder and be readily diagnosed using a standard 12-lead ECG (Figure 6.15) [32].

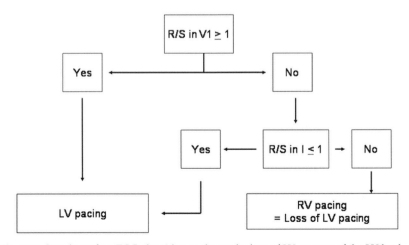

Fig. 6.15 Simple surface ECG algorithm to detect the loss of LV capture of the LV lead.

Perioperative incidence of loss of capture or lead dislodgement is around 3% [44]. Another 6–10% of patients will experience loss of capture or lead dislodgement during the first 3–6 months [34,44].

The principal reason for loss of capture or rise in pacing threshold is a macrodislodgement or microdislodgement of the LV lead. If the lead becomes completely dislodged, the patient needs to undergo re-operation. It is important to identify the reason for the dislodgement in order to avoid the same mistake. One possible solution is the use of a smaller unipolar lead that may be readily wedged in a small side branch over a wire. If one has used a non–preshaped lead, a preshaped LV lead that becomes anchored in a middle-sized vein, could be used in the second attempt. Finally, there should not be too much slack on the LV lead in the right atrium and proper fixation of the sleeve should be ascertained (Figure 6.10).

In the case of microdislodgement, change of the stimulation configuration can often mend the problem [37]. Otherwise, one may want to accept higher pacing threshold. However, this will obviously lead to premature battery depletion, tends to be associated with less stable thresholds and can at times result in extracardiac stimulation.

Device infection

There is cumulating evidence that antibiotic prophylaxis reduces the incidence of device infections [16,17]. A sample of 6,319 patients with pacemaker or ICD implantation revealed an incidence of device-related infections of 0.68% after one year [16]. The occurrence of infection was positively correlated to early re-intervention, fever within 24 hours before device placement, and use of a temporary pacing wire before implantation. De-novo device implantation and use of antibiotic prophylaxis were negatively correlated with device infection. Because the strongest prediction of infection was the need for early re-intervention, great care must be taken to avoid a pocket hematoma, particularly because many of the CRT-patients are on anticoagulation or antiplatelet therapy, and lead dislodgement. In our own experience, extraction of the coronary sinus lead causes surprisingly little problems. In the case of difficult LV lead extraction, the use of laser-lead extraction systems has been shown to be feasible and safe [45]. After the extraction of chronic LV-pacing leads, the affected CS branch was occluded in 50% of the patients. Even in the absence of infection, we re-evaluate the LV-pacing lead position in nonresponders and consider explanation of the old and re-implantation of a new LV-pacing lead into a more suitable vein.

Surgical placement of LV leads

With the advent of better LV lead delivery systems and the growing experience of operators, successful transvenous LV lead placement is now possible in more than the 91.6% reported in over 2,000 patients from a multicenter study program

[44]. In the former study, 8% of the patients required re-operation in the first 6 months for LV lead dislodgement, loss of LV capture, or uncorrectable extracardiac stimulation. Surgery remains an option if the venous tree does not allow optimal lead placement for anatomical reasons or due to scar at the target site, unavoidable stimulation of the phrenic nerve, inability to enter the coronary sinus, or to keep the LV lead in a stable position.

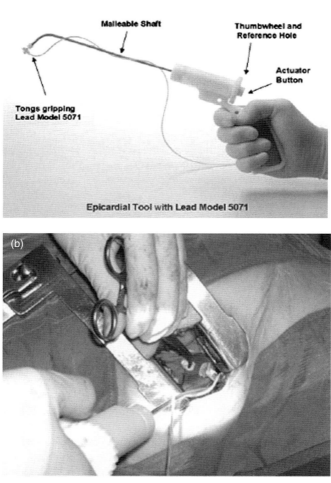

Fig. 6.16 (a) The epicardial implant tool (Medtronic, Minneapolis, MN); (b) Positioning of the epicardial screw lead. (From Doll et al. [48].)

Several surgical approaches have been described [46,47]. The epicardial approach lends itself to more freedom in positioning the LV lead. One has to bear in mind, though, that the postero-lateral wall is also not readily accessible with minimally invasive techniques. Furthermore, the patient is exposed to the risk associated with general anesthesia and single lung ventilation.

For minithoracotomy a 3-cm skin incision is performed over the fourth and fifth left intercostals space [47]. During single lung ventilation the pericardium is incised just anteriorly to the phrenic nerve. By using stay suture in the pericardium, the posterior wall can be better exposed and screw-in pacing leads can be placed in the posterior wall. Lead placement on the posterolateral aspect of the left ventricular wall can be further facilitated by using the epicardial lead placement tool (Medtronic, Minneapolis). This consists of a malleable shaft and gripping tongs that allow implantation of a mounted screw-in lead perpendicular to the LV wall (Figure 6.16) [48]. In some medical centers, two LV leads are implanted in case one fails in the future.

Video-assisted thorascopic surgery (VATS) and robotically assisted procedures have been decribed [47]. Studies comparing the LV lead placement via the coronary venous approach with left lateral thoracotomy revealed a lower incidence for the need of re-interventions in the surgical approach [49,50]. This was mainly driven by a very high implantation failure rate in one early series [50] and a 5% lead dislodgement rate with the transvenous approach [49]. On the other hand, the hospitalization was longer, the increase in functional capacity smaller and the mortality at 1-year higher in the surgically placed group [49]. Under normal circumstances, the transvenous approach should therefore be chosen. As surgical placement of LV leads becomes more commonplace, a surgeon may consider placement for future use in selected patients at the time of bypass or valve surgery.

Minimally invasive subxiphoid epicardial approaches are used by electro-physiologists for ablation procedures and are potential future routes for LV lead placement [24,27,51].

Summary

CRT has become an important therapeutic option for symptomatic heart failure patients with a wide QRS complex. Consequently, the number of implantations continues to rise, and many implanting physicians who perform pacemaker and defibrillator operations are faced with the challenge to position a left ventricular pacing lead. With the advent of modern LV lead delivery systems, cannulation of the coronary sinus is possible in the vast majority of patients. Knowledge of the cardiac venous anatomy is paramount to choose an optimal pacing site. Although it has not been precisely determined how to choose the optimal LV-pacing site, it is evident that placement in the posterolateral and lateral veins yields the best results. Complications typical for the LV lead placement occur in the realm of 5–8% and consist of coronary sinus dissections, phrenic nerve stimulation, and lead dislodgement. Nevertheless, the implantation procedure is remarkably safe and becomes even safer with the growing experience of the implanting physician.

Finally, although other techniques are more invasive and require general anaesthesia, there are viable surgical options to place an epicardial LV-pacing lead in the case of a failed transvenous approach or concomitant to coronary bypass or valve surgery.

References

1. Abraham WT, Fisher WG, Smith AL, Delurgio DB, Leon AR, Loh E, Kocovic DZ, Packer M, Clavell AL, Hayes DL, Ellestad M, Trupp RJ, Underwood J, Pickering F, Truex C, McAtee P, Messenger J. Cardiac resynchronization in chronic heart failure. *N Engl J Med.* 2002;346(24):1845–53.
2. Auricchio A, Stellbrink C, Sack S, Block M, Vogt J, Bakker P, Huth C, Schondube F, Wolfhard U, Bocker D, Krahnefeld O, Kirkels H. Long-term clinical effect of hemodynamically optimized cardiac resynchronization therapy in patients with heart failure and ventricular conduction delay. *J Am Coll Cardiol.* 2002;39(12):2026–33.
3. Cazeau S, Leclercq C, Lavergne T, Walker S, Varma C, Linde C, Garrigue S, Kappenberger L, Haywood GA, Santini M, Bailleul C, Daubert JC. Effects of multisite biventricular pacing in patients with heart failure and intraventricular conduction delay. *N Engl J Med.* 2001;344(12):873–80.
4. Bristow MR, Saxon LA, Boehmer J, Krueger S, Kass DA, De Marco T, Carson P, DiCarlo L, DeMets D, White BG, DeVries DW, Feldman AM. Cardiac-resynchronization therapy with or without an implantable defibrillator in advanced chronic heart failure. *N Engl J Med.* 2004;350(21):2140–50.
5. Young JB, Abraham WT, Smith AL, Leon AR, Lieberman R, Wilkoff B, Canby RC, Schroeder JS, Liem LB, Hall S, Wheelan K. Combined cardiac resynchronization and implantable cardioversion defibrillation in advanced chronic heart failure: the MIRACLE ICD Trial. *JAMA.* 2003;289(20):2685–94.
6. Cleland JG, Daubert JC, Erdmann E, Freemantle N, Gras D, Kappenberger L, Tavazzi L. The effect of cardiac resynchronization on morbidity and mortality in heart failure. *N Engl J Med.* 2005;352(15):1539–49.
7. Strickberger SA, Conti J, Daoud EG, Havranek E, Mehra MR, Pina IL, Young J. Patient selection for cardiac resynchronization therapy: from the Council on Clinical Cardiology Subcommittee on Electrocardiography and Arrhythmias and the Quality of Care and Outcomes Research Interdisciplinary Working Group, in collaboration with the Heart Rhythm Society. *Circulation.* 2005;111(16):2146–50.
8. Vardas PE, Auricchio A, Blanc JJ, Daubert JC, Drexler H, Ector H, Gasparini M, Linde C, Morgado FB, Oto A, Sutton R, Trusz-Gluza M. Guidelines for cardiac pacing and cardiac resynchronization therapy: the task force for cardiac pacing and cardiac resynchronization therapy of the European Society of Cardiology. Developed in collaboration with the European Heart Rhythm Association. *Eur Heart J.* 2007;28(18):2256–95.
9. McAlister FA, Ezekowitz J, Hooton N, Vandermeer B, Spooner C, Dryden DM, Page RL, Hlatky MA, Rowe BH. Cardiac resynchronization therapy for patients with left ventricular systolic dysfunction: a systematic review. *JAMA.* 2007;297(22):2502–14.

10. Singh JP, Houser S, Heist EK, Ruskin JN. The coronary venous anatomy: a segmental approach to aid cardiac resynchronization therapy. *J Am Coll Cardiol.* 2005;46(1):68–74.
11. Chou CC, Kim DT, Fishbein MC, Chen PS. Marshall bundle and the valve of Vieussens. *J Cardiovasc Electrophysiol.* 2003;14(11):1254.
12. Meisel E, Pfeiffer D, Engelmann L, Tebbenjohanns J, Schubert B, Hahn S, Fleck E, Butter C. Investigation of coronary venous anatomy by retrograde venography in patients with malignant ventricular tachycardia. *Circulation.* 2001;104(4):442–7.
13. Karaca M, Bilge O, Dinckal MH, Ucerler H. The anatomic barriers in the coronary sinus: implications for clinical procedures. *J Interv Card Electrophysiol.* 2005;14(2): 89–94.
14. Giudici MC, Paul DL, Bontu P, Barold SS. Pacemaker and implantable cardioverter defibrillator implantation without reversal of warfarin therapy. *Pacing Clin Electrophysiol.* 2004;27(3):358–60.
15. Fox DJ, Davidson NC, Royle M, Bennett DH, Clarke B, Garratt CJ, Hall MC, Zaidi AM, Patterson K, Fitzpatrick AP. Safety and acceptability of implantation of internal cardioverter-defibrillators under local anesthetic and conscious sedation. *Pacing Clin Electrophysiol.* 2007;30(8):992–7.
16. Klug D, Balde M, Pavin D, Hidden-Lucet F, Clementy J, Sadoul N, Rey JL, Lande G, Lazarus A, Victor J, Barnay C, Grandbastien B, Kacet S. Risk factors related to infections of implanted pacemakers and cardioverter-defibrillators: results of a large prospective study. *Circulation.* 2007;116(12):1349–55.
17. Bertaglia E, Zerbo F, Zardo S, Barzan D, Zoppo F, Pascotto P. Antibiotic prophylaxis with a single dose of cefazolin during pacemaker implantation: incidence of long-term infective complications. *Pacing Clin Electrophysiol.* 2006;29(1):29–33.
18. Leon AR, Delurgio DB, Mera F. Practical approach to implanting left ventricular pacing leads for cardiac resynchronization. *J Cardiovasc Electrophysiol.* 2005;16(1): 100–5.
19. Sticherling C, Chough SP, Baker RL, Wasmer K, Oral H, Tada H, Horwood L, Kim MH, Pelosi F, Michaud GF, Strickberger SA, Morady F, Knight BP. Prevalence of central venous occlusion in patients with chronic defibrillator leads. *Am Heart J.* 2001;141(5):813–16.
20. Corcoran SJ, Lawrence C, McGuire MA. The valve of Vieussens: an important cause of difficulty in advancing catheters into the cardiac veins. *J Cardiovasc Electrophysiol.* 1999;10(6):804–8.
21. Jongbloed MR, Lamb HJ, Bax JJ, Schuijf JD, de Roos A, van der Wall EE, Schalij MJ. Noninvasive visualization of the cardiac venous system using multislice computed tomography. *J Am Coll Cardiol.* 2005;45(5):749–53.
22. Chiribiri A, Kelle S, Gotze S, Kriatselis C, Thouet T, Tangcharoen T, Paetsch I, Schnackenburg B, Fleck E, Nagel E. Visualization of the cardiac venous system using cardiac magnetic resonance. *Am J Cardiol.* 2008;101(3):407–12.
23. Butter C, Auricchio A, Stellbrink C, Fleck E, Ding J, Yu Y, Huvelle E, Spinelli J. Effect of resynchronization therapy stimulation site on the systolic function of heart failure patients. *Circulation.* 2001;104(25):3026–9.
24. Leon AR. New tools for the effective delivery of cardiac resynchronization therapy. *J Cardiovasc Electrophysiol.* 2005;16 Suppl 1:S42–S47.
25. Rivero-Ayerza M, Thornton AS, Theuns DA, Scholten MF, Mekel JM, Res J, Jordaens LJ. Left ventricular lead placement within a coronary sinus side branch using remote

magnetic navigation of a guidewire: a feasibility study. *J Cardiovasc Electrophysiol.* 2006;17(2):128–33.

26. Rivero-Ayerza M, van Belle Y, Mekel J, Jordaens LJ. Left ventricular lead implantation assisted by magnetic navigation in a patient with a persistent left superior vena cava. *Int J Cardiol.* 2007;116(1):E15–E17.

27. Burkhardt JD, Wilkoff BL. Interventional electrophysiology and cardiac resynchronization therapy: delivering electrical therapies for heart failure. *Circulation.* 2007;115(16):2208–20.

28. Singh JP, Fan D, Heist EK, Alabiad CR, Taub C, Reddy V, Mansour M, Picard MH, Ruskin JN, Mela T. Left ventricular lead electrical delay predicts response to cardiac resynchronization therapy. *Heart Rhythm.* 2006;3(11):1285–92.

29. Auricchio A, Fantoni C, Regoli F, Carbucicchio C, Goette A, Geller C, Kloss M, Klein H. Characterization of left ventricular activation in patients with heart failure and left bundle-branch block. *Circulation.* 2004;109(9):1133–9.

30. Vannan MA, Pedrizzetti G, Li P, Gurudevan S, Houle H, Main J, Jackson J, Nanda NC. Effect of cardiac resynchronization therapy on longitudinal and circumferential left ventricular mechanics by velocity vector imaging: description and initial clinical application of a novel method using high-frame rate B-mode echocardiographic images. *Echocardiography.* 2005;22(10):826–30.

31. Murphy RT, Sigurdsson G, Mulamalla S, Agler D, Popovic ZB, Starling RC, Wilkoff BL, Thomas JD, Grimm RA. Tissue synchronization imaging and optimal left ventricular pacing site in cardiac resynchronization therapy. *Am J Cardiol.* 2006;97(11): 1615–21.

32. Ammann P, Sticherling C, Kalusche D, Eckstein J, Bernheim A, Schaer B, Osswald S. An electrocardiogram-based algorithm to detect loss of left ventricular capture during cardiac resynchronization therapy. *Ann Intern Med.* 2005;142(12) Pt 1:968–73.

33. Hoffmeister P, Chaudhry GM, Orlov MV, Shukla G, Haffajee CI. Sheathless implantation of permanent coronary sinus-LV pacing leads. *Pacing Clin Electrophysiol.* 2006;29(2):117–23.

34. Knight BP, Desai A, Coman J, Faddis M, Yong P. Long-term retention of cardiac resynchronization therapy. *J Am Coll Cardiol.* 2004;44(1):72–7.

35. Alonso C, Leclercq C, d'Allonnes FR, Pavin D, Victor F, Mabo P, Daubert JC. Six year experience of transvenous left ventricular lead implantation for permanent biventricular pacing in patients with advanced heart failure: technical aspects. *Heart.* 2001;86(4):405–10.

36. Albertsen AE, Nielsen JC, Pedersen AK, Hansen PS, Jensen HK, Mortensen PT. Left ventricular lead performance in cardiac resynchronization therapy: impact of lead localization and complications. *Pacing Clin Electrophysiol.* 2005;28(6):483–8.

37. Gurevitz O, Nof E, Carasso S, Luria D, Bar-Lev D, Tanami N, Eldar M, Glikson M. Programmable multiple pacing configurations help to overcome high left ventricular pacing thresholds and avoid phrenic nerve stimulation. *Pacing Clin Electrophysiol.* 2005;28(12):1255–9.

38. Chalil S, Stegemann B, Muhyaldeen SA, Khadjooi K, Foley PW, Smith RE, Leyva F. Effect of posterolateral left ventricular scar on mortality and morbidity following cardiac resynchronization therapy. *Pacing Clin Electrophysiol.* 2007;30(10):1201–9.

39. Bleeker GB, Kaandorp TA, Lamb HJ, Boersma E, Steendijk P, de Roos A, van der Wall EE, Schalij MJ, Bax JJ. Effect of posterolateral scar tissue on clinical and

echocardiographic improvement after cardiac resynchronization therapy. *Circulation.* 2006;113(7):969–76.

40. Maya ID, Saddekni S, Allon M. Treatment of refractory central vein stenosis in hemodialysis patients with stents. *Seminars in dialysis.* 2007;20(1):78–82.

41. Sticherling C, Osswald S. Implantation of a biventricular defibrillator system in a patient with persistent left and absent right superior vena cava. *Heart.* 2006;92(10):1424.

42. Higgins SL, Hummel JD, Niazi IK, Giudici MC, Worley SJ, Saxon LA, Boehmer JP, Higginbotham MB, De Marco T, Foster E, Yong PG. Cardiac resynchronization therapy for the treatment of heart failure in patients with intraventricular conduction delay and malignant ventricular tachyarrhythmias. *J Am Coll Cardiol.* 2003;42(8):1454–9.

43. Medina-Ravell VA, Lankipalli RS, Yan GX, Antzelevitch C, Medina-Malpica NA, Medina-Malpica OA, Droogan C, Kowey PR. Effect of epicardial or biventricular pacing to prolong QT interval and increase transmural dispersion of repolarization: does resynchronization therapy pose a risk for patients predisposed to long QT or torsade de pointes? *Circulation.* 2003;107(5):740–6.

44. Leon AR, Abraham WT, Curtis AB, Daubert JP, Fisher WG, Gurley J, Hayes DL, Lieberman R, Petersen-Stejskal S, Wheelan K. Safety of transvenous cardiac resynchronization system implantation in patients with chronic heart failure: combined results of over 2,000 patients from a multicenter study program. *J Am Coll Cardiol.* 2005;46(12):2348–56.

45. Burke MC, Morton J, Lin AC, Tierney S, Desai A, Hong T, Kim S, Salem Y, Alberts M, Knight BP. Implications and outcome of permanent coronary sinus lead extraction and reimplantation. *J Cardiovasc Electrophysiol.* 2005;16(8):830–7.

46. Navia JL, Atik FA. Minimally invasive surgical alternatives for left ventricle epicardial lead implantation in heart failure patients. *Ann Thorac Surg.* 2005;80(2):751–4.

47. Navia JL, Atik FA, Grimm RA, Garcia M, Vega PR, Myhre U, Starling RC, Wilkoff BL, Martin D, Houghtaling PL, Blackstone EH, Cosgrove DM. Minimally invasive left ventricular epicardial lead placement: surgical techniques for heart failure resynchronization therapy. *Ann Thorac Surg.* 2005;79(5):1536–44; discussion 1536–44.

48. Doll N, Opfermann UT, Rastan AJ, Walther T, Bernau H, Gummert JF, Mohr FW. Facilitated minimally invasive left ventricular epicardial lead placement. *Ann Thorac Surg.* 2005;79(3):1023–5; discussion 1025.

49. Koos R, Sinha AM, Markus K, Breithardt OA, Mischke K, Zarse M, Schmid M, Autschbach R, Hanrath P, Stellbrink C. Comparison of left ventricular lead placement via the coronary venous approach versus lateral thoracotomy in patients receiving cardiac resynchronization therapy. *Am J Cardiol.* 2004;94(1):59–63.

50. Mair H, Sachweh J, Meuris B, Nollert G, Schmoeckel M, Schuetz A, Reichart B, Daebritz S. Surgical epicardial left ventricular lead versus coronary sinus lead placement in biventricular pacing. *Eur J Cardiothorac Surg.* 2005;27(2):235–42.

51. Schweikert RA, Saliba WI, Tomassoni G, Marrouche NF, Cole CR, Dresing TJ, Tchou PJ, Bash D, Beheiry S, Lam C, Kanagaratnam L, Natale A. Percutaneous pericardial instrumentation for endo-epicardial mapping of previously failed ablations. *Circulation.* 2003;108(11):1329–35.

52. Sauer WH, Bristow MR. The Comparison of Medical Therapy, Pacing, and Defibrillation in Heart Failure (COMPANION) trial in perspective. *J Interv Card Electrophysiol.* 2008;21:3–11.

Chapter 7

Programming CRT devices

Bengt Herweg, Arzu Ilercil, and S. Serge Barold

Key Points:

1. *The lower rate* of cardiac resynchronization therapy (CRT) devices should be programmed to permit atrial sensing because atrial pacing produces a lesser hemodynamic benefit and may predispose to atrial fibrillation. The *upper rate* should be relatively fast ($\geq$140 ppm) to prevent loss of atrial tracking with resultant inhibition of ventricular synchronization during sinus tachycardia and during exercise.

2. The postventricular atrial refractory period (PVARP) should be relatively short ($\leq$250 ms) to minimize or prevent migration of the sinus P wave into the PVARP, where it cannot be tracked. As atrio-ventricular (AV) conduction is often normal in CRT patients, functional atrial undersensing promotes spontaneous AV conduction that inhibits the delivery of biventricular pacing. It is important to turn off PVARP extension after a pacemaker-defined premature ventricular complex and algorithms that use PVARP prolongation for the automatic termination of pacemaker-mediated tachycardia. A short PVARP is safe because endless loop tachycardia is rare in CRT patients

3. Electrical desynchronization can occur as an upper-rate response but also at atrial rates *below* the programmed upper when P waves are continually trapped in the PVARP. A relatively slow upper rate, a long PVARP and a long PR interval predispose to the latter. A special pacemaker function can detect this form of electrical desynchronization *below* the upper rate and can restore P-wave tracking by automatic PVARP abbreviation for one cycle.

4. In selected patients, the left ventricular output can be programmed to ×1.5 the threshold voltage at the same pulse duration to conserve battery life

Pacing to Support the Failing Heart, 1st edition. Edited by K. Ellenbogen and A. Auricchio.
© 2008 American Heart Association, ISBN: 978-1-4051-7534-0

because CRT systems require a much higher current drain the battery than from conventional devices.

5. Atrial fibrillation and atrial tachyarrhythmias should be treated aggressively in CRT patients and if long-term sinus rhythm cannot be achieved, atrio-ventricular (AV) junctional ablation should be performed. With conservative therapy, the presence of CRT should be confirmed with Holter recordings and an exercise stress test.

6. In the presence of a bipolar left ventricular (LV) lead, some devices provide "electrical repositioning" whereby the two electrodes in each ventricle can be configured in a variety of combinations. This function can be useful in eliminating phrenic nerve stimulation and in lowering the LV output for pacing.

7. Availability of the 12-lead ECG during programming is essential. A negative complex (lack of a dominant R wave) in lead V_1 during biventricular pacing can occur in uncomplicated CRT, but commonly reflects a suboptimal balance between LV and right ventricular (RV) activation. Several problematic situations should be ruled out including lack of LV capture, suboptimal LV lead position, ventricular fusion with the conducted complex, LV latency and/or slowed intraventricular conduction. In contrast, CRT with RV outflow tract pacing often generates a negative complex in V_1.

8. Optimizing the AV delay should be done in most, if not all patients. The optimal AV delay changes with the passage of time. Methodology varies, and there is no gold standard. A degree of fusion with spontaneous right ventricular activity may be acceptable in some patients particularly if the intrinsic interval is short.

9. Both intra-atrial and inter-atrial conduction delay complicate AV optimization and occasionally may require AV junctional ablation to provide effective CRT. Inter-atrial conduction delay should be recognized before CRT implantation whereupon the atrial lead can be placed on the inter-atrial septum to prevent programming difficulties.

10. Despite the negative results of two trials, VV interval optimization may be beneficial in selected patients with a suboptimal CRT response. Patients with slow intra-ventricular conduction in the area of myocardial scar, LV latency, or less than satisfactory lead position may benefit from VV interval optimization. VV programming attempts to restore the balance of right and left ventricular depolarization. Most commonly, the left ventricle is pre-excited often by only 20 ms. Anodal stimulation cancels the VV delay to zero.

General considerations

The goal of cardiac resynchronization therapy (CRT) programming is to ensure ventricular resynchronization in virtually 100% of the time and to optimize and inter-ventricular timing. As heart failure patients represent a heterogeneous group, optimal CRT device performance can only be achieved by tailored programming on an individual basis. It is important to evaluate the patient as well as the device. One should assess the patient's New York Heart Association functional class, physical activity, current medications, and special problems, such as phrenic nerve stimulation. Heart rate histograms, the percentage of atrial and ventricular pacing, underlying atrial and ventricular rhythm abnormalities, and the 12-lead ECG should be studied before any programming activity. CRT programming requires careful attention to the patient's hemodynamic problem, knowledge of CRT device technology, and the electrocardiographic manifestations of normal and abnormal device function.

Twelve-lead electrocardiography

A 12-lead ECG is essential for CRT evaluation and should be available during device programming. A single-channel rhythm strip from a pacemaker programmer is inappropriate. During evaluation of CRT devices the 12-lead ECG yields important information about the presence or absence of fusion with the intrinsic conducted QRS complex, the balance between right ventricular (RV) and left ventricular (LV) activation, and the presence of RV anodal capture in patients with unipolar LV leads [1,2]. Complete assessment requires comparison of the QRS morphology during native conduction, single-chamber RV, single-chamber LV, and biventricular pacing.

QRS morphology during right ventricular pacing

Pacing from the RV, regardless of site, virtually always produces a left bundle branch block (LBBB) pattern in the precordial leads. RV apical pacing produces negative paced QRS complexes in the inferior leads (II, III, and aVF) because depolarization begins in the inferior part of the heart and travels superiorly away from the inferior leads. The mean paced QRS frontal-plane axis is always superior (Figure 7.1), usually in the left, or less commonly in the right superior quadrant. Pacing from the RV outflow tract or septum, shifts the frontal-plane–paced QRS axis to the left inferior quadrant, a site considered normal for spontaneous supraventricular QRS complexes. The inferior leads become positive. The axis then shifts to the right inferior quadrant as the stimulation site moves more superiorly toward the pulmonary valve. With the backdrop of dominant R waves in the inferior leads, RV outflow tract pacing may generate qR, QR, or Qr complexes in leads I and aVL but not in leads V_5 and V_6.

QRS morphology during left ventricular pacing from the coronary venous system

Single-site pacing from the posterior or postero-lateral coronary vein (the traditional sites for CRT) results in a right bundle branch block (RBBB) pattern in

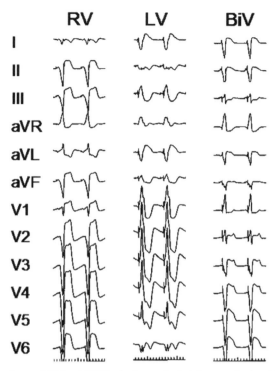

Fig. 7.1 Comparison of 12-lead ECGs during apical right ventricular (RV) pacing, left ventricualar (LV) pacing, and biventricular (BiV) pacing in a patient with a CRT device. During RV pacing, there is a left bundle branch pattern with a negative QRS complex in lead V_1, and the frontal-plane axis points toward the right superior quadrant. During LV pacing there is a dominant R wave in lead V_1 and right axis deviation. During BiV pacing there is also a dominant R wave in V_1, and the axis typically points to the right superior quadrant.

a correctly positioned lead V_1 [1–3] (Figure 7.1). Leads V_2 and V_3 may or may not be positive. With apical lead position, ECG leads V_4–V_6 are typically negative. With basal lead position, ECG leads V_4–V_6 are usually positive as with the concordant positive R waves during overt pre-excitation in left-sided accessory pathway conduction in the Wolff–Parkinson–White syndrome. Pacing from the middle or the great (anterior) cardiac vein (unsatisfactory sites for CRT) produces a LBBB pattern of depolarization [3].

Thus, when lead V_1 during LV pacing shows a negative QRS complex during LV pacing, one should consider incorrect ECG lead placement, lead location in the middle or great (anterior) cardiac vein or rarely an undefined mechanism involving a severe intra-myocardial conduction abnormality related to substantial scarring [4,5]. The frontal-plane axis during LV pacing from the lateral and

infero-lateral wall often points to the right inferior quadrant (right axis deviation), (Figure 7.1), less commonly to the right superior quadrant and only
occasionally the axis may point to the left inferior or left superior quadrant.

QRS morphology during biventricular pacing

Biventricular pacing with the RV lead located at the apex

Biventricular pacing often shifts the frontal-plane vector to the right superior
quadrant in an anticlockwise fashion (as if starting with RV pacing) although the
frontal-plane axis may occasionally reside in the left superior quadrant during
uncomplicated biventricular pacing [1,2].

The QRS is often positive in lead V_1 during biventricular pacing when the RV
is paced from the apex (Figure 7.1). A negative QRS complex in lead V_1 may
occur during uncomplicated biventricular pacing but its presence mandates a
thorough investigation to rule out the following situations:

- Incorrect placement of lead V_1 (too high on the chest) [1,2], lack of LV capture,
- LV lead displacement, marked LV latency (exit block) [5],
- Major conduction delay from a scarred LV stimulation site [4],
- Ventricular fusion with the conducted QRS complex, coronary venous pacing
  via the middle cardiac vein (also the anterior cardiac vein) [3], or
- Unintended placement of two leads in the RV.

A negative QRS complex in lead V_1 during uncomplicated biventricular pacing probably reflects different activation of a heterogeneous biventricular substrate (ischemia, scar, His–Purkinje participation in view of the varying patterns
of LV activation in spontaneous LBBB, etc.) and does not necessarily indicate a
poor (electrical or mechanical) contribution from LV stimulation.

Biventricular pacing with the RV lead in the outflow tract

During biventricular pacing with the RV lead in the outflow tract, the paced
QRS in lead V_1 is often negative and the frontal–plane–paced QRS axis is often
directed to the right inferior quadrant (right axis deviation) (Figure 7.2) [2].

Frontal-plane axis of the paced QRS complex

Figure 7.2 shows the importance of the frontal-plane axis of the paced QRS
complex in the evaluation of pacing during single-chamber (RV and LV) pacing
and biventricular pacing.

Ventricular fusion

Ventricular fusion with the intrinsic conducted QRS complex may decrease the
effectiveness of CRT in some patients while others with a short PR interval may
actually benefit from it. The clinical and hemodynamic impact of fusion in the
individual patient can only be determined by trial and error [6]. The presence
of ventricular fusion should be suspected in the presence of marked QRS

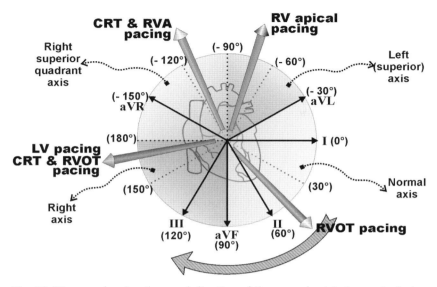

Fig. 7.2 Diagram showing the usual direction of the mean frontal-plane axis during RV apical pacing, RV outflow tract pacing, LV pacing from the coronary venous system, and biventricular pacing (RV at the apex and outflow tract). LV = left ventricular, RV = right ventricular, RVOT = right ventricular outflow tract. (Modified with permission from Barold SS, Stroobandt RX, Sinnaeve AF. *Cardiac Pacemakers Step By Step. An Illustrated Guide*, Malden MA, Blackwell-Futura, 2004.)

narrowing, especially in patients with a short spontaneous PR interval (Figure 7.3). It should be ruled out by observing the paced QRS morphology during progressive shortening of the AS–VP (atrial sensing–ventricular pacing) interval in the VDD mode or the AP–VP (atrial pacing–ventricular pacing) interval in the DDD mode.

QRS duration

Measurement of QRS duration during follow-up is helpful in the analysis of appropriate biventricular capture and the presence of fusion with intrinsic conduction. Chronic studies have shown that the degree of narrowing of the paced QRS duration is a poor predictor of the mechanical CRT response [2,7]. In this context, it is interesting that single-chamber LV pacing with a paced QRS complex is wider than that of biventricular pacing, which can produce CRT virtually as effective as that of biventricular pacing [8]. Loss of capture in one ventricle will cause a change in the paced QRS morphology and duration in the 12-lead ECG similar to that of either single- chamber RV or LV pacing. As the paced QRS during biventricular pacing is often narrower than that of single-chamber RV or LV pacing, widening of the paced QRS complex may reflect loss of capture in one chamber with effectual capture in the other.

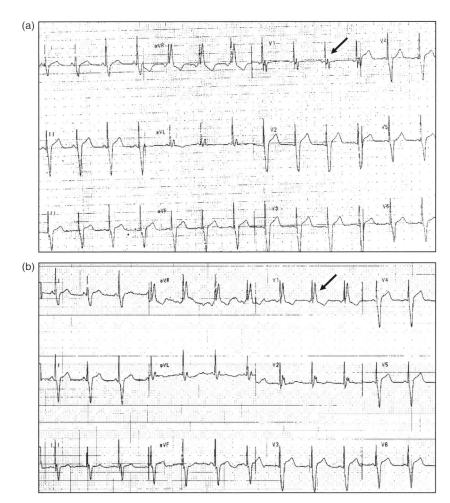

Fig. 7.3 Fusion with spontaneous ventricular activation in a patient with a short PR interval. (a). This 12-lead ECG was acquired immediately on the arrival of the patient in the pacemaker clinic. There is marked narrowing of the paced QRS complex (well-seen in V_1) due to ventricular fusion with spontaneous right ventricular activity. AV delay = 100 ms. (b) This tracing was acquired after the patient rested in a supine position(sympathetic tone now decreased) for 10 minutes. The dominant R wave in lead V1 indicates an increased LV contribution to ventricular activation. The QRS complex is still relatively narrow. AV delay = 100 ms. (Modified with permission from [1].)

Upper-rate response

Upper-rate behavior of CRT devices differs from that of conventional pacemakers because the majority of CRT patients have relatively normal sinus node function and AV conduction [9]. When the atrial rate exceeds the programmed upper-rate, biventricular pacemakers exhibit two forms of upper-rate behavior according to the location of the P wave in the pacemaker cycle.

Pre-empted Wenckebach upper-rate response

In the setting of a relatively short postventricular atrial refractory period (PVARP) when the spontaneous ventricular cycle shortens beyond the programmed upper-rate interval, the AV interval of each pacemaker cycle becomes partially or incompletely extended (greater than the programmed AS–VP interval) creating an attempted Weckenbach type upper-rate response (Figure 7.4). There are no pacemaker stimuli because the P wave and the spontaneous QRS complex are both sensed by the device. This form of upper-rate response based on a sinus rate faster than the programmed (atrial-driven) upper rate, tends to occur in patients with relatively normal AV conduction, a short programmed AV delay, a short PVARP, and a relatively slow programmed (atrial-driven) upper rate [9].

Upper-rate limitation with P wave in the PVARP

When the PP interval during biventricular pacing becomes shorter than the total atrial refractory period (TARP) (in the setting of relatively normal sinus node function), spontaneous P waves fall into the PVARP where they cannot be tracked. The conducted QRS complex (VS) linked to the preceding P wave (in the PVARP) initiates a PVARP that will contain the succeeding P wave [9]. This sequence ensures the perpetuation of functional atrial undersensing with loss of biventricular pacing. The prevailing AV delay (or the spontaneous PR interval or AR–VS) is longer than the programmed AS–VP. There are no pauses and no pacemaker stimuli. This form of upper response is therefore quite different from 2:1 fixed-ratio block produced by conventional pacemakers because all the P waves remain in the PVARP

Programming the upper rate

Because patients with heart failure are susceptible to sinus tachycardia (particularly during heart failure exacerbation with elevated sympathetic tone), it is important to program a relatively fast upper rate to avoid an upper-rate response manifested by the emergence of spontaneous conducted QRS complexes. In patients with normal sinus and AV nodal function the risk of tracking rapid atrial rates with a biventricular device is not an important issue. Therefore, it is appropriate to program the upper rate to ≥ 140 bpm. If necessary the tendency toward sinus tachycardia may be attenuated by larger doses of beta-blockers, an important consideration in patients with an ICD and slow ventricular

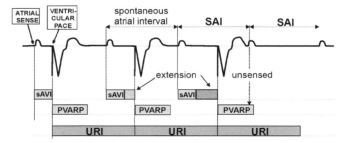

(a) **Normal upper rate response of the Wenckebach type**

(b) **The pre-empted Wenckebach behavior with short sAVI**

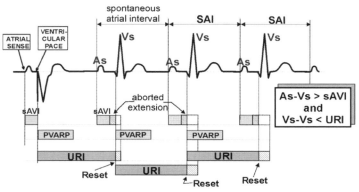

Fig. 7.4 (a) Traditional Wenckebach upper-rate response in an antibradycardia DDD pace-maker. The spontaneous atrial interval (SAI) is shorter than the programmed upper- rate interval but *longer* than the total atrial refractory period (TARP). The AV delay (AS–VP) lengthens gradually until a P wave falls in the PVARP where it cannot be tracked. A pause then occurs and the next P wave restarts the same sequence. When the SAI becomes *shorter* than the TARP, the pacemaker responds with a fixed-ratio (such as the 2:1 block) upper-rate behavior. (b) When the spontaneous ventricular rate exceeds the programmed upper rate (VS-VS < URI), a pre-empted Wenckebach upper-rate response supervenes. The device senses all of the P waves (AS) and spontaneous QRS complexes (VS). There are no pacemaker stimuli or pauses typical of a traditional Wenckebach upper-rate response. AS conducts and generates VS so that the AV delay (AS–VS interval, which is the spon-taneous PR interval) becomes longer than the programmed AS–VP interval. Note that all the sinus P waves are sensed beyond the PVARP and SAI > TARP. AS initiates an AV delay. The AS–VP interval is extended to conform to the URI because the device cannot release VP until the URI has timed out. VS occurs when the AV delay is only partially extended (i.e. before completion of the URI). The device senses VS so that VS pre-empts the release of VP expected at the termination of the URI. AS = atrial sensed event, VS = ventricular sensed event, When the SAI becomes shorter than the TARP, all of the P waves will be confined to the PVARP and AR–VS (AR = atrial refractrory sensed event) sequences will occur in contrast to the traditional fixed-ratio block response. VP = ven-tricular paced event, PVARP = postventricular atrial refractory period, URI = upper-rate interval, sAVI = sensed AV delay initiated by atrial sensing. (Reproduced with permission from Barold SS, Stroobandt RX, Sinnaeve AF. *Cardiac Pacemakers Step By Step. An Illustrated Guide*, Malden MA, Blackwell-Futura, 2004).

tachycardia (VT) where the VT detection rate must be faster then the programmed upper rate.

Loss of resynchronization below the programmed upper rate and optimal programming of PVARP

Desynchronized fast AR–VS sequences containing trapped or locked P waves within the PVARP can occur in an upper-rate response but also in some circumstances below the programmed upper rate [9–11]. There are numerous causes of electrical desynchronization at rates slower than the programmed upper rate especially in association with a relatively long PVARP. For example, during sinus rhythm (below the upper rate), a sensed ventricular premature complex wave (or an oversensed T wave) initiates a regular PVARP. This event shifts pacemaker timing so that the succeeding undisturbed sinus P wave now falls into the PVARP. This refractory-sensed P wave inside the PVARP conducts to the ventricle producing a spontaneous QRS complex sensed by the device. The sinus P waves will remain trapped in the PVARP as long as the PP interval is shorter than the prevailing TARP equal to [(AR–VS) + PVARP]. Hence, biventricular pacing will remain inhibited until either the occurrence of a non-refractory sensed atrial depolarization (when the PP intervals becomes longer than the prevailing TARP) or an atrial pacing pulse occurs outside the TARP. Similarly, when a fast atrial rate (above the programmed upper rate) gradually drops below the programmed upper rate, biventricular pacing will remain inhibited for some time according to the above prevailing TARP formula. Based on these considerations, one should program a short PVARP of 250 ms or less. The PVARP extension after a ventricular premature complex should be turned off as well as the pacemaker-mediated tachycardia termination algorithm based on PVARP prolongation for one cycle. A short PVARP is safe because endless loop tachycardia is rare in CRT patients without conduction system disease apart from left bundle branch block or its equivalent.

Some devices provide a programmable option to record ventricular sensing episodes. Such recordings are useful in reprogramming CRT devices. Many such episodes are due to AF or unsustained slow VT. The latter is very common and often of no important clinical significance. These ventricular sensing recordings may provide a clue to the mechanism of electrical desynchronization, such as an unsuspected upper-rate response requiring reprogramming of the upper rate to a faster value.

Programming automatic unlocking of P waves from the PVARP

Locking of the P wave in the PVARP is facilitated by a long spontaneous PR interval, a long PVARP and a relatively slow programmed upper rate [11,12]. Special algorithms can be programmed to restore 1:1 atrial tracking when P waves are locked in the PVARP at rates slower than the programmed upper rate. A device can detect AR–VS sequences, a situation suggestive of electrical ventricular desynchronization whereupon temporary PVARP abbreviation permits the device to sense a sinus P wave beyond the PVARP promoting atrial tracking and ventricular resynchronization (Figure 7.5). These algorithms do not function when the atrial rate is faster than the programmed upper rate or during automatic mode switching. They are particularly useful in patients with sinus tachycardia and first-degree AV block in whom prolonged locking of P waves inside the PVARP can be an important problem [12].

Programming the lower rate

The optimal lower rate in CRT patients is unknown and may exhibit great variability according to the presence and severity of heart failure. One should always aim for atrial sensing, which is hemodynamically more favorable than atrial pacing [13]. There is evidence that atrial pacing may increase the risk of atrial fibrillation [14]. Thus, the lower rate should be programmed to maintain sinus rhythm. In the occasional patient an accelerated idioventricular or junctional rhythm may compete with biventricular pacing and require an increase in the lower rate limit to overdrive and suppress the interfering rhythm.

Far-field, R-wave oversensing

Far-field, R-wave oversensing on the atrial channel impairs dual-chamber, supra-ventricular tachycardia–(VT) discrimination but it does not cause inappropriate detection of VT when the ventricular rate remains in the sinus zone. It may also cause inappropriate mode switching and loss of electrical desynchronization in the DDI mode. Far-field, R-wave oversensing often shows a pattern of alternating short and long atrial cycle lengths because the marker depicting the oversensed R wave remains close to the ventricular electrogram. Control of far-field, R-wave sensing can be achieved by programmability in several ways:

1 Prolongation of the postventricular atrial blanking period, which carries the risk of undersensing atrial fibrillation.
2 Decrease of atrial sensitivity, which can also jeopardize sensing of atrial fibrillation.
3 Algorithmic rejection by identifying a specific pattern of atrial and ventricular events (Medtronic PR Logic).
4 Programmable automatic decrease of atrial sensitivity after ventricular events. This function is similar to the dynamic ventricular sensitivity in implantable cardioverter-defibrillator (ICD) devices.

Atrial fibrillation and atrial tachyarrhythmia

Many patients undergoing CRT have a history of paroxysmal atrial tachyarrhythmias, which are often associated with a rapid ventricular response that

(a)

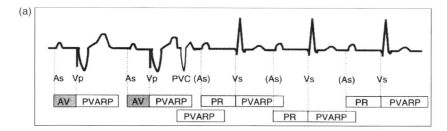

(b)

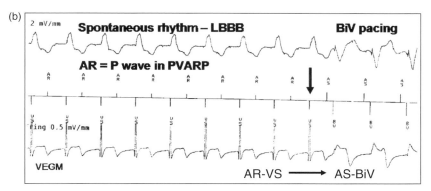

Fig. 7.5 (a) Diagrammatic representation of loss of ventricular synchronization induced by a premature ventricular complex (PVC). The sinus P wave following the PVC falls in the PVARP initiated by the PVC. The device does not track this P wave, which conducts to the ventricle giving rise to a QRS complex sensed by the pacemaker. The timing cycles are altered so that the sinus P waves now fall within the PVARP initiated by sensing the spontaneous QRS complex. Note that desynchronization or locking of the P waves within the PVARP occurs at a rate slower than the programmed upper rate. AS = atrial sensed event, (AS) = atrial sensed event within the pacemaker atrial refractory period, VS = ventricular sensed event, AV = atrioventricular delay, PVARP = postventricular atrial refractory period, PR = PR interval. (b) Automatic restoration of ventricular resynchronization. On the left there is ventricular desynchronization (AR–VS sequences) in a patient with first-degree AV block. The CRT device restores ventricular resynchronization with an algorithm that detects a specific number of AR–VS sequences (interpreted by the device as loss of resynchronization) and then temporarily abbreviates the PVARP (arrow). The shorter PVARP permits P wave tracking and restores ventricular resynchronization (AS–VP sequences at the programmed AV delay) on the right of the recording. AS = atrial sensed event, AR = atrial sensed event in the pacemaker atrial refractory period, VS = ventricular sensed event, VP = ventricular paced event, PVARP = postventricular atrial-refractory period, LBBB = left bundle branch block, BiV = biventricular, CRT = cardiac resynchronization therapy. (Reproduced with permission from Barold et al. [9] and Barold et al. [12].)

inhibits the delivery of CRT. Heart rate may be controlled at rest but not during exercise, and even if the mean heart rate is pharmacologically controlled, pronounced RR variability of conducted beats may decrease the number of resynchronized beats. Atrial fibrillation (AF) and atrial tachyarrhythmias should be treated aggressively, and if long-term sinus rhythm cannot be achieved, AV junctional ablation should be performed. In this respect, one should not be mislead by what appears to be a satisfactory percentage of stored paced beats because many stored beats could be fusion and/or pseudofusion beats unrelated to effective electrical resynchronization. Gasparini et al. [15] reported that heart failure patients with permanent AF treated with CRT showed sustained long-term improvements of LV function and functional capacity similar to patients in sinus rhythm, only if AV junctional ablation was performed.

Some devices have programmable algorithms that increase the percentage of biventricular pacing during AF so as to promote some degree of rate regularization and CRT (without an overall increase in the ventricular rate) by dynamic matching with the patient's own ventricular responses (up to the programmed maximum tracking rate) [11]. Activation of this algorithm does not result in ventricular rate control and should not be a substitute for AV junctional ablation. Automatic mode switching should be activated and is particularly important in patients with relatively slow conduction to the ventricle. Some devices have a lower rate interval that may be set separately during mode switching with the intent of increasing the percentage of biventricular pacing by virtue of a relatively fast pacing rate during the DDI mode. There is no need to program mode switching in patients without a history of atrial tachyarrhythmias because far-field, R-wave sensing may cause repeated automatic mode switching and electrical desynchronization in some devices when the base rate in the DDI mode is not particularly fast.

Programming of left ventricular pacing output

Traditionally, a safety margin of twice the voltage threshold is recommended for LV capture. Battery longevity is an important consideration in CRT devices where two ventricles are being paced continuously and LV pacing may require a high output as the pacing threshold is generally twice that of RV pacing. Thus, an LV safety margin of 1.5 times the voltage threshold may be reasonable without increasing the risk of asystole [16]. Such a lower safety margin must be individualized. Battery longevity may be enhanced by future algorithms that automatically measure the LV threshold and may help maintain LV capture while reducing output.

Phrenic nerve stimulation and electrical repositioning

Phrenic nerve stimulation is a common problem and may become evident only when the patient becomes active and changes body position. This complication is related to the anatomic vicinity of the left phrenic nerve to the LV pacing site, especially when the LV lead is placed into a posterior or postero-lateral coronary vein. During implantation in the sedated and supine patient, phrenic nerve stimulation can be difficult to demonstrate. It may also be related to LV lead microdislodgment. Phrenic nerve stimulation can often be controlled by lowering the LV voltage (maintaining capture) provided the capture threshold for phrenic nerve stimulation is much higher than that of LV capture. Programming the pulse duration is generally ineffective.

With bipolar LV leads, some device manufacturers provide innovative programming options that allow a change in pacing configuration from true bipolar RV and LV pacing to a variety of pacing arrangements between the electrodes of both ventricular leads [17]. Such "electrical repositioning" alters the LV–RV pacing vector noninvasively, and the multiple LV pacing configurations are clinically useful in patients undergoing CRT system implantation by helping to overcome high LV pacing thresholds and phrenic nerve stimulation, and by providing more flexibility in placing the LV lead.

Gurevitz et al. [17] compared CRT systems capable of multiple LV pacing configurations implanted in 43 patients with a control group of 49 patients who received CRT systems lacking this feature. Acute high (≥ 2.5 V/0.5 ms) LV pacing thresholds were encountered in 13 (30%) of the study group and in 25 (50%) of the control group patients ($p = 0.03$). Phrenic nerve stimulation was encountered in 5 (12%) of the study group and in 12 (24%) of the control group patients ($p = 0.13$). All cases of high LV pacing thresholds and phrenic nerve stimulation in the study group were managed by switching to a different LV pacing configuration, while high thresholds remained in control group patients, and phrenic nerve stimulation was managed by replacing or repositioning the lead.

Anodal stimulation in biventricular pacemakers

Although anodal capture may occur with high output traditional bipolar RV pacing, this phenomenon is almost always not discernible electrocardiographically. Biventricular pacing systems that use a unipolar lead for LV pacing via a coronary vein may create RV anodal pacing. The tip electrode of the LV lead is the cathode and the proximal electrode of the bipolar RV lead often provides the anode for LV pacing. This arrangement creates a common anode for RV and LV pacing. A high current density (from two sources) at the common anode during biventricular pacing may cause anodal capture manifested as a paced QRS complex with a somewhat different configuration from that derived from standard biventricular pacing [16].

A different form of anodal capture involving the proximal electrode of the bipolar RV lead can also occur with contemporary biventricular pacemakers with separately programmable ventricular outputs. During monochamber LV pacing at a relatively high output, RV anodal capture produces a paced QRS

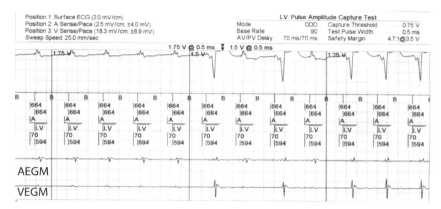

Fig. 7.6 Anodal capture during left ventricular (LV) pacing in a patient with a CRT system with a unipolar LV lead. The paced QRS morphology during LV pacing is shown on the left side. This is identical to the pattern that was previously recorded with biventricular pacing. This response was due to ventricular capture at the common anodal site in the right ventricle (RV) (proximal or ring electrode of the RV lead) with consequent capture of both the LV and the RV simultaneously. Intermittent capture of the isolated LV occurred only after the LV output was decreased to 1.5 V at 0.5 ms. Monochamber LV pacing became continual at 1.25 V and 0.5 ms. Thus, the RV anodal threshold was 1.75 V at 0.5ms. A = atrial paced event, AEGM = atrial electrogram, LV = LV paced event, VEGM = ventricular electrogram. (Reproduced with permission from Barold et al. [2].)

complex identical to that registered with biventricular pacing (Figure 7.6) [18,19]. Occasionally this type of anodal capture prevents electrocardiographic documentation of pure LV pacing if the LV pacing threshold is higher than that of RV anodal stimulation. Such anodal stimulation may complicate threshold testing and should not be misinterpreted as pacemaker malfunction. Furthermore, if the LV threshold is not too high, appropriate programming of the LV output should eliminate anodal stimulation in most cases. It is important to understand that in the presence of anodal capture it is impossible to advance the LV activation by VV interval programming because the effective VV interval remains at zero. The use of true bipolar LV leads eliminates all forms of RV anodal stimulation [20].

Triggered ventricular pacing

The triggered ventricular pacing mode, available in some devices, is a programmable option that attempts resynchronization by triggering a biventricular output immediately when the CRT device senses a spontaneous QRS complex within the programmed AV delay or it senses a pacemaker-defined ventricular premature complex. Because ventricular sensing in modern CRT devices is limited to the RV channel, only rhythms arising from the RV will be sensed relatively early to possibly allow resynchronization by triggered LV pacing. Ectopic rhythms arising remotely from the RV lead will be sensed relatively late, and, therefore, the delivered triggered stimuli may occur too late for effective electrical resynchronization. There are no data about the efficacy of triggered biventricular pacing: Does pacing-induced LV depolarization actually occur, and if it does, to what degree?

Verification of programmed settings by exercise testing

Exercise testing in CRT patients is now technically less difficult with the advent of wireless device telemetry. Exercise testing is helpful in the overall evaluation of CRT particularly in patients with a suboptimal CRT response where no obvious cause is found at rest [21]. An exercise test may reveal loss of capture, atrial undersensing, various arrhythmias, and the development of spontaneous AV conduction because of PR shortening or upper-rate limitation. In the latter, the upper rate should be reprogrammed to ensure consistent biventricular capture with effort. Exercise testing is vital in CRT patients with permanent atrial fibrillation who have not undergone ablation of the AV junction.

In CRT patients with severe chronotropic incompetence (defined by the failure to achieve 85% of the age-predicted heart rate (determined as 220—the patient's age) rate-adaptive pacing DDDR may provide incremental benefit on exercise capacity [22]. An exercise test facilitates programming the rate-adaptive mode and its related parameters.

Programming the AV interval

Although optimization of the left-sided AV interval timing is important, the majority of acute and long-term CRT benefit depends mostly on reliable ventricular resynchronization (with the proper choice of the LV pacing site) and less on AV optimization [23,24]. Nevertheless, programming of the left-sided AV interval in CRT patient is important and should be aimed primarily toward maintenance of LV pre-excitation to assure delivery of CRT and secondarily toward optimization of atrio-ventricular timing. In patients with intact AV conduction and short PR intervals, both goals *may not be* achievable. Optimization rarely, if ever will convert a nonresponder to a responder, but may convert an underresponder to improved status. The optimal AV delay in CRT patients exhibits great variability from patient to patient [23,25]. Therefore, empiric programming of the AV interval is suboptimal in many patients and is generally not recommended.

The optimal AV relationship

Optimized AV synchrony is achieved by the AV delay setting that provides the best left atrial contribution to LV filling, the maximum stroke volume, shortening

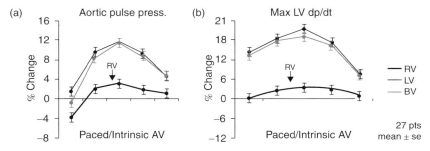

Fig. 7.7 AV delay optimization. Average percentage change in systolic parameters as a function of 5 normalized AV delays for each pacing chamber (RV, LV, and BiV) in 20 patients with a QRS complex 180 ± 22 ms. Tested AV delays were normalized to the patient's PR interval minus 30 ms. Data points are shown with SE bars. Solid points are significantly different from 0 (paired t test, $p < 0.0001$). (a) Changes in aortic pulse pressure. (b) Changes in LV + dP/dt. BiV = biventricular, LV = left ventricle, RV = right ventricle. (Reproduced with permission from Auricchio et al. [23].)

of the isovolumic contraction time, and the longest diastolic filling time in the absence of diastolic mitral regurgitation (in patients with a long PR interval) (Figures 7.7 and 7.8) [26,27]. At optimal AV delay settings, late diastolic filling by atrial contraction is complete, diastolic mitral regurgitation is absent, and the LV diastolic filling time is maximized, which results in maximal stroke volume and cardiac output. At the optimal AV delay, there is maximum time for early diastolic LV filling without compromise of late diastolic filling, and the end of atrial contraction coincides with onset of rise in LV pressure (Figure 7.9). As a rule of thumb, one should program the shortest AV delay that does not compromise the transmitral Doppler A wave.

Prolonged AV conduction and too-long AV delay

Prolonged AV conduction is not uncommon in heart failure patients. In this situation, atrial contraction occurs too early in diastole causing an ineffective or decreased atrial contribution to cardiac output. Atrial depolarization begins too early resulting in superimposition of atrial contraction on the early diastolic LV filling phase. On the transmitral Doppler signal a relatively early A wave fuses with a relatively late E wave, which results in a shortening of the LV diastolic filling time (Figure 7.9). A prolonged PR interval or a too-long AV delay induces diastolic mitral regurgitation. Following atrial contraction, the mitral valve remains open because LV contraction is delayed and LV diastolic pressure exceeds left atrial pressure during atrial relaxation, thereby producing diastolic mitral regurgitation, a decrease in preload (LV end diastolic pressure) at the onset of LV systole and, ultimately, a decrease in the peak rate of rise of LV pressure

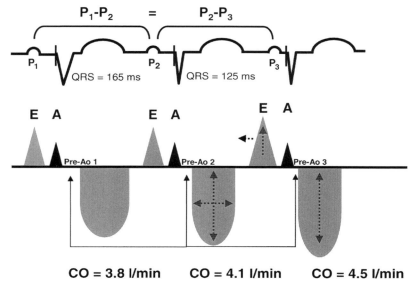

Fig. 7.8 Consequences of optimization of AV delay during biventricular pacing at stable heart rate. The QRS complex resulting from P_1 is wide due to apical right ventricular pacing (165 ms). The aortic pre-ejection time interval (Pre-Ao1) d is long; the aortic systolic phase is also long due to the wide QRS complex. The second QRS complex resulting from P_2 is narrowed due to biventricular pacing leading to a shorter aortic pre-ejection time interval (Pre-Ao2) compared with Pre-Ao1. Consequently, time duration of the aortic systolic phase is reduced, and the E-wave corresponding to P_3 occurs earlier (compared to P_1 and P_2) with a greater amplitude, indicating a better LV filling phase. Pre-Ao3 is even shorter than Pre-Ao2 due to the addition of an AV delay optimization during P_3, resulting in a greater cardiac output (CO) during P_3 compared with the one obtained during P_2, in which biventricular pacing was delivered without AV delay optimization. (Reproduced with permission from Bax et al. [26].)

during isovolumetric contraction (LV dP/dt_{max}) and cardiac output. The subsequent decreased cardiac output is poorly tolerated in heart failure patients.

Short AV delay

A short AV delay results in premature LV contraction that causes premature mitral valve closure, which, in turn, compromises the left atrial contribution to LV filling. LV filling during atrial contraction is interrupted by LV contraction (early mitral valve closure) resulting in truncation of the relatively late A wave on the transmitral Doppler signal and a relatively early E-wave, and therefore, a longer LV filling time with widely separated E and A waves (Figure 7.9). The

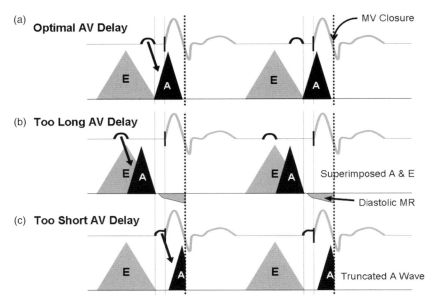

Fig. 7.9 Schematic diagram of the effect of AV delay duration on Doppler echocardiographic recordings of transmitral flow. (a) Note that when the AV interval is optimal, the mitral valve closes at the end of the A wave. (b) If the AV delay is too long (middle panel), the E and A waves fuse and the duration of diastolic filling is reduced. Late diastolic mitral regurgitation (MR) may occur. (c) If the AV delay is too short (bottom panel), E and A waves are widely separated and the A wave is truncated by early mitral valve (MV) closure prior to completion of left ventricular filling during atrial contraction.

low LV end-diastolic pressure and loss in preload is reflected in a decreased LV dP/dt_{max} and LV stroke volume.

Invasive and noninvasive methods of AV optimization

In clinical practice, there are many techniques for AV interval optimization in CRT patients as well as great variability in their use. The best method of measuring or assessing the effects of AV interval programming in terms of accuracy, cost, rapidity, ease and perhaps full automaticity remains to be defined but a recently developed semi-automatic method holds great promise.

Echocardiography

Currently, there is no universally accepted gold standard method for AV optimization; the method used often depends on local expertise and resources (Figures 7.10 and 7.11).

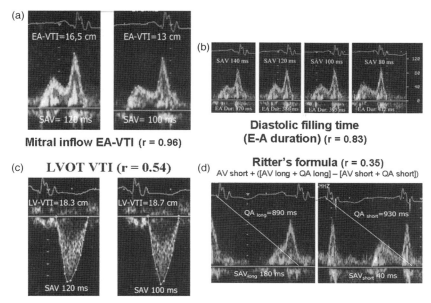

Fig. 7.10 Comparison of several echocardiographic techniques for AV delay optimization. (a) Velocity-time integral (VTI) of transmitral flow (EA VTI) at 2 consecutive sensed AV delays (SAV). The values are the average of four heart beats. Note the clear difference in EA VTI value with change in the sensed AV delay. (b) EA duration of four different sensed AV delays (SAV). Shortening of the sensed AV delay increased the EA duration by progressively separating the E and A waves. At 80 ms, the A wave is abbreviated, therefore the optimal AV delay by EA duration is 100 ms. This example illustrates the difficulty in judging the A-wave abbreviation. (c) Example of the VTI of the left ventricular outflow tract (LVOT VTI) at two adjacent sensed AV delays (SAV). The LVOT VTI is averaged from four beats. (d) Pulsed-wave Doppler signals of transmitral flow at long and short sensed AV delays (SAV) (180 ms and 40 ms, respectively). The corresponding QA time (time from the onset of electrical activation until the end of the A wave) is using. Ritter's formula for optimizing AV delay. The left-sided optimal AV delay is calculated as $AV_{short} + ([AV_{long} + QA_{long}] - [AV_{short} + QA_{short}])$. In this example, the derived optimal AV delay is 140 ms. (Reproduced with permission from Jansen et al. [31].)

Mitral inflow (Ritter) method

AV delay optimization of conventional and CRT devices is commonly performed by the Ritter method [28,29] that evaluates transmitral flow using pulsed wave Doppler. The method assumes that LV diastolic filling is optimized when mitral valve closure due to LV systole, coincides with the end of the Doppler A wave. This approach provides the longest diastolic filling time and allows completion of LV end-diastolic filling prior to LV contraction. The method does not assess forward output.

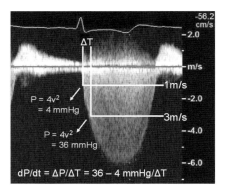

Fig. 7.11 Doppler derived dP/dt determined by measuring the time difference (ΔT) between two points of the continuous wave mitral regurgitation spectral signal corresponding, as indicated, to 1 m/s and 3 m/s. These points correspond to pressure gradients between the LV and LA of 4 mm and 36 mmHg according to the modified Bernoulli equation ($\Delta P = 4v^2$). dP/dt is determined by this change in pressure (32 mmHg) divided by the time difference. P = pressure, T = time, v = velocity. (Reproduced with permission from Barold et al. [73].)

Limitations of the Ritter method in CRT patients

Ritter's method has been evaluated in patients with normal LV ejection fractions and dual-chamber pacemakers for AV block [28,29]. In a study evaluating 40 CRT patients with severe heart failure, the optimized AV delay by the aortic velocity time integral (VTI) method was significantly longer than that calculated from the Ritter method [30]. In CRT patients with normal or short PR interval (<150 ms), the Ritter method cannot ensure biventricular pacing with the long AV delay used for the second part of the protocol. Furthermore, it is difficult to determine whether the A wave is abbreviated or not as increased LV end diastolic pressure in heart failure promotes mitral valve closure immediately after the A wave. The Ritter method is also difficult to carry out at high heart rates. Moreover, there is evidence that it may not represent the maximum achievable hemodynamic benefit [31].

Iterative method

This method involves programming a long AV delay then shortening it by 20 ms increments while monitoring pulse wave Doppler transmitral inflow until truncation of the A wave is noted [32]. Optimal AV delay is then identified by lengthening the AV delay in 10-ms increments until A-wave truncation is no longer present.

Velocity–time integral (VTI) methods

AV delay (and VV) optimizations with Doppler echocardiography are often done by assessing the VTI [26,31,33–38] of flow across the LV outflow tract, aortic valves, or mitral valves. Such VTI measures are directly proportional to LV stroke volume. The optimal AV delay is associated with the largest VTI. LV stroke volume can be estimated by measuring the diameter of the LV outflow tract (in the parasternal long-axis view) to calculate its area (assumed circular) and by using pulsed wave Doppler to interrogate LV outflow tract (in the apical five-chamber view) to obtain its VTI. The product of LV outflow tract area and its VTI estimates stroke volume. Small changes in the angle of incidence between the outflow jet and ultrasound beam or a small measurement error of LV outflow tract diameter can introduce significant inaccuracy into the calculated stroke volume. Thoroughly trained sonographers are needed to maintain consistency in methodology.

Aortic VTI obtained by continuous wave Doppler is more reproducible than LV outflow tract VTI measured by pulsed wave Doppler. Changes in aortic VTI can serve as a surrogate for changes in stroke volume as it is directly proportional to the LV outflow tract VTI. The mitral VTI is usually obtained from the apical four-chamber view using pulsed wave Doppler to sample at the tip of the mitral valve leaflets. Diastolic flow including both the E and A waves are included in the VTI. Stroke volume cannot be derived from the mitral VTI.

A randomized, prospective, single-blind clinical trial, compared AV optimization–guided by aortic VTI at AV intervals between 60 ms and 200 ms ($n = 20$) to an empirically programmed AV interval of 120 ms ($n = 20$) [39]. Both groups were programmed in the biventricular VDD mode. When comparing echo-Doppler–guided optimization to an empiric AV delay, aortic VTI improved by 4.0 ± 1.7 cm versus 1.8 ± 3.6 cm ($p<0.02$), LV ejection fraction increased by $7.8 \pm 6.2\%$ versus $3.4 \pm 4.4\%$ ($p<0.02$), and after 3 months, New York Heart Association (NYHA) functional class improved by 1.0 ± 0.5 versus 0.4 ± 0.6 class points ($p<0.01$).

AV delay optimization guided by LV dP/dT determination

The LV dP/dt_{max} is a sensitive index of LV contractility [23,25,31,40–43]. It is measured during cardiac catheterization but can also be estimated noninvasively from the continuous-wave Doppler mitral regurgitation velocity envelope (Figure 7.11) [44]. Invasive measurement of LV dP/dt_{max} at the time of CRT implantation can be used to guide AV delay programming but noninvasive methods are preferable.

Morales et al. [45] compared echo-Doppler–derived LV dP/dt_{max} at AV delays of 60 ms, 80 ms, 100 ms, 120 ms, 140 ms, 160 ms, 180 ms (Group I, $n = 23$) to an empiric AV delay of 120 ms (Group II, $n = 15$). There were no clinical differences between the groups and all devices were programmed to atrio-synchronous pacing mode with synchronous VV stimulation. At the 6-month follow-up, Group I had significantly lower NYHA class (2.1 ± 0.1 vs. 3 ± 0.2, $p <0.01$) and higher LV ejection fraction ($32.1 \pm 1\%$ vs. $27.5 \pm 1.6\%$, $p<0.05$) as compared to Group II.

The maximal difference in LV dP/dt_{max} values in each patient during the entire sequence of AV delays ranged from 27% to 100%.

VTI of transmitral flow

Jansen et al. [31] evaluated various echocardiographic methods of AV delay optimization to determine which resulted in the highest LV dP/dt_{max} measured with a sensor-tipped pressure guide wire in 30 heart failure patients <24 hours after CRT device implantation. Echocardiographic methods included VTI of transmitral flow, diastolic filling time, VTI of the LV outflow tract or aorta, and Ritter's method. The maximal VTI of mitral inflow was found to be the most accurate method based on invasive LV dP/dt_{max}.

Alternative AV optimization techniques apart from echocardiography

There are limited but promising data about simpler and faster noninvasive AV optimization techniques such as plethysmography [46–48], impedance cardiography [49,50] and a semi-automatic techniques with the device programmer [51–54].

Semi-automatic optimization of the AV interval

QuickOpt™ Timing Cycle Optimization (St. Jude Medical) runs an automatic sequence of intracardiac electrogram measurements and displays on the programmer the optimal AV and VV intervals in 90 seconds. The first step of the algorithm [51] first measures the intrinsic atrio-ventricular depolarization delay in RV and LV during atrial sensing or pacing. It is assumed that the ventricle that is depolarized latest will have to be stimulated first. The device assigns a "sign" to the measured difference (Δ) (positive if LV has to be paced first, negative in case of RV first). The second step of the algorithm then determines the RV–LV and LV–RV interventricular conduction time by pacing one ventricle and sensing the response in the opposite ventricle. Epsilon (ε) is the difference between the LV–RV and RV–LV interventricular conduction intervals. Thus, if the interventricular conduction is slower during pacing from the LV lead, ε will be positive. Finally the optimal VV delay is determined as half the sum of the intrinsic depolarization delay and the interventricular conduction delay. VV Opt formula: $0.5 \times (\Delta + \varepsilon)$. These values are then programmed manually into the CRT device. QuickOpt optimization was found to be consistently comparable to a traditional echocardiographic procedure for determining optimal AV and VV delays [51–54].

Another system (SmartAVDelay™) recently introduced by Boston Scientific (which also designed the Guidant system) also permits rapid programmer-based determination of the AV delay. The algorithm also uses a formula based on intracardiac electrograms that accurately predicts the AV delay associated with the maximum LV dP/dt [52]. This approach is based on the original method, by Auricchio et al. [55], demonstrated that the AV delay can be reliably predicted from the intrinsic AV interval. It was used for AV optimization in the COM-PANION trial [56], and it was recently refined and verified by Gold et al. [52]. The device measures the sensed and paced AV delays (AS–VS and AP–VS). It also measures the interventricular conduction interval between the RV and LV electrograms in the case of a bipolar LV lead whereupon the system provides the optimal AV delay automatically. The duration of the surface QRS complex is used in the semi-automatic function if the LV lead is unipolar. A further programming adjustment is required if the LV lead is not in the correct site. This system does not evaluate the VV delay, which has to be programmed before determining the optimal AV delay. The sensed and paced AV delays are individually determined in contrast to the St. Jude Medical system that calculates the paced AV delay by adding 50 ms to the optimal sensed AV delay [54].

Most CRT patients do not undergo AV and VV optimization by traditional methods because echocardiographic optimization typically takes a long time and is expensive. These new systems based on intracardiac electrograms allow efficient and frequent optimization of AV and VV interval can even be used when the device is being programmed before leaving the surgical suite. Although preliminary data are encouraging, further study of these automatic or semi-automatic AV optimization based on intracardiac electrograms is needed.

Fusion with the spontaneously conducted QRS complex

Van Gelder et al. [6] investigated the hemodynamic effect of intrinsic conduction during LV pacing as compared to biventricular pacing in 34 patients with NYHA functional Class III or Class IV, sinus rhythm with normal AV conduction, left bundle branch block, QRS >130 ms, and optimal medical therapy. LV dP/dt$_{max}$ index was measured invasively during LV and simultaneous biventricular pacing. The AV interval was varied in four steps starting with an AV interval 40 ms shorter than the intrinsic PQ time and increased with 25% for each step causing progressive fusion between paced complexes and intrinsic AV conduction via the His–Purkinje system. LV dP/dt$_{max}$ was higher with LV than biventricular pacing provided that LV pacing was associated with ventricular fusion caused by intrinsic activation via the right bundle branch.

The clinical implications of the study of Van Gelder et al. [6] are unclear. It is currently impossible to obtain sustained LV stimulation with a stable degree of fusion due to perturbation of intrinsic conduction related to autonomic factors. As present, it's best to program the AV delay to minimize ventricular fusion with spontaneous ventricular activity until more data are available, and a reliable way is found to synchronize right bundle branch activity or unpaced RV sensed events with LV stimulation. The hemodynamic impact of fusion as yet cannot be predicted. It may be beneficial and inevitable in some patients with a short PR interval, but it may also carry the risk of incomplete resynchronization. In these patients optimization of the AV interval may be suboptimal or impossible at short AV delays without fusion. Therefore, a relatively longer (possibly hemodynamically more favorable) AV interval associated with fusion may be programmed on a trial basis in a patient with suboptimal response to CRT.

Rate adaptation of the AV interval and exercise

Exercise testing in CRT patients is technically difficult and inconvenient. There is preliminary evidence in acute studies suggesting that the short AV delay at rest should be prolonged during exercise to achieve optimal LV systolic performance [57]. This is in contrast to the proven benefit of programming rate-adaptive shortening of the AV delay in patients with conventional DDDR pacemakers. The dynamic changes of LV dyssynchrony during exercise may partially explain what appears to be paradoxical behavior of the AV delay on exercise in CRT patients [57,58]. If the AV delay behavior is confirmed by other studies, it would be desirable to provide CRT devices with dynamic lengthening of the AV delay on exercise. In the meantime, it might be wise to program CRT devices first without dynamic shortening of the AV delay in patients with normal sinus node function. There are no chronic data available that provide insight regarding the optimal AV interval during activity states. In the future, it might be possible to predict the optimal AV delay on exercise from the value of the optimal resting AV delay [59].

In some CRT patients with severe chronotropic incompetence, DDDR pacing with a rate-adaptive AV delay may provide incremental benefit on exercise capacity [22]. Therefore, if atrial pacing is likely to occur during exercise, a treadmill test can be performed to demonstrate optimal adjustment of the rate-adaptive AV delay.

Long-term evaluation of the AV delay

The optimal follow-up and long-term programming of the AV delay is uncertain. There is preliminary evidence suggesting that the optimal AV and VV intervals changes with time in patients undergoing CRT [60–62]. Biventricular stimulation will result in LV reverse remodeling with changes in LV end-diastolic and end-systolic volumes and pressures over time. This dynamic process also includes autonomic changes and may take several months before a new steady state of maximum improvement in LV function is reached. The status of AV interval optimization should therefore be assessed periodically. Further studies are needed to determine how often the AV interval needs to be optimized.

Intra-atrial and Inter-atrial conduction delay

Intra-atrial and inter-atrial conduction delays are now being recognized as important abnormalities in patients with heart failure who are considered to be candidates for CRT [63]. These abnormalities of conduction should be suspected in patients with extensive atrial myocardial disease, absent atrial electrical activity or low electrogram amplitudes, and in patients who underwent surgical procedures, such as mitral valve replacement and a maze procedure.

Inter-atrial conduction delay

Inter-atrial conduction delay is characterized by a wide and notched P wave (>120 ms) traditionally in ECG lead II, associated with a wide terminal negative deflection in lead V_1 [64]. The latter is commonly labeled left atrial enlargement though it reflects left atrial conduction disease. Inter-atrial conduction time is also measured as the activation time from the high right atrium or the onset of the P wave to the distal coronary sinus (60–85 ms) [64]. In the presence of inter-atrial conduction delay with late left atrial activation, left atrial contraction occurs late and even during LV systole. Consequently, the need to program a long AV delay to adjust for delayed left atrial contraction can preclude ventricular resynchronization because of the emergence of competing spontaneous AV conduction. The incidence of inter-atrial conduction delay in patients who are candidates for CRT is unknown. When the ECG suggests inter-atrial conduction delay, it would be wise to look for delayed left atrial activation at the time of CRT implantation by showing that the conduction time from the right atrium to the left atrium is longer than the conduction time from right atrium to the ventricles (onset of the QRS complex) [65]. In the presence of inter-atrial conduction delay, the surgeon should consider placing the atrial lead in the inter-atrial septum where pacing produces a more simultaneous activation of both atria and abbreviates total atrial activation time judged by a decrease in P wave duration [66,67]. In the presence of established CRT with an atrial lead in the right atrial appendage, restoration of mechanical left-sided AV synchrony requires simultaneous bi-atrial pacing performed by the implantation of a second atrial lead either in the proximal coronary sinus or low atrium near the coronary sinus to preempt left atrial systole [68,69]. Ablation of the AV junction permits control of the AV delay to promote mechanical left-sided AV synchrony [70].

Intra-atrial conduction delay (late atrial sensing)

In some patients with right intra-atrial conduction delay, conduction from the sinus node to the right atrial appendage (site of atrial sensing) is delayed in the absence of significant conduction delay from sinus node to the AV junction or to the left atrium. The clinical incidence of this entity and its association with inter-atrial conduction delay are unknown. In this situation, left atrial activation may take place or may even be complete by the time the device senses the

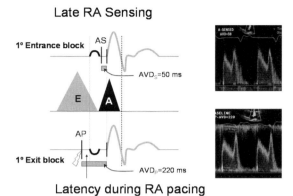

Fig. 7.12 Schematic representation of recordings from a CRT patient with intra-atrial conduction block. Intra-atrial conduction block is manifested by late right atrial sensing due to delayed conduction from the sinus node to the right atrial appendage (top). This produces a very short atrial sensed– ventricular sensed interval that can interfere with the establishment of satisfactory CRT. During right atrial pacing there is a prolonged atrial latency interval (pacemaker exit block) (bottom). A short sensed AV delay and long paced AV delay achieved similar satisfactory hemodynamic results as depicted in the corresponding mitral inflow patterns shown on the right side. AP = atrial pacing, AS = atrial sensing, AVD_S = AV delay sensed, AVD_P = AV delay paced, RA = right atrial (Reproduced and modified with permission from Herweg et al. [70].)

right atrial electrogram. The AS–VS interval (AS = atrial sensed event, VS = ventricular sensed event) becomes quite short because AS is delayed but VS is not (Figure 7.12). Thus, in CRT patients it may be impossible to program an optimal AV delay without interference from a comparatively early VS event due to emergence of competing spontaneous conduction. In such cases, VS produces potentially harmful ventricular fusion or incomplete cardiac resynchronization. Thus, one is often forced to program unphysiologically short-sensed AV delays and possibly long paced AV delays to adjust for the delay associated with first-degree pacemaker exit block (Figure 7.12). In a difficult situation ablation of the fast pathway of the AV node or complete AV junctional ablation can be performed with satisfactory results [70]. This approach is similar to the use of pacing in patients with hypertrophic obstructive cardiomyopathy and a short PR interval where AV junctional ablation is the only way to ensure complete pacemaker-induced ventricular depolarization [71].

Programming the inter-ventricular (V–V) interval

The usefulness of programming the V–V interval is controversial in view of two recent trials showing no benefit [35,72]. Despite the negative results in these recent trials, we believe that VV interval optimization may prove beneficial in some heart failure patients with a suboptimal CRT response. In most patients V–V interval optimization produces a rather limited improvement in LV function and/or stroke volume [72], but, in individual patients, it can lead to significant benefit. V–V interval optimization should decrease LV dyssynchrony, provide more simultaneous LV activation with faster LV emptying and longer diastolic filling, may increase LV ejection fraction, and reduce mitral regurgitation in some patients [58]. VV programmability may also partially compensate for less than optimal LV lead position by tailoring ventricular timing and may correct for individual heterogeneous ventricular activation patterns commonly found in patients with LV dysfunction and heart failure. VV interval optimization can be viewed as the individual adjustment of left and right ventricular AV intervals and its benefit is additive to AV interval optimization.

Programming of the VV interval is guided by the same techniques as AV delay optimization. Determination of the extent of residual LV dyssynchrony after VV programming requires more sophisticated echocardiographic techniques, such as tissue Doppler imaging. Contemporary biventricular ICD devices permit programming of the VV interval usually in steps from +80 ms (LV first) to-80 ms (RV first) to optimize LV hemodynamics (Figure 7.13). This design is based on evidence that CRT with sequential rather than simultaneous pacing of the two ventricles yields the best mechanical efficiency [42].

Optimized VV intervals show great patient to patient variability and usually cannot be identified clinically in the majority of patients [34–41,43,44,73–76]. Consequently, the adjustment of the VV interval like the AV interval must be individualized. The range of optimal VV intervals is relatively narrow and most commonly involves LV pre-excitation by 20 ms. RV pre-excitation should be used cautiously because advancing RV activation may cause a decline of LV function. Consequently RV pre-excitation should be reserved for patients with LV dyssynchrony in the septal and inferior segments provided there is hemodynamic proof of benefit (Figure 7.13) [76]. Patients with ischemic cardiomyopathy (with slower conducting scars) may require more pre-excitation than those with idiopathic dilated cardiomyopathy [44]. VV programming is of particular benefit in patients with a previous myocardial infarction [75].

Prior to performing VV interval optimization consideration should be given to pacing lead configuration, the presence of anodal capture (which forces the VV interval to 0), and manufacturer related differences of VV timing. Further, careful analysis of the 12-lead ECG during RV, LV and biventricular pacing is crucial.

Impact of V–V interval programming on the effective AV delay: Differences between device manufacturers

V–V interval programming allows separate programming of the RV and LV–AV delays. In most devices (all American manufacturers except Boston

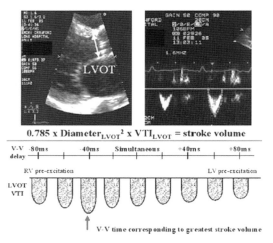

$$0.785 \times \text{Diameter}_{LVOT}^2 \times \text{VTI}_{LVOT} = \textbf{stroke volume}$$

Fig. 7.13 Interventricular interval delay using left ventricular outflow tract (LVOT) measurements of blood flow velocities for estimation of stroke volume (SV). SV is exponentially related to the LVOT diameter and directly to the velocity time integral (VTI) of the LVOT. Variation of the interventricular interval (VV) interval, affects the SV as evidenced by varying VTI measurements that can serve as surrogate markers for resynchronisation. The optimal VVinterval in this example is derived from pacing the right ventricle (RV) 40 msec before the left ventricle (LV). The optimal AV delay becomes equal to (optimal AS-LVP) minus the 40-ms VV interval. This example is unusual because RV pre-excitation is used infrequently. LVP = monochamber LV pacing (Reproduced with permission from Gassis S, Leon AR. Cardiac resynchronization therapy: strategies for device programming, troubleshooting and follow-up. *J Interv Card Electrophysiol.* 2005;13:209–22.)

Scientific–Guidant) the ventricular channel advanced by V–V interval programming will be paced at the programmed PV–AV delay. In Boston Scientific (Guidant) devices PV–AV timing seen on the programmer applies to the RV channel and if LV activation is advanced by V–V interval programming, the LV–AV delay can be calculated by subtracting the V–V interval from the PV–AV delay (Figure 7.14) [74].

Latency and delayed intraventricular, and interventricular conduction

In some CRT patients, lack of hemodynamic improvement may be due to imbalance between RV and LV electrical activation related to variations of electrical excitability and impulse propagation, such as electrical latency, slow impulse propagation in proximity of the lead (due to scar tissue) or, more globally, delayed intra- ventricular and inter-ventricular conduction [5,77,78].

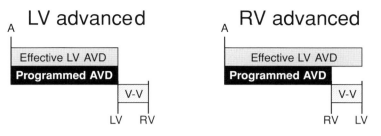

Effective AVD = Programmed AV D   Effective AVD = Programmed AVD + V-V

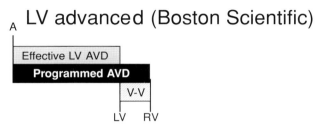

Effective AVD = Programmed AVD − V-V

Fig. 7.14 Impact of programming the VV interval on the effective AV delay. In the case of left ventricular (LV) pre-excitation, the effective LV–AV interval will be equal to the programmed AV interval, except for Boston Scientific (Guidant) devices (where the AV delay is based only on RV timing). In the latter, the programmer will display the RV–AV delay so that the LV–AV delay (with LV pre-excitation) becomes equal to the RV–AV delay minus the programmed VV interval. With RV pre-excitation in Boston Scientific devices, the effective LV–AV interval = programmed AV interval + VV interval. (Modified with permission from Burri et al. [74].)

The interval from the pacemaker stimulus to the onset of the earliest paced QRS complex on the 12-lead ECG is called "latency," and, during RV pacing, this interval normally measures <40 ms. We measured latency intervals on the 12-lead ECG acquired at a speed of 100 mm/s in 37 consecutive patients with CRT devices. Latency intervals were longer during LV pacing (30 ± 10 ms) when compared to RV pacing 13 ± 11 ms, $p < 0.001$) and shortened with increased stimulus strength ($p < 0.05$) independent of the site of pacing. Five of 37 (14%) patients exhibited prolonged LV latency intervals >40 ms. In a series of 150 patients, we have observed latency (>50 ms) during LV pacing on seven occasions.

Prolonged LV latency intervals during stimulation from within epicardial cardiac veins may be due to interposed venous tissue and epicardial fat that prevent direct contact between electrode and LV myocardium and/or an overlying scar. We have observed infero-lateral akinesis or severe hypokinesis in some patients with prolonged LV latency intervals involving the area of the LV lead

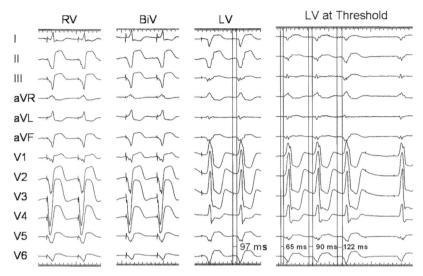

Fig. 7.15 Twelve-lead ECGs showing comparison of QRS morphology during right, biventricular, and left ventricular pacing in the VVI mode at 80 ppm during complete AV block (excluding fusion with the spontaneous QRS complex). Right and left ventricular outputs were each at twice the threshold voltage. During biventricular pacing (VV delay = 0) the QRS morphology is identical to that of right ventricular pacing (no evidence of biventricular fusion). During LV pacing the stimulus to QRS latency interval measures 97 ms. Right panel: 12-lead ECG during LV pacing at 90 bpm near the pacing threshold (2.5V @ 0.1 ms) shows a type I, second-degree (Wenckebach) exit block from the pacing site characterized by progressive prolongation of the latency interval culminating in total exit block. BiV = biventricular, LV = left ventricular, RV = right ventricular. (Reproduced with permission from Herweg et al. [5].)

implantation site [5]. This is concordant with recent reports about low response rates to CRT in patients with LV dyssynchrony and postero-lateral scar as demonstrated by echocardiography and contrast enhanced magnetic resonance imaging [79,80]. Delayed LV depolarization related to latency during simultaneous biventricular pacing (VV = 0 ms) generates an ECG pattern dominated by RV stimulation (Figure 7.15). Advancing LV stimulation via a programmable inter-ventricular (VV) delay or programming the device to single-chamber LV pacing can result in immediate hemodynamic and symptomatic improvement (Figure 7.16). Increased LV ventricular stimulus output decreases inter-ventricular conduction time in patients with biventricular pacing systems [81–83]. Increasing output strength in all likelihood depolarizes larger volumes of myocardium by creating a larger virtual electrode and this may be of particular importance during pacing of diseased myocardium.

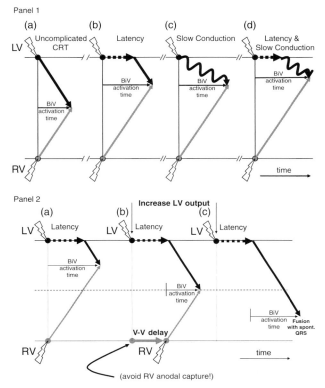

Fig. 7.16 Diagrammatic representation of the significance of left ventricular (LV) latency and slow conduction during simultaneous biventricular pacing. Panel 1(a): During uncomplicated cardiac resynchronization therapy (CRT) undisturbed impulse propagation from both pacing sites produces balanced fusion of right ventricular (RV) and LV wavefronts. Panel 1(b): In the presence of a prolonged LV latency interval (dashed black arrow) LV activation occurs late and the RV wavefront depolarizes more myocardium causing a longer biventricular activation time. Panel 1(c). Slow conduction in the proximity to the LV pacing site (due to scar tissue or myocardial fibrosis) produces a similar effect as in Panel 1(B). Panel 1(d): Coexistence of a long LV latency interval and slow conduction in the proximity to the LV pacing site may coexist in some patients. Major portions of the LV are then depolarized by the RV wavefront with minimal contribution from LV pacing and further prolongation of the biventricular activation time. Panel 2: Compensatory programming for LV latency. Panel 2(a). Simultaneous activation of both ventricles (on the left) results in late LV activation and more myocardium depolarized by the RV wavefront. Panel 2(b). VV programming permits LV pre-excitation to compensate for the prolonged LV latency interval. Both ventricles are activated synchronously resulting in a shorter biventricular activation time. Panel 2(c). Pacing the LV only may result in some degree of fusion with native conduction on the right side depending on the programmed AV delay. This approach may yield satisfactory hemodynamic results in patients with a markedly prolonged LV latency interval. (BiV = biventricular, LV = left ventricular, RV = right ventricular) (Modified with permission from Barold SS, Ilercil A, Herweg B. Programmability of the interventricular interval during cardiac resynchronization therapy. In: Barold SS, Ritter P eds., *Devices for Cardiac Resynchronization. Technologic and Clinical Aspects*, New York, NY, Springer, 2008:237–51.)

BiV at triple threshold (2.5 V @ 0.3 ms)

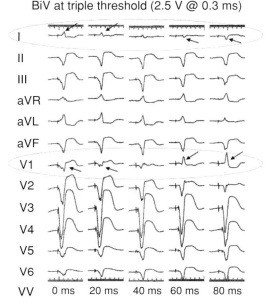

Fig. 7.17 Impact of progressive left ventricular (LV) pre-excitation during biventricular pacing (80 bpm at 2.5V @ 0.3 ms) on QRS morphology in a patient with an increased LV latency interval. Programming of incremental left to right ventricular (VV) delays (left ventricular pre-excitation) can bring out a dominant R wave in lead V_1 during biventricular pacing and may guide the selection of a VV interval to produce balanced left and right ventricular fusion. BiV = biventricular pacing (Reproduced with permission from Herweg et al. [5].)

Optimization of V–V timing using the electrocardiogram

We measure RV and LV latency intervals on the ECG at a speed of 50–100 mm/s and use the difference between LV and RV latency intervals as the value to program the VV interval. In patients with long LV latency intervals programming of incremental left to right ventricular (VV) delays can bring out a dominant R wave in lead V_1 during biventricular pacing and may guide the selection of a VV delay that yields more balanced left and right ventricular depolarization (Figure 7.17) [5]. The accuracy and validity of these electrocardiographic methods for VV interval optimization require further investigation.

Vidal et al. [84] described a simple ECG method comparing the time difference of the interval from the pacing spike to the beginning of the fast deflection of the QRS complex in leads V_1, V_2 during pacing from the LV (T1), and from the RV (T2) in a cohort of 31 consecutive patients treated with CRT. The T2–T1 interval was considered as a surrogate measurement of inter-ventricular delay and defined as the best VV, which was compared to three echocardiographic measurements of LV synchrony at VV interval setting of −30 ms, 0 m, and +30 ms. Echo results had an 83% coincidence with the ECG method ($r = 0.81$, $p < 0.001$). The investigators concluded that the time difference in the fast ventricular depolarization observed between RV and LV stimulation on the surface ECG shows a good correlation with echocardiographic VV optimization.

References

1. Barold SS, Herweg B, Giudici, M. Electrocardiographic follow-up of biventricular pacemakers. *Ann Noninvasive Electrocardiol.* 2005;10:231–55.
2. Barold SS, Giudici MC, Herweg B, Curtis AB. Diagnostic value of the 12-lead electrocardiogram during conventional and biventricular pacing for cardiac resynchronization. *Cardiol Clin.* 2006;24:471–90.
3. Giudici MC, Tigrett DW, Carlson JI, Lorenz TD, Paul DL, Barold SS. Electrocardiographic patterns during: pacing the great cardiac and middle cardiac veins. *Pacing Clin Electrophysiol.* 2007;30:1376–80.
4. Grimley SR, Suffoletto MS, Gorcsan J, III, Schwartzman D. Electrocardiographically concealed variation in left ventricular capture: a case with implications for resynchronization therapy in ischemic cardiomyopathy. *Heart Rhythm.* 2006;3:739–42.
5. Herweg B, Ilercil A, Madramootoo C, Krishnan S, Rinde-Hoffman D, Weston M, Curtis AB, Barold SS. Latency during left ventricular pacing from the lateral cardiac veins: a cause of ineffectual biventricular pacing. *Pacing Clin Electrophysiol.* 2006;29:574–81.
6. van Gelder BM, Bracke FA, Meijer A, Pijls NH. The hemodynamic effect of intrinsic conduction during left ventricular pacing as compared to biventricular pacing. *J Am Coll Cardiol.* 2005;46:2305–10.
7. Kashani A, Barold SS. Significance of QRS complex duration in patients with heart failure. *J Am Coll Cardiol.* 2005;46:2183–92.
8. Leclercq C, Faris O, Tunin R, Johnson J, Kato R, Evans F, Spinelli J, Halperin H, McVeigh E, Kass DA. Systolic improvement and mechanical resynchronization does not require electrical synchrony in the dilated failing heart with left bundle-branch block. *Circulation.* 2002;106: 1760–3.
9. Barold SS, Herweg B. Upper rate response of biventricular pacing devices. *J Interv Card Electrophysiol.* 2005;12:129–36.
10. Kay GN. Troubleshooting and programming of cardiac resynchronization therapy. In: Ellenbogen KA, Kay GN, Wilkoff BL, eds., *Device therapy for congestive heart failure.* Philadelphia, PA, Saunders, 2004;232–93.
11. Sweeney MO. Programming and follow-up of CRT and CRT-D devices. In: Barold SS, Ritter P, eds., *Devices for cardiac resynchronization technologic and clinical aspects.* New York, NY, Springer, 2008;317–423.
12. Barold SS, Ilercil A, Leonelli F, Herweg B. First-degree atrioventricular block. Clinical manifestations, indications for pacing, pacemaker management and consequences during cardiac resynchronization. *J Interv Card Electrophysiol.* 2006;17:139–52.
13. Bernheim A, Ammann P, Sticherling C, Burger P, Schaer B, Brunner-La Rocca HP, Eckstein J, Kiencke S, Kaiser C, Linka A, Buser P, Pfisterer M, Osswald S. Right atrial pacing impairs cardiac function during resynchronization therapy: acute effects of DDD pacing compared to VDD pacing. *J Am Coll Cardiol.* 2005;45:1482–87.

14. Adelstein E, Saba S. Right atrial pacing and the risk of postimplant atrial fibrillation in cardiac resynchronization therapy recipients. *Am Heart J.* 2008;155: 94–9.

15. Gasparini M, Auricchio A, Regoli F, Fantoni C, Kawabata M, Galimberti P, Pini, D, Ceriotti C, Gronda E, Klersy C, Fratini S, Klein HH. Four-year efficacy of cardiac resynchronization therapy on exercise tolerance and disease progression: the importance of performing atrioventricular junction ablation in patients with atrial fibrillation. *J Am Coll Cardiol.* 2006;48:734–43.

16. Luria D, Gurevitz O, Glikson, M. Programming and diagnostic features of cardiac resynchronization therapy devices. In: Yu CM, Hayes DL, Auricchio A, eds., *Cardiac resynchronization therapy*, Malden, MA, Blackwell-Futura, 2008; in press.

17. Gurevitz O, Nof E, Carasso S, Luria D, Bar-Lev D, Tanami N, Eldar M, Glikson M. Programmable multiple pacing configurations help to overcome high left ventricular pacing thresholds and avoid phrenic nerve stimulation. *Pacing Clin Electrophysiol.* 2005;28:1255–9.

18. Herweg B, Barold SS. Anodal capture with second-generation biventricular cardioverter-defibrillator. *Acta Cardiol.* 2003;58:435–6.

19. Tamborero D, Mont L, Alanis R, Berruezo A, Tolosana JM, Sitges M, Vidal B, Brugada J. Anodal capture in cardiac resynchronization therapy implications for device programming. *Pacing Clin Electrophysiol.* 2006;29:940–5.

20. van Gelder BM, Bracke FA, van der Voort PH, Meijer A. Right ventricular anodal capture during left ventricular stimulation in CRT-implantable cardioverter defibrillators (ICD). *Pacing Clin Electrophysiol.* 2006;29:337–8.

21. Leclercq C, Mabo P, Daubert JC. Troubleshooting. In: Yu CM, Hayes DL, Auricchio A, eds., *Cardiac resynchronization therapy*, Malden, MA, Blackwell-Futura, 2006; 259–90.

22. Tse HF, Siu CW, Lee KL, Fan K, Chan HW, Tang MO, Tsang V, Lee SW, Lau CP. The incremental benefit of rate-adaptive pacing on exercise performance during cardiac resynchronization therapy. *J Am Coll Cardiol.* 2005;46:2292–7.

23. Auricchio A, Stellbrink C, Block M, Sack S, Vogt J, Bakker P, Klein H, Kramer A, Ding J, Salo R, Tockman B, Pochet T, Spinelli J. Effect of pacing chamber and atrioventricular delay on acute systolic function of paced patients with congestive heart failure. The Pacing Therapies for Congestive Heart Failure Study Group. The Guidant Congestive Heart Failure Research Group. *Circulation.* 1999;99:2993–3001.

24. Kass DA, Chen CH, Curry C, Talbot M, Berger R, Fetics B, Nevo E. Improved left ventricular mechanics from acute VDD pacing in patients with dilated cardiomyopathy and ventricular conduction delay. *Circulation.* 1999;99: 1567–73.

25. Auricchio A, Ding J, Spinelli JC, Kramer, AP, Salo RW, Hoersch, W, KenKnight BH, Klein HU. Cardiac resynchronization therapy restores optimal atrioventricular mechanical timing in heart failure patients with ventricular conduction delay. *J Am Coll Cardiol.* 2002;39:1163–9.

26. Bax JJ, Abraham T, Barold SS, Breithardt OA, Fung JW, Garrigue S, Gorcsan J, III, Hayes DL, Kass DA, Knuuti J, Leclercq C, Linde C, Mark DB, Monaghan MJ, Nihoyannopoulos P, Schalij MJ, Stellbrink C, Yu CM. Cardiac resynchronization therapy: Part 2—issues during and after device implantation and unresolved questions. *J Am Coll Cardiol.* 2005;46:2168–82.

27. Panidis IP, Ross J, Munley B, Nestico P, Mintz GS. Diastolic mitral regurgitation in patients with atrioventricular conduction abnormalities: a common finding by Doppler echocardiography. *J Am Coll Cardiol.* 1986;7:768–74.

28. Kindermann M, Frohlig G, Doerr T, Schieffer H. Optimizing the AV delay in DDD pacemaker patients with high degree AV block: mitral valve Doppler versus impedance cardiography. *Pacing Clin Electrophysiol.* 1997;20:2453–62.

29. Ritter P, Dib JC, Mahaux V, Lelievre T, Soyeur D, Lavergne T, Cazeau S, Guize L, Rabine LM, Daubert JC. New method for determining the optimal atrio-ventricular delay in DDD mode for complete atrio-ventricular block. *Pacing Clin Electrophysiol.* 2008;18:237(abstract).

30. Kerlan JE, Sawhney NS, Waggoner AD, Chawla MK, Garhwal S, Osborn JL, Faddis MN. Prospective comparison of echocardiographic atrioventricular delay optimization methods for cardiac resynchronization therapy. *Heart Rhythm.* 2006;3: 148–54.

31. Jansen AH, Bracke FA, van Dantzig JM, Meijer A, van der Voort PH, Aarnoudse W, van Gelder BM, Peels KH. Correlation of echo-Doppler optimization of atrioventricular delay in cardiac resynchronization therapy with invasive hemodynamics in patients with heart failure secondary to ischemic or idiopathic dilated cardiomyopathy. *Am J Cardiol.* 2006;97:552–7.

32. Cleland JG, Daubert JC, Erdmann E, Freemantle N, Gras D, Kappenberger L, Tavazzi L. The effect of cardiac resynchronization on morbidity and mortality in heart failure. *N Engl J Med.* 2005;352:1539–49.

33. Bax JJ, Ansalone G, Breithardt OA, Derumeaux G, Leclercq C, Schalij MJ, Sogaard P, St. John SM, Nihoyannopoulos P. Echocardiographic evaluation of cardiac resynchronization therapy: ready for routine clinical use? A critical appraisal. *J Am Coll Cardiol.* 2004;44:1–9.

34. Bordachar P, Lafitte S, Reuter S, Sanders P, Jais P, Haissaguerre M, Roudaut R, Garrigue S, Clementy J. Echocardiographic parameters of ventricular dyssynchrony validation in patients with heart failure using sequential biventricular pacing. *J Am Coll Cardiol.* 2004;44:2157–65.

35. Boriani G, Muller CP, Seidl KH, Grove R, Vogt J, Danschel W, Schuchert A, Djiane P, Biffi M, Becker T, Bailleul C, Trappe HJ. Randomized comparison of simultaneous biventricular stimulation versus optimized interventricular delay in cardiac resynchronization therapy. The Resynchronization for the HemodYnamic Treatment for Heart Failure Management II implantable cardioverter defibrillator (RHYTHM II ICD) study. *Am Heart J.* 2006;151:1050–8.

36. Mortensen PT, Sogaard P, Mansour H, Ponsonaille J, Gras D, Lazarus A, Reiser W, Alonso C, Linde CM, Lunati M, Kramm B, Harrison EM. Sequential biventricular pacing: evaluation of safety and efficacy. *Pacing Clin Electrophysiol.* 2004;27:339–45.

37. Porciani MC, Dondina C, Macioce R, Demarchi G, Pieragnoli P, Musilli N, Colella A, Ricciardi G, Michelucci A, Padeletti L. Echocardiographic examination of atrioventricular and interventricular delay optimization in cardiac resynchronization therapy. *Am J Cardiol.* 2005;95:1108–10.

38. Riedlbauchova L, Kautzner J, Fridl P. Influence of different atrioventricular and interventricular delays on cardiac output during cardiac resynchronization therapy. *Pacing Clin Electrophysiol.* 2005;28 Suppl 1:S19–S23.

39. Vanderheyden M, De Backer T, Rivero-Ayerza M, Geelen P, Bartunek J, Verstreken S, De Zutter M, Goethals M. Tailored echocardiographic interventricular delay programming further optimizes left ventricular performance after cardiac resynchronization therapy. *Heart Rhythm*. 2005;2:1066–172.

40. Hay I, Melenovsky V, Fetics BJ, Judge DP, Kramer A, Spinelli, J, Reister C, Kass DA, Berger RD. Short-term effects of right-left heart sequential cardiac resynchronization in patients with heart failure, chronic atrial fibrillation, and atrioventricular nodal block. *Circulation*. 2004;110:3404–10.

41. Kurzidim K, Reinke H, Sperzel J, Schneider HJ, Danilovic D, Siemon G, Neumann T, Hamm CW, Pitschner HF. Invasive optimization of cardiac resynchronization therapy: role of sequential biventricular and left ventricular pacing. *Pacing Clin Electrophysiol*. 2005;28:754–61.

42. Perego GB, Chianca R, Facchini M, Frattola A, Balla E, Zucchi S, Cavaglia S, Vicini I, Negretto M, Osculati G. Simultaneous vs. sequential biventricular pacing in dilated cardiomyopathy: an acute hemodynamic study. *Eur J Heart Fail*. 2003;5:305–13.

43. Sawhney NS, Waggoner AD, Garhwal, S, Chawla, MK, Osborn J, Faddis MN. Randomized prospective trial of atrioventricular delay programming for cardiac resynchronization therapy. *Heart Rhythm*. 2004;1:562–7.

44. van Gelder BM, Bracke FA, Meijer A, Lakerveld LJ, Pijls NH. Effect of optimizing the VV interval on left ventricular contractility in cardiac resynchronization therapy. *Am J Cardiol*. 2004;93:1500–3.

45. Morales MA, StartariU, Panchetti L, Rossi A, Piacenti M. Atrioventricular delay optimization by Doppler-derived left ventricular dP/dt improves 6-month outcome of resynchronized patients. *Pacing Clin Electrophysiol*. 2006;29:564–8.

46. Butter C, Stellbrink C, Belalcazar A, Villalta D, Schlegl M, Sinha A, Cuesta F, Reister C. Cardiac resynchronization therapy optimization by finger plethysmography. *Heart Rhythm*. 2004;1:568–75.

47. Whinnett ZI, Davies JE, Willson K, Manisty CH, Chow AW, Foale RA, Davies DW, Hughes AD, Mayet J, Francis DP. Haemodynamic effects of changes in atrioventricular and interventricular delay in cardiac resynchronisation therapy show a consistent pattern: analysis of shape, magnitude and relative importance of atrioventricular and interventricular delay. *Heart*. 2006;92: 1628–34.

48. Whinnett ZI, Davies JE, Willson K, Chow AW, Foale RA, Davies DW, Hughes AD, Francis DP, Mayet J. Determination of optimal atrioventricular delay for cardiac resynchronization therapy using acute non-invasive blood pressure. *Europace*. 2006;8:358–66.

49. Braun MU, Schnabel A, Rauwolf T, Schulze M, Strasser RH. Impedance cardiography as a noninvasive technique for atrioventricular interval optimization in cardiac resynchronization therapy. *J Interv Card Electrophysiol*. 2005;13:223–9.

50. Tse HF, Yu C, Park E, Lau CP. Impedance cardiography for atrioventricular interval optimization during permanent left ventricular pacing. *Pacing Clin Electrophysiol*. 2003;26:189–91.

51. Baker JH II, McKenzie J 3rd, Beau S, Greer GS, Porterfield J, Fedor M, Greenberg S, Daoud EG, Corbisiero R, Bailey JR, Porterfield L. Acute evaluation of programmer-guided AV/PV and VV delay optimization comparing an IEGM method and echocardiogram for cardiac resynchronization therapy in heart failure patients and dual-chamber ICD implants. *J Cardiovasc Electrophysiol*. 2007;18:185–91.

52. Gold MR, Niazi I, Giudici M, Leman RB, Sturdivant JL, Kim MH, Yu Y, Ding J, Waggoner AD. A prospective comparison of AV delay programming methods for hemodynamic optimization during cardiac resynchronization therapy. *J Cardiovasc Electrophysiol.* 2007;18:490–6.

53. Meine M, Min X, Paris M, Park E. An intracardiac EGM method for VV optimization during cardiac resynchronization. *Heart Rhythm.* 2006;3(Suppl):S63–S64.

54. Min X, Meine M, Baker JH, Pires LA, Turk KT, Horn EM, Kowal RC, Paris M, Park E, Fain ES. Estimation of the optimal VV delay by an IEGM-based method in cardiac resynchronization therapy. *Pacing Clin Electrophysiol.* 2007;30 Suppl 1:S19–S22.

55. Auricchio A, Kramer A, Spinelli J. Path CHF I and II Investigator Groups. Can the optimum dosage of resynchronization therapy be derived from the intracardiac electrogram. *J Am Coll Cardiol.* 2002;39(Suppl A):124A (abstract).

56. Bristow MR, Saxon LA, Boehmer, J, Krueger, S, Kass DA, De Marco T, Carson P, DiCarlo L, DeMets D, White BG, DeVries DW, Feldman AM. Cardiac-resynchronization therapy with or without an implantable defibrillator in advanced chronic heart failure. *N Engl J Med.* 2004;350:2140–50.

57. Scharf C, Li P, Muntwyler J, Chugh A, Oral H, Pelosi F, Morady F, Armstrong WF. Rate-dependent AV delay optimization in cardiac resynchronization therapy. *Pacing Clin Electrophysiol.* 2005;28:279–84.

58. Bordachar P, Lafitte S, Reuter, S, Serri K, Garrigue S, Laborderie, J, Reant P, Jais P, Haissaguerre M, Roudaut R, Clementy J. Echocardiographic assessment during exercise of heart failure patients with cardiac resynchronization therapy. *Am J Cardiol.* 2006;97:1622–5.

59. Whinnett ZI, Davies JE, Briscoe CA. Optimal hemodynamic AV delay during exercise can be predicted by performing optimization at rest with an elevated pacing rate. *Heart Rhythm.* 2008;3 Suppl:S249.

60. O'Donnell D, Nadurata V, Hamer A, Kertes P, Mohamed W. Long-term variations in optimal programming of cardiac resynchronization therapy devices. *Pacing Clin Electrophysiol.* 2008;28 Suppl 1:S24–S26.

61. Porciani MC, Dondina C, Macioce R, Demarchi G, Cappelli F, Lilli A, Pappone A, Ricciardi G, Colombo PC, Padeletti M, Jelic S, Padeletti L. Temporal variation in optimal atrioventricular and interventricular delay during cardiac resynchronization therapy. *J Card Fail.* 2006;12:715–19.

62. Zhang Q, Fung JW, Chan YS, Chan HC, Lin H, Chan S, Yu CM. The role of repeating optimization of atrioventricular interval during interim and long-term follow-up after cardiac resynchronization therapy. *Int J Cardiol.* 2008;124:211–17.

63. Van Beeumen K, Duytschaever, M, Tavernier R, Van DV, De Sutter J. Intra- and interatrial asynchrony in patients with heart failure. *Am J Cardiol.* 2007;99:79–83.

64. Daubert JC, Pavin D, Jauvert G, Mabo P. Intra- and interatrial conduction delay: implications for cardiac pacing. *Pacing Clin Electrophysiol.* 2004;27:507–25.

65. Levin V, Nemeth M, Colombowala I, Massumi A, Rasekh A, Cheng J, Coles JA, Jr, Ujhelyi MR, Razavi M. Interatrial conduction measured during biventricular pacemaker implantation accurately predicts optimal paced atrioventricular intervals. *J Cardiovasc Electrophysiol.* 2007;18:290–5.

66. Di Pede F, Gasparini G, De Piccoli B, Yu Y, Cuesta F, Raviele A. Hemodynamic effects of atrial septal pacing in cardiac resynchronization therapy patients. *J Cardiovasc Electrophysiol.* 2005;16:1273–8.

67. Porciani MC, Sabini A, Colella A, Michelucci A, Musilli N, Pieragnoli P, Padeletti L. Interatrial septum pacing avoids the adverse effect of interatrial delay in biventricular pacing: an echo-Doppler evaluation. *Europace.* 2002;4:317–24.

68. Doi A, Takagi M, Toda I, Yoshiyama M, Takeuchi K, Yoshikawa J. Acute haemodynamic benefits of biatrial atrioventricular sequential pacing: comparison with single atrial atrioventricular sequential pacing. *Heart.* 2004;90:411–18.

69. Doi A, Takagi M, Toda I, Yoshiyama M, Takeuchi K, Yoshikawa J. Acute hemodynamic benefits of bi-atrial atrioventricular sequential pacing with the optimal atrioventricular delay. *J Am Coll Cardiol.* 2005;46:320–6.

70. Herweg B, Ilercil A, Madramootoo C, Ali R, Barold SS. AV junctional ablation allowing more effective delivery of cardiac resynchronization therapy in patients with intra- and inter-atrial conduction delay. *Pacing Clin Electrophysiol.* 2008;in press.

71. Jeanrenaud X, Schlapfer J, Fromer M, Aebischer N, Kappenberger L. Dual chamber pacing in hypertrophic obstructive cardiomyopathy: beneficial effect of atrioventricular junction ablation for optimal left ventricular capture and filling. *Pacing ClinElectrophysiol.* 1997;20:293–300.

72. Rao RK, Kumar UN, Schafer J, Viloria E, De Lurgio D, Foster E. Reduced ventricular volumes and improved systolic function with cardiac resynchronization therapy: a randomized trial comparing simultaneous biventricular pacing, sequential biventricular pacing, and left ventricular pacing. *Circulation.* 2007;115:2136–44.

73. Barold SS, Ilercil A, Garrigue S, Herweg B. Optimization of the interventricular (V-V) delay during cardiac resynchronization. In: St. John Sutton M, Bax JJ, Jessup M, Brugada J, Schalij MJ, eds., *Cardiac resynchronization therapy.* London, England, Informa Healthcare, 2007;165–76.

74. Burri H, Sunthorn H, Shah D, Lerch R. Optimization of device programming for cardiac resynchronization therapy. *Pacing Clin Electrophysiol.* 2006;29:1416–25.

75. Leon AR, Abraham WT, Brozena S, Daubert JP, Fisher WG, Gurley JC, Liang CS, Wong G. Cardiac resynchronization with sequential biventricular pacing for the treatment of moderate-to-severe heart failure. *J Am Coll Cardiol.* 2005;46:2298–2304.

76. Sogaard P, Egeblad H, Pedersen AK, Kim WY, Kristensen BO, Hansen PS, Mortensen PT. Sequential versus simultaneous biventricular resynchronization for severe heart failure: evaluation by tissue Doppler imaging. *Circulation.* 2002;106:2078–84.

77. Fung JW, Yu CM, Yip G, Zhang Y, Chan H, Kum CC, Sanderson JE. Variable left ventricular activation pattern in patients with heart failure and left bundle branch block. *Heart.* 2004;90:17–19.

78. Rodriguez LM, Timmermans C, Nabar A, Beatty G, Wellens HJ. Variable patterns of septal activation in patients with left bundle branch block and heart failure. *J Cardiovasc Electrophysiol.* 2003;14:135–41.

79. Bleeker GB, Schalij MJ, Van Der Wall EE, Bax JJ. Postero-lateral scar tissue resulting in non-response to cardiac resynchronization therapy. *J Cardiovasc Electrophysiol.* 2006;17:899–901.

80. Bleeker GB, Kaandorp TA, Lamb HJ, Boersma E, Steendijk P, de Roos A, Van Der Wall EE, Schalij MJ, Bax JJ. Effect of posterolateral scar tissue on clinical and

echocardiographic improvement after cardiac resynchronization therapy. *Circulation.* 2006;113:969–76.

81. Sauer WH, Sussman JS, Verdino RJ, Cooper JM. Increasing left ventricular pacing output decreases interventricular conduction time in patients with biventricular pacing systems. *Pacing Clin Electrophysiol.* 2006;29:569–73.

82. Tedrow U, Maisel WH, Epstein LM, Soejima K, Stevenson WG. Feasibility of adjusting paced left ventricular activation by manipulating stimulus strength. *J Am Coll Cardiol.* 2004;44:2249–52.

83. Tedrow UB, Stevenson WG, Wood MA, Shepard RK, Hall K, Pellegrini CP, Ellenbogen KA. Activation sequence modification during cardiac resynchronization by manipulation of left ventricular epicardial pacing stimulus strength. *Pacing Clin Electrophysiol.* 2007;30:65–9.

84. Vidal B, Tamborero D, Mont L, Sitges M, Delgado V, Berruezo A, Diaz-Infante E, Tolosana JM, Pare C, Brugada J. Electrocardiographic optimization of interventricular delay in cardiac resynchronization therapy: a simple method to optimize the device. *JCardiovasc Electrophysiol.* 2007;18:1252–7.

Chapter 8

Troubleshooting CRT devices and clinical outcomes

Dusan Kocovic

Key Points

1. Cardiac resynchronization therapy (CRT) provides clinical benefit in the majority of patients, and its effects should best be assessed 3–6 months after device implantation.
2. Despite the absence of widely accepted definitions of response to CRT, echocardiographic measurements of LV volumes are a useful measure of response.
3. Response to CRT as measured by changes in ejection fraction and LV volume tend to be larger in magnitude in patients with nonischemic cardiomyopathy compared to patients with ischemic cardiomyopathy.
4. Patients who do not respond to CRT should undergo evaluation for potential cause(s) that can be identified and corrected.
5. In our experience, the most important potential causes for failure to respond to therapy include:
   - Lack of dyssynchrony at the baseline
   - LV lead implanted in suboptimal position
   - Loss of LV lead capture or an inadequate percentage of LV lead pacing
   - Development of Atrial fibrillation
   - Suboptimal programming of AV and VV intervals
   - Progression of disease or development of new inter current diseases
6. Many of the causes for CRT nonresponse to CRT are correctable.
7. A better understanding of patterns of conduction abnormalities unique to individual patients are necessary to better predict pre-operatively where LV leads should be placed.

Pacing to Support the Failing Heart, 1st edition. Edited by K. Ellenbogen and A. Auricchio.
© 2008 American Heart Association, ISBN: 978-1-4051-7534-0

8. At this time, measurement of QRS width best defines the group of patients expected to respond to CRT. Measurement of dyssynchrony is an evolving field, and its precise role in determining patient selection is unclear.
9. Scar burden and scar location may significantly reduce response to CRT.
10. Most manufacturers have developed algorithms that automatically determine optimal AV and VV intervals.

Introduction

Ventricular dyssynchrony is an abnormal pattern of ventricular contraction that results in paradoxical, septal wall motion, reduction in left ventricular contractility, suboptimal ventricular filling, and prolonged duration (or degree) of mitral regurgitation, which conspire to reduce stroke volume and thus the ability of the failing heart to eject blood [1–4]. Approximately one-third of patients with systolic heart failure exhibit ventricular dyssynchrony, which is often defined (or approximated) as a QRS duration that is greater than 120 ms on the surface ECG [5–7]. The adverse consequences of ventricular dyssynchrony have been reviewed in detail in Chapters 4 and 7. The presence of ventricular dyssynchrony or QRS prolongation has been associated with increased morbidity and mortality in heart failure patients [8–14]. Thus, in the mid-1990s, pacing therapy was explored. CRT, or atrial-synchronized biventricular pacing, emerged as the most promising approach for the treatment of ventricular dyssynchrony [15–21].

More than 5,000 patients have been now been evaluated in randomized controlled trials of cardiac resynchronization therapy (CRT). These studies have been reviewed in Chapter 5. They have demonstrated that CRT, with or without an implantable cardioverter defibrillator (ICD), consistently improves quality of life, functional status, exercise capacity, and cardiac structure and function and reduces morbidity and mortality in heart failure patients with ventricular dyssynchrony. The magnitude of benefit seen with CRT is comparable to or exceeds that seen with evidence-based drug therapies for heart failure, but occurs in patients who are already receiving such medications. Thus, CRT has been added to the list of evidence-based therapies that make heart failure patients feel better and live longer [5,6,10,11].

Collectively, these trials have studied virtually all the clinically meaningful endpoints that are routinely evaluated in clinical trials of heart failure, including endpoints that measure quality of life, functional status, exercise capacity, morbidity, and mortality. The beneficial effects of CRT on such endpoints have been striking. Moreover, these trials have provided convincing evidence that CRT produces reverse remodeling of the failing heart. That is, CRT makes the failing heart smaller and stronger, an effect that is generally associated with improved survival in heart failure clinical trials. Although most patients respond favorably to biventricular pacing, some do not respond. The nonresponder rate for

CRT appears to vary from 25% to 35%, a rate similar to the nonresponder rate for heart failure drug therapies [23,24]. Suboptimal left ventricular lead placement, suboptimal AV and VV timing, ventricular scaring, heart failure disease progression, and a variety of other factors have been proposed as contributing to the nonresponder rate associated with CRT [10,11,23–25]. To date, however, no prospective predictors of responsiveness to CRT have been identified from the major clinical trials. The PROSPECT attempted to identify echocardiographic predictors of CRT response. The results of this study were disappointing because of the relatively high inter-corelab variability in determining echocardiographic measures of dyssynchrony. As a result, the presence of a single measure of dyssynchrony added only 11–13% additional predictive value to the QRS width. The authors concluded that no single measure of dyssynchrony may be recommended to improve patient selection for CRT is better than measurement of QRS duration. Ongoing and future studies with multiple imaging techniques may facilitate a better understanding of the limitations of CRT and aid in better patient selection.

Defining clinical outcomes after implantation of resynchronization device

Response to CRT can be divided into acute and chronic responses. Acute response was measured in several early studies by using pressure catheters. These studies show that left ventricular pacing and biventricular pacing acutely cause a dramatic and significant increase in contractility measured by improvements in the peak rate of rise of LV pressure during isovolumetric contraction LV dP/dt_{max} by 20%, increases in stroke volume by 40%, and increases in stroke work by up to 66% [3,4,16,18,20,26] (Figure 8.1). Despite significant improvements, acute measurements at the time of implantation have not been successfully used to determine long-term outcome [27]. Some early studies have indicated that lack of acute hemodynamic response does not preclude long term CRT response and that mechanism of chronic CRT response may be more complex than the effects represented by acute hemodynamic measurements. An alternative explanation is that the wrong acute parameters were measured to predict long-term outcome. At this point in time, the acute response is not universally accepted as an objective measure of a patient's response to therapy, and most investigators wait some period of time to observe for a chronic response to CRT.

The first assessment of the time period necessary for a chronic response was provided in the late 1990s, when it was observed that patients responding to CRT often required a period of at least 3 months of therapy. Some patients continued to improve after the initial 3 months, but at 6 months about 90% of benefit is usually reached. The earliest description of the response rate came from MIRACLE trial. MIRACLE was the first large prospective, randomized, double-blind, parallel-controlled clinical trial to evaluate the risks and

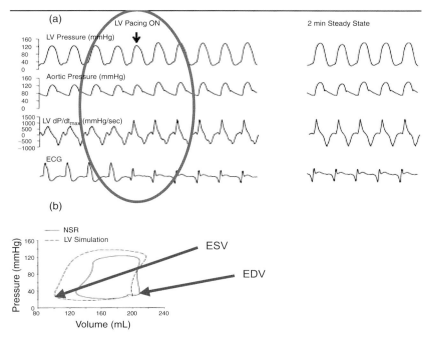

Fig. 8.1 (a) Stimulation of LV free-wall rapidly increased aortic and ventricular systolic pressures, aortic pulse amplitude, and maximal dP/dt. These increases changed very little after 2 minutes of steady-state stimulation. Please note circle highlights onset of LV pacing. (b) Pressure–volume loops measured under baseline conditions and during LV stimulation. Both stroke work (loop area) and stroke volume (width) increased, whereas end-systolic volume (left side of loop) decreased. End-diastolic volume and corresponding end-diastolic pressure were unchanged.

benefits of CRT [23,24]. Four hundred and fifty-three patients with moderate to severe symptoms of heart failure associated with a left ventricular ejection fractio 35% and a QRS duration of 130 ms were randomized (double-blind) to CRT ($n = 228$) or to a control group ($n = 225$) for 6 months while their conventional therapy for heart failure was maintained [24]. Primary endpoints were NYHA class, quality-of-life score (using the Minnesota Living with Heart Failure questionnaire), and 6-minute hall walk distance. Compared with the control group, patients randomized to CRT demonstrated a significant improvement in all three primary endpoints [24]. Moreover, treadmill exercise time (81 seconds vs. 19 seconds; $p = 0.001$), peak VO_2 (1.1 vs. 0.1 mL $\cdot$ kg^{-1} $\cdot$ min^{-1}; $p < 0.01$), and left ventricular ejection fraction (4.6% vs. −0.2%; $p < 0.001$), as well as other measures of ventricular structure and function, were significantly improved. Patients randomized to CRT demonstrated a highly significant improvement in a composite clinical heart failure response endpoint compared with controls, suggesting an overall improvement in heart failure clinical status. In addition, approximately 50% fewer patients in the CRT group required hospitalization or intravenous medications for worsening heart failure (both $p<0.05$). The major limitation of therapy was the unsuccessful implantation of the device in 8% of patients and the fact that 33% of patients who underwent device implantation either did not change or got worse according to composite response. Several other studies have demonstrated the nonresponse rate to be slightly higher or lower. The dilemma of one who is assessing the true response rate is best illustrated by a review published in *JAMA* [24]. Survival over time in recipients of CRT or combined CRT-ICD devices was similar in the 95 observational studies that reported this outcome as in the 14 randomized controlled trials (RCTs). Only one observational study [28] compared outcomes in patients with CRT with outcomes in contemporaneous controls without CRT; these findings of improved LVEF (weighted mean difference, 4.6%; 95% CI, 2.9–6.3%) and lower mortality rates (RR, 0.64; 95% CI, 0.26–1.56%) in the CRT group were consistent in magnitude to the findings from the meta-analysis of the CRT trials. The pooled effectiveness estimates from the observational studies for functional outcomes were consistent with those estimates from the efficacy RCTs. For example, in the RCTs, 59% of patients implanted with a CRT device improved by at least one NYHA class, and in the observational studies between 63% and 82% of patients improved by at least one NYHA class. Determining the true response rate with CRT was hampered by the lack of a universally accepted definition for *response* [29] and the fact that patients may demonstrate a response clinically but not echocardiographically or vice versa (with only 76% agreement in the classification of responder/nonresponder between definitions) [30]. No covariates were consistently shown across studies to predict CRT response. To complicate the situation even more is the fact that response to therapy clearly differs with different etiologies of heart failure. Patients with nonischemic etiology have significantly better outcomes with the regard to remodeling-echocardiographic parameters [29–31].

Defining failing resynchronization and causes for failure (nonresponders)

After implantation and testing of the CRT device, the patient is discharged to follow-up. Evaluation of response to therapy should be assessed at a visit typically 3–6 months after implantation. The main question to be answered at that time is whether the patient has responded to CRT. As previously mentioned no standard definition exists for the definition of responders versus nonresponders. Certainly, the main component is the patient's subjective assessment, but CRT, as with any device therapy, has an important placebo effect and distinguishing a true response from this effect can be difficult. Objective measures, such are echo-based parameters, including improvement in ejection fraction, left

Table 8.1 Definition of response to CRT.

Subjective criteria for a nonresponder:
Improvement of less than 1 NYHA class is not sufficient for improvement.
Patient notes no improvement in symptoms after device was implanted.
Patient initially got better but after 3–6 months is getting worse.

Objective criteria:
LV EF improved <5% in a nonischemic patient, <2–3% in an ischemic patient or reduction of end systolic volume <15% in anonischemic patient or <10% in an ischemic patient.
Once patient is identified as a nonresponder a search for reversible causes should be undertaken.

ventricular dimensions or left ventricular volume or an exercise evaluation, may yield additional useful information. As we stated previously, most of the benefit appears to occur by 3 months and persists thereafter. Some improvement can be seen even 6 months after implantation, but, in general, remodeling in nonischemic patients typically is stable 6 months after implantation [29,32,33].

The degree of remodeling is significantly different in ischemic versus nonischemic patient population. That has been observed in all randomized studies from MIRACLE and when we discuss nonresponse to therapy that should be taken in account [24,29–33]. For the purpose of this review, nonresponders may be defined according to subjective and objective criteria (Table 8.1).

Absence of dyssynchrony at the baseline

In the beginning of this chapter, we defined ventricular dyssynchrony as an abnormal ventricular contraction that results in suboptimal ventricular filling, a reduction in left ventricular contractility, prolonged duration or magnitude of mitral regurgitation, and paradoxical septal wall motion, which all conspire to reduce stroke volume and subsequently ability of the failing heart to eject blood. This definition refers to mechanical dyssynchrony, and, for almost all of the clinical trials, ventricular dyssynchrony, was defined as a QRS duration >120 ms on the surface ECG. What that means is that we are using a surrogate electrical definition for mechanical dyssynchrony. It has been recently accepted based on echocardiography that in up to 40% of patients with prolonged QRS complexes, mechanical dyssynchrony may not be present. In other words, this surrogate definition does not work for up to 40% of patients. Thus, it seems that enough electrical delay exists in some patients to cause a left bundle block pattern on the surface ECG, but mechanical delay may not be present or of sufficient magnitude to cause deleterious hemodynamic consequences.

Patients with an increased QRS duration, but without dyssynchrony on the basis of echocardiographic criteria may be less likely to respond to CRT. Current indications only use an increased QRS duration as a rough marker for dyssynchrony. To date several studies have demonstrated that baseline QRS duration is a reliable marker for long-term hemodynamic improvement. Auricchio and associates [23] showed that there was a positive correlation between QRS duration, percentage of change of LV dP/dt_{max} and pulse pressure during CRT. By combining the baseline QRS duration and change in LV dP/dt_{max}, these authors concluded that more than 80% of patients with QRS>150 ms and >25% change in LV dP/dt_{max} will benefit from resynchronization.

Another controversial issue is the presence of a right bundle branch block pattern on EKG. The majority of patients with chronic heart failure (CHF) and abnormal QRS duration have a left bundle branch block pattern that activates the left lateral wall later than it activated the interventricular septum. It is on the basis of this premise that CRT seems to be beneficial by activating the left lateral wall earlier or synchronously with the septum [1,34,35]. A patient with right ventricular delay and intact LV lateral wall timing would seem to be less likely to benefit from this type of pacing. In fact, some studies have shown that patients with right bundle branch block are less likely to benefit from CRT; however, the original trials included a small number of patients with EKGs showing a right bundle branch block pattern. Others argue that CRT should still be offered to this population, because some patients with a RBBB were included in clinical trials [34,35] (Figures 8.2 and 8.3).

Another consideration is that either a left bundle branch block or right bundle branch block pattern does not truly represent the conduction in patients with cardiomyopathy. These patients have conduction abnormalities and complex wall motion abnormalities in addition to "simple" bundle branch blocks [35]. Severing the right bundle branch in a man leads to a QRS duration of about 120 ms. Severing the left bundle branch results in a QRS duration of about 150 ms. CHF patients may have QRS durations >200 ms. The remainder of the delay is intraventricular and interventricular, so classification of a patient as right bundle branch block or left bundle branch block may not truly represent one pure type of dyssynchronous pattern. Overall, no other criteria for dyssynchrony other than QRS duration have been used in major trials, and no consensus exists on the optimal echocardiographic parameters to further define dyssynchrony. It is not unexpected that patients may not respond to therapy if they did not have an abnormality of contraction to begin with or if their wall motion abnormality is not corrected because of the LV lead misplacement. It should be emphasized that if the LV ventricular lead is not implanted in an appropriate position, LV pacing may cause dyssynchrony and in fact *worsen* the patient's hemodynamics and clinical condition (Figures 8.2 and 8.3). There aredata in the literature as well as case reports that support this position. This may account for the observation that some patients in the MIRACLE trial worsened after LV lead implantation [31,33,34]. Some investigators

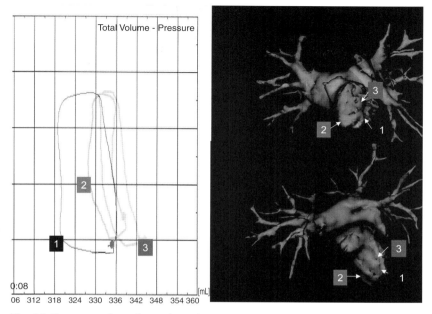

Fig. 8.2 Pressure–volume loops from the same patient obtained by coronary vein LV pacing from the three different sites. Left ventricle is illustrated with three-dimensional reconstruction from the CT scan in two different projections. The first projection shows the left side of the heart from the apex and the second projection shown straight down from above. CT scan image is given with attached left atrium and pulmonary veins. Pacing from the site 1: infero-lateral-apical LV has the largest stroke volume and stroke work with the LV dP/dt_{max}, that is, just smaller than one from site 3. Site 2, is closest to the pacing from the RV apex has the smallest dP/dt_{max}, and the stroke volume and the stroke work. (See color plate section).

feel that some additional evaluation of dyssynchrony may reduce the rate of nonresponders, however as stated earlier, the PROSPECT (PRedictors Of reSPonse to CrT) trial failed to confirm these findings [36–39]. None of the evaluated echocardiographic measures of dyssynchrony provided much additional predictive value above that provided from the QRS width. Moreover, use of the optimal pacing strategy for heart failure patients with bradycardia or heart block without evidence of ventricular dyssynchrony remains controversial. Right ventricular pacing produces "iatrogenic" left ventricular dyssynchrony and may worsen heart failure, as demonstrated in some acute hemodynamic studies and Dual Chamber and VVI Implantable Defibrillator (DAVID) trial [40].

The QRS width-based definition of dyssynchrony may also limit patients who may benefit from CRT. Some patients with normal QRS duration (less <120 ms) have been found to exhibit dyssynchrony. The recently published

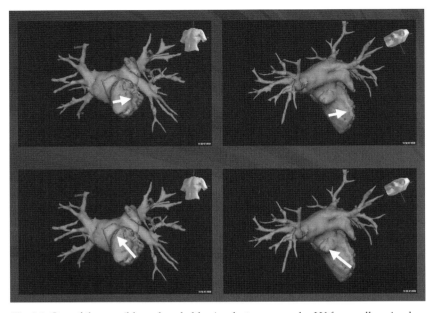

Fig. 8.3 One of the possible and probably simplest reasons why LV free-wall pacing has significantly higher stroke volume and stroke work when compared to RV septal pacing is illustrated here. The left ventricle is illustrated with three-dimensional reconstruction from the CT scan in two different projections. The first projection shows the left side of the heart from the apex and the second projection shown straight down from above. Arrows indicate the vector of initial electrical and mechanical activation in the case of left-free wall pacing (right bundle branch block with right superior axis on ECG) in the two lower pictures. Two upper pictures are illustrating initial vector of electrical and mechanical activation in the case of intraventricular-septal pacing that would give a left bundle branch block appearance on ECG. Note the aortic position in comparison to vector of electrical/mechanical activation. In case of a LBBB septal pacing, vector points straight away from aorta but in case of RBBB and left free-wall pacing vector points in the direction of aorta-LV outflow tract. One can easily recognize that in the case of the LBBB first 40–60 ms of LV activation are mechanically wasted due to the fact that blood is pushed away from the LV outflow tract aortic knob. The completely reversed situation exists with RBBB and LV free-wall pacing. This fact also explains why LV free-wall pacing increases stroke volume and stroke work within just one beat. See pressure tracings from Figure 8.1 and volume loops from Figures 8.2 and 8.10. (See color plate section).

RethinQ trial [41] addressed this issue. Biventricular ICDs were implanted in 172 patients who had a standard indication for an ICD and a narrow QRS with echocardiographic evidence for dyssynchrony. Patients received the CRT device and then were randomly assigned to the CRT group or to a control group (no CRT) for 6 months. The primary endpoint was the proportion of patients with an increase in peak oxygen consumption of at least 1.0 ml per kilogram of body weight per minute during cardiopulmonary exercise testing at 6 months. At 6 months, the CRT group and the control group did not differ significantly in the proportion of patients who achieved the primary endpoint (46% and 41%, respectively). There were 24 heart failure events requiring intravenous therapy in 14 patients in the CRT group (16.1%) and 41 heart failure events in 19 patients in the control group (22.3%), but the difference was not significant [42]. Authors concluded that CRT did not improve peak oxygen consumption in patients with moderate-to-severe heart failure, providing evidence that patients with heart failure and narrow QRS intervals may not benefit from CRT. This is in contrast with previously published, smaller nonrandomized studies [43,44].

One procedure that is frequently performed is the upgrade of an existing pacemaker or defibrillator to a CRT device. Patients that are paced in the RV may have a normal QRS at baseline, but with pacing they develop LBBB and dyssynchrony. This was not addressed in the initial clinical trials; however subsequent smaller studies have shown that these patients seem to benefit from CRT [43–46]. These patients may be excellent candidates because right ventricular apical pacing causes a dyssynchronous activation pattern [47]. Animal studies have shown that long-term right ventricular pacing leads to myofibrillar disarray, asymmetric hypertrophy, and dilatation of the left ventricle [47–49]. In humans, echocardiographic studies confirm the dyssynchronous activation and reduced efficiency, and others have found elevated serum markers of CHF and stress [50–52]. Major trials, such as the Mode Selection Trial (MOST) and the Dual Chamber and VVI Implantable Defibrillator (DAVID) trial, have determined that this type of pacing is detrimental in terms of CHF symptoms, and the current practice is to avoid unnecessary ventricular pacing [40,53–56]. Methods to reduce unnecessary right ventricular pacing are discussed in detail in Chapter 9. Pacing the right ventricle from a site other than the apex, such as using direct His-bundle pacing, may reduce dyssynchrony and CHF as well [57]. Otherwise, CHF patients with an indication for pacing, who may require a great deal of ventricular pacing, could benefit from a strategy that employs CRT, but this indication is not yet approved. BLOCK-HF is a trial addressing this issue and the HOBIPACE study revealed that patients with AV block and left ventricular dysfunction had improved quality of life, left ventricular ejection fraction, and exercise duration with CRT compared with standard dual-chamber pacing [58].

Dyssynchrony present at the baseline but not corrected at implantation—Normal device function

LV lead position

As discussed previously in this chapter, response rates to CRT have been less than ideal and that most trials report response rates in the range of 60– 70%

[25,59]. Assessment of response to therapy should be done at 3-month and 6-month follow-up visits. At the 3-month follow-up, the patient should be questioned about heart failure symptoms and specific activity limitations compared with before pacing therapy. Failure to improve at least one NYHA class should be taken as a warning sign for lack of a response to therapy. First, electrocardiography should be performed. Appropriate biventricular pacing can be confirmed by EKG or by device interrogation. A well-placed left ventricular lead yields a paced complex in which the forces in leads V_1 and V_2 are positive and the leads 1 and aVL are negative (rightward axis shift). This EKG should be compared with the postimplant and baseline EKG [60,61]. Shortening of QRS duration is not mandatory for successful CRT and in a review of many studies, a decrease or increase of the QRS duration does not appear to be predictive of a response [62]. Specifically, some acute studies indicate that LV lead should pace 30–40 ms before the RV lead in which case QRS duration may be longer than simultaneous RV-LV pacing [63,64]. However, there is a great deal of individual variability for optimal timing of LV and RV pacing.

At the 3-month and 6-month follow-up, the device should be completely evaluated for normal function of sensing and pacing parameters. Echocardiography may be performed at 3 months or 6 months to evaluate ejection fraction, left ventricular dimensions, volumes and mitral regurgitation, and possibly dyssynchrony, especially in clinical nonresponders. If a patient is responding to therapy as expected, echocardiography is considered optional by some investigators. Others however, perform routine echocardiography for all CRT patients. If any ventricular remodeling has occurred, then the previously optimized values are likely to have changed [65]. If the patient has not responded to therapy as expected, optimization of AV and VV intervals should be performed at 3-month and/or 6-month follow- up. The methodology of optimization is discussed in Chapters 4 and 7.

When the implanted device is functioning properly and patient had dyssynchrony at baseline, the most likely reason for lack of response is the LV lead position. The LV lead must first be delivered in an appropriate position to be effective. There are several possible obstacles to optimal LV lead position. The first is coronary venous anatomy. The second most common reason for inappropriate LV lead position would be myocardial scarring that was a result of coronary artery disease or an inflammatory process (Figures 8.4–8.8). The third most common problem is phrenic nerve stimulation with diaphragmatic capture. At the time of implantation once the coronary sinus has been cannulated, balloon occlusive venography is performed to identify the existing anatomy and possible target vessels. Contrary to coronary artery anatomy, coronary venous anatomy differs greatly from patient to patient. The venogram should be performed in at least two oblique projections to fully understand the anatomy. The vessels are analyzed for location, size, and angulation and tortuosity of the initial segments. The target vessel is identified, and a plan for placement of the

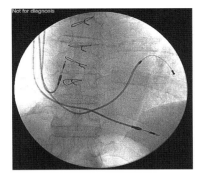

Fig. 8.4 This lead position is not optimal. The lead was initially placed closer to the mid heart level, however diaphragmatic stimulation required the implanter to pull the lead to a more basal position.

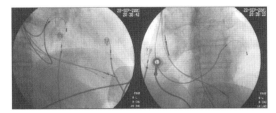

Fig. 8.5 Lead placement in two projections. LAO 30 projection shows that lead is located in a lateral position. RAO 20 projection clearly shows that lead is basal. This is not optimal. This patient may not fully respond to therapy.

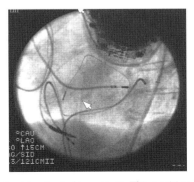

Fig. 8.6 Left ventricular lead implanted in septum. This position is suboptimal. It is separated from the RV-pacing lead by only few centimeters and minimal to no hemodynamic benefit is likely to result from this position.

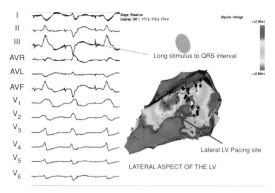

Fig. 8.7 LV endocardial electrogram voltage map of a patient with lateral wall myocardial infarction. Pacing from the lower edge of scar produces two different QRS morphologies. One with right inferior axis and other with left superior axis. Both morphologies have RBBB and long pacing stimulus to QRS interval. This illustrates difficulties of LV pacing inside and at the edge of the scar. Long delays like these may cause significant delays in LV activation and cause hemodynamically ineffective pacing. (See color plate section).

lead, which includes the decision of what vessel to use, is formulated based on the anatomy. At this time, there is no definitive consensus of the optimal LV lead position. The coronary sinus typically has several branches: middle cardiac vein, posterior vein, posterolateral vein, lateral vein, anterolateral vein, and anterior vein [66]. The preferred site of the coronary sinus lead is in the posterolateral

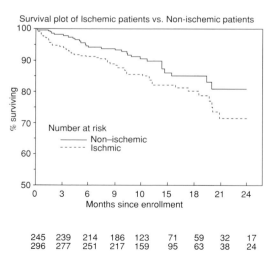

Fig. 8.8 Survival of patients with ischemic versus nonishemic cardiomyopathy from the MIRACLE trial. There is a statistically significant difference $p<0.05$ between the two groups. The nonischemic group is doing better over a 24-month period.

and lateral location. This can be achieved from the venous branches of the same name, but the venous system is variable, and the distal segments of many of the branches may lead to the posterolateral position. Evidence suggests that lateral locations are associated with the greatest response rates [67].

There are only a few original studies that compare the limited number of LV lead positions in the coronary venous system with outcome from CRT. These studies can be divided in acute studies with direct invasive measurements and noninvasive indirect measurement studies. The disadvantage of direct measurements with invasive studies is that they have a risk of vascular injury and stroke, and, so far, experience with them has been limited and the results mixed. Noninvasive measurements have blossomed in the last few years, but despite very significant investments in many different echocardiographic-derived measurement results are not very promising. In my personal experience, with 100 patients that had acute hemodynamic optimization at the time of implant with pressure impedance catheters, mid-lateral and apical lateral positions result in the best response rates (Figures 8.9 and 8.10). Another investigator using acute Millar measurements of changes in LV dP/dT reports that if the left ventricular electrogram is located in the latter half of the QRS complex, or at least 100 ms from QRS onset then response rates to CRT are high [61,62]. If multiple vessels are available in this location, then we test multiple positions to avoid possible diaphragmatic pacing.

Several technologies are being evaluated to help refine optimal lead positioning. Both echocardiographic and computed tomographic evaluation of delayed mechanical activation are being tested to identify the individual lead placement that maximizes resynchronization. The benefit of computed tomography is that coronary sinus anatomic information is obtained in addition to

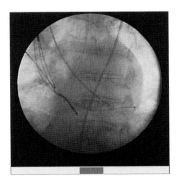

Fig. 8.9 Final hemodynamically optimal position with best stroke volume and LV dP/dt$_{max}$. Note the pressure–volume catheter in the LV of this patient. This was the best position in 80% of our series of 100 patients tested with a pressure–volume catheter. Using this testing method to determine optimal LV lead position, AV interval, and VV interval, we have achieved 93% response rate.

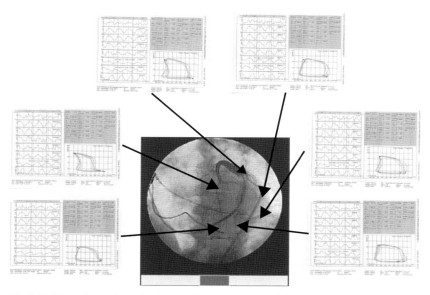

Fig. 8.10 Hemodynamic testing in one of our patients. Six different LV-pacing positions are presented here. Highest dP/dt max was achieved in anterior and anterolateral positions, but the highest stroke volume was achieved closer to the apex of the LV. Different positions in the LV may vary by up to 20% of dP/dt_{max} and up to 50% of maximal stroke volume.

mechanical information [68]. Use of transthoracic echocardiography in the electrophysiology laboratory is not a realistic option. Image quality may be suboptimal as a result of the flat position of the patient, ambient lighting, and the limitations of the sterile field. Intracardiac echocardiography shows promise as an adjunctive tool. Vector velocity imaging has been tested in conjunction with intracardiac echocardiography to refine lead position. The lead can be placed into several positions and a visual or graphic evaluation can be performed with pacing at that location. The best parameters may result in a better selection of an optimal LV lead position [69].

After the lead is advanced, the site is tested for capture thresholds and presence or absence of phrenic nerve stimulation. Phrenic nerve stimulation is a frequent complication of LV pacing, especially when the leads are positioned at the apical lateral sites. The choice of lead depends on the anatomy of the branch and diaphragmatic pacing threshold. Smaller bipolar leads are used most frequently because of the ability to program different configurations to overcome phrenic nerve stimulation or elevated pacing thresholds.

The minimally invasive subxiphoid epicardial approach is being used by cardiac electrophysiologists for epicardial ablation. This approach uses a spinal needle placed under the xiphoid process and advanced toward the cardiac border. A small puff of contrast is used to confirm position. The pericardial sac is punctured with the needle, and a wire is advanced into the space. After the needle is withdrawn, a sheath may be placed over the wire for access into the space. This technique lends itself to the placement of an epicardial left ventricular lead, and possibly other leads, without the constraint of venous anatomy. Placement of leads in this manner allows a great deal of freedom in lead positioning. This could be combined with methods of rapid lead position evaluation and timing that result in a completely optimized system. Another possible benefit of this approach is the avoidance of the intravascular system, which could reduce the risk of venous occlusion and possibly system extraction. One of the major limitations of this approach is the mechanism of lead fixation. The epicardial space allows for nearly free movement of objects. A lead system would need to be developed that allows for fixation to occur against the myocardium preferentially. Epicardial leads and delivery systems for this approach are being developed. Also, not every pericardial space is easily accessible. Patients with previous open-heart surgery may develop fibrosis in the pericardial space that does not allow access [26].

Surgical placement of epicardial leads is becoming more commonplace. These leads may be placed at the time of bypass or valve surgery for future use. Minimally invasive and robot-assisted surgeries are also performed to place leads after attempts through the venous system have been unsuccessful. This method does not require full sternotomy and reduces patient recovery time [26,64].

If patient had dyssynchrony at the time of implantation, lead position is probably the most important factor predicting response to therapy. The mid lateral and apical lateral positions have been shown to be associated with improved response rates, However, response is individual and dependent on multiple variables. At this time we do not have a universally accepted easy to use tool for optimal lead positioning. The presence of scar tissue in the posterolateral left ventricle and lack of viable myocardium has been found to be associated with reduced response rates [70]. This has been demonstrated using MRI to define transmural scar, as well as contrast echocardiography.

A chest x-ray for evaluation of lead position should be performed. If the lead is in a suboptimal position, then repositioning or adding the second LV lead based on the limitations of anatomy could be considered (Figures 8.11–8.13). Surgical epicardial lead placement is another option because there are no limitations based on venous anatomy. Optimization of AV intervals and VV interval timing should also be performed in the nonresponder, although technology advancements will allow this to be performed in all patients after implant.

Atrial fibrillation

The presence of atrial fibrillation with a rapid ventricular response also prevents CRT from being delivered. Atrial fibrillation with a rapid rate will prevent the

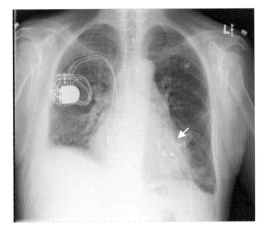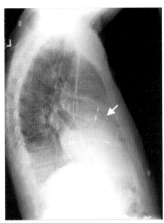

Fig. 8.11 PA and lateral chest x-ray of a 55-year-old patient with nonishemic cardiomy-opathy and an implanted biventricular pacemaker. Patient did not respond to therapy after 2 years of follow-up. He did not increase his LVEF from baseline of 15% or have a decrease in LV volume. His left ventricular lead is positioned antero-laterally. Compare this LV lead position with LV lead position at Figure 8.4.

device from pacing, if the ventricular response is above the programmed lower rate and according to some studies this may account for up to 18% of loss of LV pacing and CRT. Management options include addition of amiodarone and cardioversion in an effort to restore sinus rhythm, pharmacologic slowing of the ventricular response to below the pacing rate, programming special algorithms that favor pacing, and ablation of the AV junction. Radio frequency ablation of the AV junction has been long established as a safe and well-investigated option and it would allow complete control of heart rate and eliminate competition with the underlying ventricular rhythm. Programming algorithms that favor ventricular pacing has met with limited success, at least partially because the pacing rate is increased and ventricular fusion from both the RV and LV paced wavefronts may be variable and inconsistent. Recently, RF ablation of the left atrium for atrial fibrillation has been advocated by several European groups, although the results in patients with both heart failure and left atrial enlarge-ment are not nearly as good as left atrial ablation in patients without CHF [71]. We recommend one (or more) attempts to restore and maintain sinus rhythm. If that fails, one approach is to try pharmacologic management with beta-blockers (e.g. especially carvedilol) to slow the heart rate and if that fails to proceed with AV junction ablation or primary ablation of the left atrium if it is not too enlarged. A reasonable goal is to achieve at least 90% pacing in LV. This should prompt the need for improved rate control and, possibly, attempts to restore sinus rhythm.

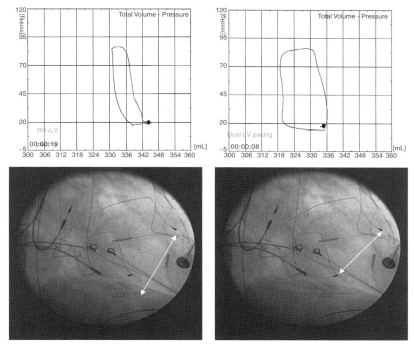

Fig. 8.12 After admission patient had implantation of the new LV lead with hemodynamic testing. We used variety of pacing configurations and in this patient two LV leads were better than any other combination. He was left with two unipolar LV leads that were connected with a bipolar adapter and were paced simultaneously. VV timing optimization demonstrated that the best stroke volume increase was achieved when the LV was paced 40 ms earlier than the RV lead. This figure demonstrates pressure volume loops achieved with two LV leads versus RV-LV lead pacing. Stroke volume with two LV leads was almost 100% higher than in the conventional LV and RV configuration.

AV interval optimization

If the AV interval is too long and the patient's intrinsic PR conduction prevents biventricular pacing, hemodynamic deterioration may occur. The AV interval may have been programmed appropriately, but accelerated intrinsic AV conduction may result in loss of effective biventricular pacing. Programmed paced AV delays differ significantly from sensed AV delays during sinus rhythm. The main reasons for this are latency in atrial sensing and capture and intra-atrial conduction delay. The magnitude of atrial capture and sensing latencies varies among patients and is influenced by multiple factors including lead design, sensing circuitry, and velocity of right-to-left atrial conduction that is partially dependent on status of the autonomic nervous system.. Most CRT devices allow

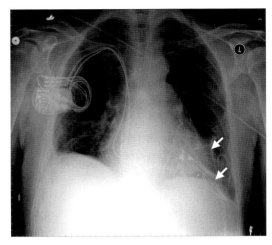

Fig. 8.13 Chest x-ray of the same patient, but this time 6 months after implantation of the second LV lead. After 6 months patients LV EF increased to 25% and after 4 years of follow-up is 35%. Patient was removed from the transplant list as well.

adjustment of the AV and VV delay. Too long an AV delay permits inefficient diastolic filling, which affects subsequent cycles. Diastolic mitral regurgitation may occur, and contractility is reduced. Echo-based evaluation of transmitral Doppler flow is frequently used for optimization. The normal transmitral pattern reveals distinct E and A waves. The E wave represents passive ventricular filling, and the A wave represents atrial contraction. Prolonged AV conduction results in fusion of these two waves. The opposite end of the spectrum is an AV delay that is too short. On transmitral Doppler, this is seen by truncation of the A wave. Patients will frequently report increased pulmonary symptoms and pacemaker syndrome type symptoms. As is seen on the transmitral flow patterns, CRT improves diastolic ventricular filling, which continues to improve over time as the ventricle remodels. It should be emphasized that benefit from optimization of AV intervals have not yet been demonstrated in large prospective clinical trials [26,63,65,69].

Nevertheless, most manufacturers have developed algorithms that are automatically programmable in their devices that automatically optimize AV intervals, either at the time of programming or at regular intervals.

VV interval optimization

Another timing variable present in most devices is alterable timing between the left and right ventricular pacing outputs. Patients vary significantly in the amount of delay between myocardial segments. Adjustable pacing intervals may improve resynchronization. Echo-based studies and acute studies using impedance pressure catheters reveal that most patients' optimal LV and RV

Table 8.2 Differential diagnosis of causes of non-response to CRT

I. Absence of dyssynchrony at the baseline

II. Dyssynchrony present at the baseline but not corrected at implantation
    A. With normal device function (normal capture and sensing)
       1. LV lead position suboptimal
       2. Atrial Fibrillation
       3. Non optimal AV delay
       4. Non optimal VV timing
       5. Inadequate percentage of LV pacing due to AF with a rapid ventricular rate, frequent ventricular ectopy, atrial rate above upper rate limit, etc.
       6. Latency or delay of conduction from LV lead
    B. Abnormal device function (inappropriate pacing and sensing function)
       1. Increase in LV or RV pacing threshold
       2. LV or RV lead dislodgement
       3. Atrial undersensing
       4. T-wave oversensing
       5. Ventricular double counting
       6. Far-field atrial sensing

III. Other reasons: progression of disease or development of new inter-current disease.

pacing is not simultaneous. In some studies, the best VV interval is typically seen with LV activation approximately 40 ms before RV pacing [72]. Several studies have shown improvement in responder rates, quality of life, exercise time, ejection fraction, direct contractile measurements, and NYHA class compared with simultaneous pacing [72–74]. Unfortunately, noninvasive optimization of ventricular timing can be tedious. It has required use of echo-based parameters such as aortic velocity time integral, tissue Doppler imaging, or M-mode evaluation. This process can be time-consuming and technically challenging; therefore, it has been mostly reserved for nonresponders. Invasive measurements using impedance volume catheters can be helpful, but the methodology is neither widely accepted nor widely available and is also tedious and is associated with a small risk. Currently, an intracardiac electrogram-based method is available. It measures the timing between all the leads and calculates the optimal settings based on a mathematical formula. This has been shown to correlate with echo-based optimization and takes only a few minutes to perform. No large controlled randomized trials have yet shown an objective benefit VV timing optimization.

Abnormal device function (inappropriate pacing and sensing function)
The treatment of nonresponders should first focus on whether the patient is receiving CRT. As previously stated the device function should be evaluated to ensure appropriate sensing and capture of all leads.

Loss of CRT may be result of intermittent or permanent loss of LV capture for various reasons. A very common problem and one of the major limitations of LV lead implantation is coronary venous anatomy and presence of myocardial scar close to the target area for implantation. The extent of scarring is clearly related to the success of LV lead implantation and was addressed earlier in this chapter and also in Chapter 7. The relationship between the extent of transmural scarring caused by coronary artery disease and success of CRT was investigated in several studies, but probably as important is the epicardial scarring that is characteristic for nonischemic cardiomyopathy. That problem has to be addressed in future investigations.

At follow-up, routine testing in the clinic should include capture thresholds to document that left ventricular capture is present. Lead dislodgement or a change in capture threshold may result in the loss of left ventricular pacing. It also is possible that left ventricular lead placement and pacing thresholds are fine, but resynchronization is lost for other reasons. Anything that frequently or consistently inhibits left ventricular stimulation can effectively inhibit CRT. Basic problems that may affect any pacing system can be classified as:

1 Undersensing
2 Oversensing
3 Loss of capture

Undersensing may be atrial and ventricular. Atrial undersensing may be divided into *true undersensing* caused by a small atrial endocardial signal *or functional undersensing* caused by atrial events falling in refractory periods. These problems may result in loss of atrial synchronous ventricular pacing and delivery of LV pacing. These problems can be addressed by device reprogramming but occasionally require surgical repositioning of the atrial lead.

Ventricular undersensing is a rare problem with CRT and typically would not cause loss of LV pacing, It can be addressed in the same way as atrial undersensing by device reprogramming to higher sensitivity or with lead repositioning.

Atrial oversensing may result in spurious mode switching, causing reversion to a nontracking mode DDI/R or VDI with loss of atrial synchronous ventricular pacing and CRT. Spurious mode switching can usually be minimized by reducing atrial sensitivity and modifying the PVAB.

Ventricular oversensing may cause inhibition of ventricular pacing and loss of CRT as well as spurious VT detection resulting in misdiagnosis of ventricular tachyarrhythmias. These problems can be addressed by reprogramming to a lower sensitivity but caution must be applied to guarantee VF detection. Occasionally, the LV lead may dislodge into or close to the mitral annulus and sensing of the far-field atrial signal result in inhibition of ventricular pacing. This may require lead revision to correct.

Loss of capture is defined as an atrial or ventricular stimulus without capture. Loss of ventricular capture is the most common cause for a lack of response. The complication rates associated with implantation of CRT have been remarkably low. The most common complication is inability to deliver coronary sinus pacing for one of the reasons mentioned above, but the overall delivery rate exceeds 90%. The need for re-operation to replace or reposition the coronary sinus lead occurs in 6% of cases. Dissection or perforation of the coronary sinus occurs in up to 4% of patients, but tamponade results in <1% of implants [75]. Overall LV lead dislodgement rate in initial studies was about 12% but currently is probably <5% in centers with a large experience [75]. Loss of LV lead capture may be sudden or gradual due to the exit block. The 12-lead ECG remains to be with the device interrogation critical tool for evaluation of LV lead capture. Lack of capture can be solved by device reprogramming to higher outputs or with LV lead repositioning. Frequent premature ventricular contractions also may inhibit ventricular pacing output, but that is relatively rare cause of loss of LV capture. However, if ventricular bigeminy or ventricular ectopy precludes CRT delivery, it may need to be suppressed with amiodarone, or even in some cases require catheter ablation to allow effective CRT delivery.

Although follow-up for the device is similar to that seen for contemporary dual-chamber pacemakers and defibrillators and is usually managed by an implanting physician, heart failure specialists, general cardiologists, and primary care providers must possess the knowledge required to recognize the aforementioned limitations of CRT and to troubleshoot the device. The benefits of CRT are substantial and unequivocal in the group of patients studied to date. CRT represents guideline-recommended, evidence-based therapy for the treatment of chronic heart failure.

References

1. Xiao HB, Brecker SJ, Gibson DG. Effects of abnormal activation on the time course of the left ventricular pressure pulse in dilated cardiomyopathy. *Br Heart J.* 1992;68:403–7.
2. Littmann L, Symanski JD. Hemodynamic implications of left bundle branch block. *J Electrocardiol.* 2000;33 Suppl:115–21.
3. Saxon LA, Kerwin WF, Cahalan MK, Kalman JM, Olgin JE, Foster E, Schiller NB, Shinbane JS, Lesh MD, Merrick SH. Acute effects of intraoperative multisite ventricular pacing on left ventricular function and activation/contraction sequence in patients with depressed ventricular function. *J Cardiovasc Electrophysiol.* 1998;9: 13–21.
4. Kerwin WF, Botvinick EH, O'Connell JW, Merrick SH, DeMarco T, Chatterjee K, Scheibly K, Saxon LA. Ventricular contraction abnormalities in dilated cardiomyopathy: effect of biventricular pacing to correct interventricular dyssynchrony. *J Am Coll Cardiol.* 2000;35:1221–1227.
5. Xaio HB, Roy C, Fujimoto S, Gibson DG. Natural history of abnormal conduction and its relation to prognosis in patients with dilated cardiomyopathy. *Int J Cardiol.* 1996;53:163–70.

6. Hunt SA, Abraham WT, Chin MH, Feldman AM, Francis GS, Ganiats TG, Jessup M, Konstam MA, Mancini DM, Michl K, Oates JA, Rahko PS, Silver MA, Stevenson LW, Yancy CW. ACC/AHA 2005 guideline update for the diagnosis and management of chronic heart failure in the adult: summary article. *Circulation.* 2005;112:1825–52; *J Am Coll Cardiol.* 2005;46:1116–43.

7. Adams KF, Lindenfeld J, Arnold JMO, Baker DW, Barnard DH, Baughman KL, Boehmer JP, Deedwania P, Dunbar SB, Elkayam U, Gheorghiade M, Howlett JG, Konstam MA, Kronenberg MW, Massie BM, Mehra MR, Miller AB, Moser DK, Patterson JH, Rodeheffer RJ, Sackner-Bernstein J, Silver MA, Starling RC, Stevenson LW, Wagoner LE. Executive summary: HFSA 2006 comprehensive heart failure practice guideline. *J Cardiac Failure.* 2006;12:10–38.

8. Unverferth DV, Magorien RD, Moeschberger ML, Baker PB, Fetters JK, Leier CV. Factors influencing the one-year mortality of dilated cardiomyopathy. *Am J Cardiol.* 1984;54:147–52.

9. Shamim W, Francis DP, Yousufuddin M, Varney S, Pieopli MF, Anker SD, Coats AJ. Intraventricular conduction delay: a prognostic marker in chronic heart failure. *Int J Cardiol.* 1999;70:171–8.

10. Abraham WT, Hayes DL. Cardiac resynchronization therapy for heart failure. *Circulation.* 2003;108:2596–2603.

11. Auricchio A, Abraham WT. Cardiac resynchronization therapy: current state of the art: cost versus benefit. *Circulation.* 2004;109:300–7.

12. Aaronson KD, Schwartz JS, Chen TM, Wong KL, Goin JE, Mancini DM. Development and prospective validation of a clinical index to predict survival in ambulatory patients referred for cardiac transplant evaluation. *Circulation.* 1997;95:2660–7.

13. Farwell D, Patel NR, Hall A, Ralph S, Sulke AN. How many people with heart failure are appropriate for biventricular resynchronization? *Eur Heart J.* 2000;21:1246–50.

14. Brophy JM, Deslauriers G, Rouleau JL. Long-term prognosis of patients presenting to the emergency room with decompensated congestive heart failure. *Can J Cardiol.* 1994;10:543–7.

15. Cazeau S, Ritter P, Bakdach S, Lazarus A, Limousin M, Henao L, Mundler O, Daubert JC, Mugica J. Four-chamber pacing in dilated cardiomyopathy. *Pacing Clin Electrophysiol.* 1994;17:1974–9.

16. Foster AH, Gold MR, McLaughlin JS. Acute hemodynamic effects of atrio-biventricular pacing in humans. *Ann Thorac Surg.* 1995;59:294–300.

17. Cazeau S, Ritter P, Lazarus A, Gras D, Backdach H, Mundler O, Mugica J. Multisite pacing for end-stage heart failure: early experience. *Pacing Clin Electrophysiol.* 1996;19:1748–57.

18. Blanc JJ, Etienne Y, Gilard M, Mansourati J, Munier S, Boschat J, Benditt DG, Lurie KG. Evaluation of different ventricular pacing sites in patients with severe heart failure: results of an acute hemodynamic study. *Circulation.* 1997;96:3273–7.

19. Leclercq C, Cazeau S, Le Breton H, Ritter P, Mabo P, Gras D, Pavin D, Lazarus A, Daubert JC. Acute hemodynamic effects of biventricular DDD pacing in patients with end-stage heart failure. *J Am Coll Cardiol.* 1998;32:1825–31.

20. Kass DA, Chen CH, Curry C, Talbot M, Berger R, Fetics B, Nevo E. Improved left ventricular mechanics from acute VDD pacing in patients with dilated cardiomyopathy and ventricular conduction delay. *Circulation.* 1999;99:1567–73.

21. Gras D, Mabo P, Tang T, Luttikuis O, Chatoor R, Pedersen AK, Tscheliessnigg HH, Deharo JC, Puglisi A, Silvestre J, Kimber S, Ross H, Ravazzi A, Paul V, Skehan D. Multisite pacing as a supplemental treatment of congestive heart failure: preliminary results of the Medtronic Inc. InSync Study. *Pacing Clin Electrophysiol.* 1998;21:2249–55.

22. Chung ES, Leon AR, Tavazzi L, Sun JP, Nihoyannopoulos P, Merlino J, Abraham WT, Ghio S, Leclercq C, Bax JJ, Yu CM, Gorsan J 3rd, St John Sutton M, De Sutter J, Murillo J. Results of the Predictors of Response to CRT (PROSPECT) trial. *Circulation.* 2008; 117: 2608–2016.

23. Auricchio A, Stellbrink C, Sack S, Block M, Vogt J, Bakker P, Mortensen P, Klein H. The Pacing Therapies for Congestive Heart Failure (PATH-CHF) Study: rationale, design, and endpoints of a prospective randomized multicenter study. *Am J Cardiol.* 1999;83:D130–D135.

24. Abraham WT, Fisher WG, Smith AL, Delurgio DB, Leon A, Loh E, Kocovic DZ, Packer M, Clavell AL, Hayes DL, Ellestad M, Messenger J (for the Multicenter InSync Randomized Clinical Evaluation (MIRACLE) Investigators and Coordinators). Double-blind, randomized controlled trial of cardiac resynchronization in chronic heart failure. *N Engl J Med.* 2002;346:1845–53.

25. McAlister FA, Ezekowitz J, Hooton N, Vandermeer B, Spooner C, Dryden DM, Page RL, Hlatky MA, Rowe BH. Cardiac resynchronization therapy for patients with left ventricular systolic dysfunction: a systematic review. *JAMA.* 2007; Jun 13;297(22):2502–14.

26. Burkhardt JD, Wilkoff BL. Interventional electrophysiology and cardiac resynchronization therapy: delivering electrical therapies for heart failure. *Circulation.* 2007; Apr 24;115(16):2208–20.

27. Auricchio A, Stellbrink C, Block M, Sack S, Vogt J, Bakker P, Klein H (for the Pacing Therapies for Congestive Heart Failure Study Group). Kramer A, Ding J, Salo R, Tockman B, Pochet T, Spinelli J (for the Guidant Congestive Heart Failure Research Group). Effect of pacing chamber and atrioventricular delay on acute systolic function of paced patients with congestive heart failure. *Circulation.* 1999; 99:2993–3001.

28. Stellbrink C, Breithardt OA, Franke A, Sack S, Bakker P, Auricchio A, Pochet T, Salo R, Kramer A, Spinelli J. PATH-CHF (PAcing THerapies in Congestive Heart Failure) Investigators; CPI Guidant Congestive Heart Failure Research Group. Impact of cardiac resynchronization therapy using hemodynamically optimized pacing on left ventricular remodeling in patients with congestive heart failure and ventricular conduction disturbances. *J Am Coll Cardiol.* 2001; Dec;38(7):1957–65.

29. Braunschweig F, Mortensen PT, Gras D, Reiser W, Lawo T, Mansour H, Sogaard P, Stegemann B, Bruns HJ, Linde C. InSync III Study Investigators. Monitoring of physical activity and heart rate variability in patients with chronic heart failure using cardiac resynchronization devices. *Am J Cardiol.* 2005; May 1;95(9):1104–7.

30. Birnie DH, Tang AS. The problem of non-response to cardiac resynchronization therapy. *Curr Opin Cardiol.* 2006; Jan;21(1):20–6.

31. Bleeker GB, Bax JJ, Fung JW, van der Wall EE, Zhang Q, Schalij MJ, Chan JY, Yu CM. Clinical versus echocardiographic parameters to assess response to cardiac resynchronization therapy. *Am J Cardiol.* 2006; Jan 15;97(2):260–3.

32. St John Sutton MG, Plappert T, Abraham WT, Smith AL, DeLurgio DB, Leon AR, Loh E, Kocovic DZ, Fisher WG, Ellestad M, Messenger J, Kruger K, Hilpisch KE,

Hill MR. Multicenter InSync Randomized Clinical Evaluation (MIRACLE) Study Group. Effect of cardiac resynchronization therapy on left ventricular size and function in chronic heart failure. *Circulation.* 2003; Apr 22;107(15):1985–90.

33. Molhoek SG, Bax JJ, Bleeker GB, Holman ER, Van Erven L, Bootsma M, Boersma E, Steendijk P, Van Der Wall EE, Schalij MJ. Long-term follow-up of cardiac resynchronization therapy in patients with end-stage heart failure. *J Cardiovasc Electrophysiol.* 2005;16:701–7.

34. Yu CM, Wing-Hong Fung J, Zhang Q, Sanderson JE. Understanding nonresponders of cardiac resynchronization therapy: current and future perspectives. *J Cardiovasc Electrophysiol.* 2005;16:1117–24

35. Aranda JM Jr, Conti JB, Johnson JW, Petersen-Stejskal S, Curtis AB. Cardiac resynchronization therapy in patients with heart failure and conduction abnormalities other than left bundle-branch block: analysis of the Multicenter InSync Randomized Clinical Evaluation (MIRACLE). *Clin Cardiol.* 2004;27:678–82.

36. Fantoni C, Kawabata M, Massaro R, Regoli F, Raffa S, Arora V, Salerno-Uriarte JA, Klein HU, Auricchio A. Right and left ventricular activation sequence in patients with heart failure and right bundle branch block: a detailed analysis using three-dimensional non-fluoroscopic electroanatomic mapping system. *J Cardiovasc Electrophysiol.* 2005;16:112–19.

37. Pitzalis MV, Iacoviello M, Romito R, Guida P, De Tommasi E, Luzzi G, Anaclerio M, Forleo C, Rizzon P. Ventricular asynchrony predicts a better outcome in patients with chronic heart failure receiving cardiac resynchronization therapy. *J Am Coll Cardiol.* 2005;45:65–9.

38. Penicka M, Bartunek J, De Bruyne B, Vanderheyden M, Goethals M, De Zutter M, Brugada P, Geelen P. Improvement of left ventricular function after cardiac resynchronization therapy is predicted by tissue Doppler imaging echocardiography. *Circulation.* 2004;109:978–83.

39. Bax JJ, Bleeker GB, Marwick TH, Molhoek SG, Boersma E, Steendijk P, van der Wall EE, Schalij MJ. Left ventricular dyssynchrony predicts response and prognosis after cardiac resynchronization therapy. *J Am Coll Cardiol.* 2004;44:1834–40.

40. Yu C-M, Abraham WT, Bax J, Chung E, Fedewa M, Ghio S, Leclercq C, Leon AR, Merlino J, Nihoyannopoulos P, Notabartolo D, Sun JP, Tavazzi L. Predictors of response to cardiac resynchronization therapy (PROSPECT) study design. *Am Heart J.* 2005;149:600–5.

41. Wilkoff BL, Cook JR, Epstein AE, Greene HL, Hallstrom AP, Hsia H, Kutalek SP, Sharma A. Dual-chamber pacing or ventricular backup pacing in patients with an implantable defibrillator: the Dual Chamber and VVI Implantable Defibrillator (DAVID) Trial. *JAMA.* 2002;288:3115–23.

42. Beshai JF, Grimm RA, Nagueh SF, Baker JH 2nd, Beau SL, Greenberg SM, Pires LA, Tchou PJ. RethinQ Study Investigators. Cardiac-resynchronization therapy in heart failure with narrow QRS complexes. *N Engl J Med.* 2007; Dec 13;357(24):2461–71

43. Turner MS, Bleasdale RA, Vinereanu D, Mumford CE, Paul V, Fraser AG, Frenneaux MP. Electrical and mechanical components of dyssynchrony in heart failure patients with normal QRS duration and left bundle-branch block: impact of left and biventricular pacing. *Circulation.* 2004;109:2544–9.

44. Yu CM, Chan YS, Zhang Q, Yip GW, Chan CK, Kum LC, Wu L, Lee AP, Lam YY, Fung JW. Benefits of cardiac resynchronization therapy for heart failure patients with narrow QRS complexes and coexisting systolic asynchrony by echocardiography. *J Am Coll Cardiol.* 2006; Dec 5;48(11):2251–7.

45. Eldadah ZA, Rosen B, Hay I, Edvardsen T, Jayam V, Dickfeld T, Meininger GR, Judge DP, Hare J, Lima JB, Calkins H, Berger RD. The benefit of upgrading chronically right ventricle-paced heart failure patients to resynchronization therapy demonstrated by strain rate imaging. *Heart Rhythm.* 2006;3:435–42.

46. Horwich T, Foster E, De Marco T, Tseng Z, Saxon L. Effects of resynchronization therapy on cardiac function in pacemaker patients "upgraded" to biventricular devices. *J Cardiovasc Electrophysiol.* 2004;15:1284–9.

47. Wyman BT, Hunter WC, Prinzen FW, McVeigh ER. Mapping propagation of mechanical activation in the paced heart with MRI tagging. *Am J Physiol.* 1999; 276:H881–H891.

48. van Oosterhout MF, Prinzen FW, Arts T, Schreuder JJ, Vanagt WY, Cleutjens JP, Reneman RS. Asynchronous electrical activation induces asymmetrical hypertrophy of the left ventricular wall. *Circulation.* 1998; 98: 588–95.

49. Adomian GE, Beazell J. Myofibrillar disarray produced in normal hearts by chronic electrical pacing. *Am Heart J.* 1986;112:79–83.

50. Prinzen FW, Peschar M. Relation between the pacing induced sequence of activation and left ventricular pump function in animals. *Pacing Clin Electrophysiol.* 2002;25:484–98.

51. Ichiki H, Oketani N, Hamasaki S, Ishida S, Kataoka T, Ogawa M, Saihara K, Okui H, Fukudome T, Shinasato T, Kubozono T, Ninomiya Y, Matsushita T, Otsuji Y, Tei C. Effect of right ventricular apex pacing on the Tei index and brain natriuretic peptide in patients with a dual-chamber pacemaker. *Pacing Clin Electrophysiol.* 2006;29:985–90.

52. Al-Hesayen A, Parker JD. Adverse effects of atrioventricular synchronous right ventricular pacing on left ventricular sympathetic activity, efficiency, and hemodynamic status. *Am J Physiol Heart Circ Physiol.* 2006;291:H2377–H2379.

53. Tops LF, Schalij MJ, Holman ER, van Erven L, van der Wall EE, Bax JJ. Right ventricular pacing can induce ventricular dyssynchrony in patients with atrial fibrillation after atrioventricular node ablation. *J Am Coll Cardiol.* 2006;48:1642–8.

54. Ichiki H, Oketani N, Hamasaki S, Ishida S, Kataoka T, Ogawa M, Saihara K, Okui H, Fukudome T, Shinasato T, Kubozono T, Ninomiya Y, Matsushita T, Otsuji Y, Tei C. Effect of right ventricular apex pacing on the Tei index and brain natriuretic peptide in patients with a dual-chamber pacemaker. *Pacing Clin Electrophysiol.* 2006;29: 985–90.

55. Al-Hesayen A, Parker JD. Adverse effects of atrioventricular synchronous right ventricular pacing on left ventricular sympathetic activity, efficiency, and hemodynamic status. *Am J Physiol Heart Circ Physiol.* 2006;291:H2377–H2379.

56. Tops LF, Schalij MJ, Holman ER, van Erven L, van der Wall EE, Bax JJ. Right ventricular pacing can induce ventricular dyssynchrony in patients with atrial fibrillation after atrioventricular node ablation. *J Am Coll Cardiol.* 2006;48:1642–8.

57. Sweeney MO, Hellkamp AS, Ellenbogen KA, Greenspon AJ, Freedman RA, Lee KL, Lamas GA. Adverse effect of ventricular pacing on heart failure and atrial fibrillation among patients with normal baseline QRS duration in a clinical trial of pacemaker therapy for sinus node dysfunction. *Circulation.* 2003;107:2932–7.

58. Kindermann M, Hennen B, Jung J, Geisel J, Bohm M, Frohlig G. Biventricular versus conventional right ventricular stimulation for patients with standard pacing indication and left ventricular dysfunction: the Homburg Biventricular Pacing Evaluation (HOBIPACE). *J Am Coll Cardiol*. 2006;47:1927–37

59. Birnie DH, Tang AS. The problem of non-response to cardiac resynchronization therapy. *Curr Opin Cardiol*. 2006;21:20–6.

60. Gassis S, Leon AR. Cardiac resynchronization therapy: strategies for device programming, troubleshooting and follow-up. *J Interv Card Electrophysiol*. 2005;13: 209–22.

61. Ammann P, Sticherling C, Kalusche D, Eckstein J, Bernheim A, Schaer B, Osswald S. An electrocardiogram-based algorithm to detect loss of left ventricular capture during cardiac resynchronization therapy. *Ann Intern Med*. 2005;142:968–73.

62. Kashani A, Barold SS. Significance of QRS complex duration in patients with heart failure. *J Am Coll Cardiol*. 2005;46:2183–92.

63. van Gelder BM, Bracke FA, Meijer A, Lakerveld LJ, Pijls NH. Effect of optimizing the VV interval on left ventricular contractility in cardiac resynchronization therapy. *Am J Cardiol*. 2004; Jun 15;93(12):1500–3.

64. Dekker A., Phelps B., Dijkman B., van Der Nagel T., van Der Veen F., Geskes G, Maessen J. Epicardial left ventricular lead placement for cardiac resynchronization therapy: optimal pace site selection with pressure-volume loops. *J Thoracic Cardiovascular Surgery*. 2004;127(6):1641–7.

65. O'Donnell D, Nadurata V, Hamer A, Kertes P, Mohammed W. Long-term variations in optimal programming of cardiac resynchronization therapy devices. *Pacing Clin Electrophysiol*. 2005;28 Suppl 1:S24–S26.

66. Ortale JR, Gabriel EA, Iost C, Marquez CQ. The anatomy of the coronary sinus and its tributaries. *Surg Radiol Anat*. 2001;23:15–21.

67. Rossillo A, Verma A, Saad EB, Corrado A, Gasparini G, Marrouche NF, Golshayan AR, McCurdy R, Bhargava M, Khaykin Y, Burkhardt JD, Martin DO, Wilkoff BL, Saliba WI, Schweikert RA, Raviele A, Natale A. Impact of coronary sinus lead position on biventricular pacing: mortality and echocardiographic evaluation during long-term follow-up. *J Cardiovasc Electrophysiol*. 2004;15:1120–5.

68. Woodard PK, Bhalla S, Javidan-Nejad C, Gutierrez FR. Non-coronary cardiac CT imaging. *Semin Ultrasound CT MR*. 2006;27:56–75.

69. McAlister FA, Ezekowitz JA, Wiebe N, Rowe B, Spooner C, Crumley E, Hartling L, Klassen T, Abraham W. Systematic review: cardiac resynchronization in patients with symptomatic heart failure. *Ann Intern Med*. 2004;141:381–90.

70. Bleeker GB, Schalij MJ, Van Der Wall EE, Bax JJ. Postero-lateral scar tissue resulting in non-response to cardiac resynchronization therapy. *J Cardiovasc Electrophysiol*. 2006; Aug;17(8):899–901.

71. Koebe J, Kirchhof P. Novel non-pharmacological approaches for antiarrhythmic therapy of atrial fibrillation. *Europace*. 2008; Apr;10(4):433–7.

72. van Gelder BM, Bracke FA, Meijer A, Lakerveld LJ, Pijls NH. Effect of optimizing the VV interval on left ventricular contractility in cardiac resynchronization therapy. *Am J Cardiol*. 2004; Jun 15;93(12):1500–3.

73. Vanderheyden M, De Backer T, Rivero-Ayerza M, Geelen P, Bartunek J, Verstreken S, De Zutter M, Goethals M. Tailored echocardiographic interventricular delay

programming further optimizes left ventricular performance after cardiac resynchronization therapy. *Heart Rhythm.* 2005;2:1066–72.

74. Bordachar P, Lafitte S, Reuter S, Sanders P, Jais P, Haissaguerre M, Roudaut R, Garrigue S, Clementy J. Echocardiographic parameters of ventricular dyssynchrony validation in patients with heart failure using sequential biventricular pacing. *J Am Coll Cardiol.* 2004;44:2157–65.

75. Leon AR, Abraham WT, Curtis AB, Daubert JP, Fisher WG, Gurley J, Hayes DL, Lieberman R, Petersen-Stejskal S, Wheelan K. Safety of transvenous cardiac resynchronization system implantation in patients with chronic heart failure: combined results of over 2,000 patients from a multicenter study program. *J Am Coll Cardiol.* 2005;46: 2348–56.

Chapter 9

Non-CRT pacing in the failing heart: Limiting ventricular pacing and searching for alternate pacing sites

C. W. Israel

Key Points

1. There is strong evidence that pacing from the right ventricular apex has deleterious hemodynamic effects which are particularly prominent in patients with heart failure.
2. The most efficient way to avoid pacing induced deterioration of cardiac function is the prevention of unnecessary right ventricular pacing.
3. This is feasible in the majority of patients, namely in those without AV conduction disturbances.
4. Implantation of atrial leads in positions that prolong intra-, interatrial, and atrioventricular conduction (right atrial appendage, atrial lateral wall), may prevent intrinsic ventricular activation.

   Implantation at atrial septal positions facilitates intrinsic atrioventricular conduction.
5. Dual-chamber pacing with very long AV delays promotes intrinsic conduction but creates several problems (limited maximum tracking rate, ventricular tachycardia detection, atrial flutter detection, endless loop tachycardia, non-reentrant ventriculo-atrial synchrony).
6. Study results and published experience strongly advocate the use of dedicated algorithms to switch from AAI to DDD pacing, allowing single P waves to remain nonconducted instead of switching rigorously to ventricular pacing if AV conduction is temporarily impaired.
7. In patients with permanent or frequent AV block where ventricular pacing cannot be avoided, pacing from the high septal RVOT may maintain a

Pacing to Support the Failing Heart, 1st edition. Edited by K. Ellenbogen and A. Auricchio.
© 2008 American Heart Association, ISBN: 978-1-4051-7534-0

normal vector of ventricular activation from basis to apex and may thus prevent unfavorable ventricular remodeling.

8. Septal RVOT pacing is better than right ventricular apical pacing but inferior to intrinsic ventricular activation if present.

Therefore, RVOT pacing may be used as an alternative to right ventricular pacing but not to intrinsic ventricular activation or biventricular pacing if the latter is indicated.

9. A promising option may be the implantation of the ventricular lead near the His bundle to use the His – Purkinje specialized conduction system for a physiologic ventricular activation.

10. In patients with heart failure and AV block where left ventricular lead implantation is not possible due to coronary sinus anatomy and a surgical approach is not feasible, bifocal right ventricular may provide an option, which is at least superior to right ventricular apical pacing.

Introduction

Left bundle branch block (LBBB) in patients with congestive heart failure is associated with significant deterioration in hemodynamic function by causing asynchronous contraction, particularly of the left ventricular lateral wall. There is emerging and compelling evidence that right ventricular pacing, particularly from the apical standard position, by producing aberrant left ventricular depolarization with an ECG pattern comparable to left bundle branch block, may cause similar left ventricular dyssynchrony with the same or even worse adverse effect on cardiac function [1–5]. This poses a problem for the large number of patients with heart failure and bradycardia, spontaneously induced by drugs, such as beta-blockers, that are indicated and should not be discontinued. Although bradycardia may worsen heart failure in these patients and should be treated, strategies are required to prevent pacing-induced deterioration.

Biventricular pacing has been advocated to replace dual-chamber pacing as a more "physiologic" way of stimulation [6]. However, it requires an additional lead, increasing the risk of hardware complication or subclavia thrombosis, and it is more complex at implantation and during follow-up. Two other options to limit adverse effects of dual-chamber pacing in patients with heart failure are discussed in this chapter: (1) programming of device algorithms to prevent unnecessary right ventricular pacing and (2) alternative right ventricular pacing sites.

Limitation of right ventricular pacing in patients with heart failure: Evidence for adverse effects

Even though right ventricular pacing has been used for five decades and evidence of detrimental effects on systolic and diastolic function were already reported in the early 1980s, recognition of the deleterious effects of right ventricular pacing became widely appreciated only after clinical studies demonstrated the extent of its deleterious effects [7,8]. Anatomic/histological, neurohumoral, hemodynamic, echocardiographic, and clinical evidence of harmful side effects of right ventricular pacing are summarized in this chapter.

Histological evidence of adverse effects of right ventricular pacing

Apical right ventricular pacing alters the ventricular contraction sequence, fiber strain and regional blood flow patterns [9,10]. In animal studies, pathological realignment of the myocardial cellular architecture has been observed to be associated with structural ventricular remodeling, characterized by cellular disarray, subendocardial fibrosis, abnormal fat deposition, calcification, and mitochondrial abnormalities [11]. Adomian et al. [12] produced an atrio-ventricular (AV) block and instituted right ventricular apical pacing in 12 dogs. After 3 months, myofibrillar disarray as a consequence of the abnormal contraction pattern during pacing was observed in nine dogs.

In 14 pediatric patients with AV block, Karpawich et al. obtained biopsies from the right ventricular septum before or after pacing from the right ventricular apex (mean duration of pacing of 5.5 years, [13]). Before pacing therapy, the only pathological change observed was myocardial cell hypertrophy, which is typically associated with bradycardia and altered stroke volume. However, all of the samples obtained after right ventricular pacing was initiated demonstrated various cellular and intracellular alterations including myofibrillar hypertrophy, mitochondrial morphological variations, diffuse intracellular vacuolization, degenerative fibrosis, and fatty deposits. Similarly, Moak et al. [14] found abnormal cellular fibrosis in 16 infants paced from the right ventricular apex for congenital AV block.

Even though these findings do not specifically address patients with heart failure, the link between abnormal contraction and structural changes on the cellular level is so convincing that it can be generalized.

Neurohumoral and autonomic evidence of adverse effects of right ventricular pacing

The impact of right ventricular pacing on brain natriuretic peptide (BNP) and other neurohumoral markers for heart failure have been investigated in some small studies. In 76 patients with an indication for permanent pacing, but no structural heart disease, ventricularly paced patients had significantly higher BNP levels than patients with no right ventricular pacing [15]. Simantirakis et al. [16] performed myocardial single-photon emission computed tomography (SPECT) in 39 patients permanently paced from the right ventricular apex for AV block and compared the images with 23 healthy controls. As a sign of impaired sympathetic activity, paced patients had regional uptake abnormalities in the inferior and apical wall. At the same time, approximately one-half of the paced patients had regional perfusion defects in the same regions. Norepinephrine spillover as a parameter of sympathetic impairment was also increased in patients with normal left ventricular function who received temporary atrio-ventricular synchronous right ventricular pacing compared with atrial pacing [17].

Although these issues are not completely understood, available data support the impression that right ventricular pacing has harmful effects at least in a subset of patients.

Hemodynamic deterioration due to right ventricular pacing

Compared to ventricular single-chamber pacing, dual-chamber pacing minimizes changes in left ventricular loading conditions, but ventricular dysynchrony persists. Some of the numerous studies that demonstrated adverse hemodynamic effects of right ventricular apical pacing (alone or in context with dual-chamber systems) during the last three decades should be mentioned. In 1984, Askenazi et al. [18] compared invasive hemodynamic parameters during dual-chamber pacing to the intrinsic rhythm and observed a deterioration of left ventricular contractility (dP/dt) and relaxation ($-$dP/dt), an increase in left ventricular end-systolic volume (LVESV), a reduction in stroke volume, and an absolute change in left ventricular ejection fraction by -10%. The negative impact of right ventricular dual-chamber pacing on left ventricular relaxation was confirmed for patients with heart failure, but pacing did not significantly affect patients with normal systolic function [19].

In 1987, Zile et al. [20] reported a disadvantageous influence of right ventricular pacing on left ventricular synchrony, loading conditions, and relaxation. This was seen in single-chamber right ventricular as well as dual-chamber pacing. Leclercq et al. [21] elegantly demonstrated the superiority of single-chamber atrial pacing over single-chamber ventricular and dual-chamber pacing in 11 patients with sinus node dysfunction and normal intrinsic conduction. AAI pacing significantly increased cardiac output at rest and during exercise, and reduced pulmonary capillary wedge pressure compared with DDD and VVI. AAI pacing demonstrated identical benefits for all other hemodynamic parameters (right atrial pressure, pulmonary artery pressure, left ventricular stroke work index, systemic vascular resistances, and left ventricular ejection fraction). Using hemodynamic and radionuclide studies, Leclercq et al. related the superiority of AAI pacing to a better septal ejection fraction and diastolic filling and pointed out that not only preservation of a normal atrioventricular synchrony, but also that a normal ventricular activation sequence is important in permanent cardiac pacing.

Newer data corroborate the negative hemodynamic effect of right ventricular pacing. A small hemodynamic study demonstrated that RV pacing caused no change in systemic arterial pressure, but a significant increase in left ventricular end-diastolic pressure and a significant slowing of isovolumic relaxation [17]. Both were associated with increased sympathetic activity. Furthermore, right ventricular pacing was accompanied by a reduction in left ventricular efficiency, expressed as a decrease in the ratio between peak positive dP/dt and myocardial oxygen consumption.

In 31 patients with ($n = 17$) or without ($n = 14$) severely impaired left ventricular function, Lieberman et al. [22] recorded pressure–volume loops during ventricular pacing using a micromanometer conductance catheter. In both patient groups, right ventricular pacing significantly impaired cardiac output, stroke work, ejection fraction, and left ventricular relaxation compared with atrial pacing. Additionally, right ventricular pacing also reduced left ventricular systolic pressure, stroke volume, LV dP/dt$_{max}$, LV dP/dt$_{min}$, and pulse pressure in patients with EF <40%.

In conclusion, hemodynamic data clearly demonstrate detrimental effects of right ventricular apical pacing, particularly in patients with heart failure.

Echocardiographic evidence of adverse effects of right ventricular pacing

It has been shown echocardiographically that right ventricular pacing impairs systolic and diastolic ventricular function. Numerous studies demonstrate a reduction of ejection fraction with right ventricular apical pacing compared to intrinsic ventricular rhythm. Tantengco et al. [1] assessed children with pacemakers by area- and Doppler flow-derived indexes of left ventricular systolic and diastolic function (fractional area of change, myocardial performance index) and described a significant time-dependent decrease in left ventricular function compared with the control subjects. Similarly, Ichiki et al. [15] reported a significantly higher Tei index (right and left ventricular) if patients with dual-chamber pacemakers were predominantly paced in the ventricle compared to patients with a low proportion of pacing. In addition, they found a larger left ventricular diastolic diameter in paced patients. The reduction in left ventricular systolic function seems to progress over time and to be, at least partly, reversible [23].

In 33 patients with a conventional single-chamber or dual-chamber pacemaker and narrow QRS, Schmidt et al. [24] assessed mechanical dyssynchrony by two-dimensional and Doppler echocardiography. Aortic pre-ejection delay, interventricular mechanical delay, activation of the posterior left ventricular wall, and septal-to-posterior wall motion delay deteriorated during right ventricular pacing in patients with an ejection fraction ≤35% while in patients with an ejection fraction >35%, only the aortic pre-ejection delay was slightly prolonged.

Thambo et al. performed echocardiography before implantation and after 5 years or more of right ventricular pacing in 23 adults with congenital AV block and a dual-chamber pacemaker [2]. Compared with 30 matched healthy control subjects, paced patients had a significantly higher intra–left ventricular asynchrony, extent of left ventricular myocardium with delayed longitudinal contraction, and septal-to-posterior wall-motion delay. The ratio between late-activated posterior and early-activated septal wall thickness was higher after long-term right ventricular pacing, as was the percentage of patients with an increased left ventricular end-diastolic diameter. As we have seen in previous studies, long-term right ventricular pacing was associated with a lower cardiac output.

In summary, echocardiography unequivocally shows impaired systolic and diastolic ventricular performance and dyssynchrony induced by right ventricular pacing, particularly in patients with pre-existing left ventricular dysfunction.

Clinical evidence of adverse effects of right ventricular pacing

Clinical studies on dual-chamber compared to single-chamber ventricular pacing were crucial because only after the unexpectedly disappointing results were published, the possibility of deleterious effects of right ventricular pacing attracted general attention.

The DAVID trial included patients with an ICD indication but without bradycardia who had a left ventricular ejection fraction ≤40%. It assessed the hypothesis that bradycardia prevention by dual-chamber pacing may be beneficial in terms of mortality and development of heart failure compared to ventricular single-chamber "back-up" pacing at 40 bpm [8]. However, the opposite result was found: Dual-chamber pacing was associated with a significantly higher cumulative event rate (death or heart failure hospitalization) than single-chamber back-up pacing. A post hoc analysis by Sharma et al. [25] clarified that it was not the dual-chamber mode itself that brought upon the adverse effects but the amount of right ventricular pacing, which was—by inclusion criteria— unnecessary in all patients. Patients with a dual-chamber device who received right ventricular pacing for >40% of the time had significantly more adverse events than patients with ventricular "back-up" pacing. In contrast, patients with ≤40% ventricular pacing in the dual-chamber mode had a strong trend ($p = 0.07$) for fewer adverse events.

These findings were confirmed for patients with severely impaired left ventricular function in the MADIT II trial [26]. If patients were divided into two equally large groups with those predominantly paced in the ventricle (median: 96% of the time) and those with prevailing intrinsic rhythm (median: 0.2% ventricular pacing), ventricular pacing was associated with a two-fold risk for new or worsened heart failure.

In a landmark study, Sweeney et al. [7] performed a retrospective analysis of the impact of ventricular pacing on heart failure and atrial fibrillation in patients enrolled into the MOST trial. They determined the cumulative percentage that patients were paced in the ventricle from pacemaker memory data. In 1,339 patients with a narrow QRS, randomization to dual-chamber pacing was associated with more ventricular pacing than randomization to single-chamber ventricular pacing (90% vs. 58%). Ventricular pacing correlated strongly with hospitalization for heart failure in the dual-chamber mode (hazard ratio: 2.99 for ventricular pacing >40%) and in the single-chamber ventricular mode (HR: 2.56 for ventricular pacing >80%). Similarly, the risk of atrial fibrillation increased with the amount of ventricular pacing in both groups. Compared to ventricular pacing in the dual-chamber mode for less than 40%, single-chamber ventricular pacing for more than 80% had a 3.6-fold increased risk of heart failure. Dual-chamber ventricular pacing >40% and single-chamber pacing >80% carried a 1.8-fold increased risk of heart failure compared to dual-chamber ventricular pacing ≤40% [27]. As we have seen in the DAVID trial, ventricular pacing was unnecessary in most patients in the MOST trial, which enrolled patients with sinus node disease and usually normal atrioventricular conduction.

In conclusion, histological, echocardiographic, and clinical evidence is firm that right ventricular pacing desynchronizes ventricular contraction, which can cause heart failure. It should be avoided whenever possible, particularly in patients with heart failure.

How to avoid unnecessary right ventricular pacing

There are several strategies to avoid unnecessary right ventricular pacing. Importantly, dual-chamber devices should always be checked carefully immediately after implantation for the possibility to reprogram AV delay, pacing mode, and special algorithms to prevent unnecessary ventricular pacing in the individual patient. Even after the devastating clinical results of ventricular pacing in the dual-chamber mode outlined above, the vast majority of dual-chamber devices are still shipped with settings that force ventricular pacing in almost all patients, almost permanently.

Strategies for reprogramming include programming to:

1 Single-chamber atrial mode (AAI, AAIR),
2 Dual-chamber modes (mainly DDD, DDDR, DDI, DDIR) with AV hysteresis,
3 Dual-chamber modes with a long AV delay, and
4 Dual-chamber mode with mode switching between AAI(R) and DDD(R).

Atrial single-chamber pacing mode

This mode of pacing definitively prevents ventricular pacing. It has been shown in the DAVID II trial that in contrast to dual-chamber pacing, single-chamber atrial pacing at 70 bpm was not associated with an increase in death or heart failure compared to ventricular single-chamber back-up pacing [28]. However, in this randomized trial, patients with a conventional pacing indication were excluded.

In patients with sinus node disease, it was shown more than 10 years ago that atrial single-chamber pacing is associated with a significantly lower mortality than ventricular single-chamber pacing [29]. Several publications have demonstrated the low incidence of AV block in sinus node disease if patients with bundle branch block are excluded [30,31]. Despite these findings, atrial

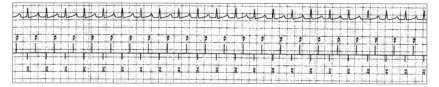

Fig. 9.1 Atrial rate-adaptive, single-chamber pacing (AAIR). In this example, an overreactive sensor causes pacemaker syndrome with atrial stimuli falling into the T wave. Surface ECG (lead II) and marker annotations (AP: atrial pacing, VS: ventricular sensing). Paper speed: 25 mm/s.

single-chamber pacing is used only rarely in most countries. Data from the German pacemaker registry indicate that AAI(R) systems currently account for only 0.9% of all implanted pacemakers. Even in sinus node disease, only 2.8% of systems are AAI(R), and 0.6% in the brady-tachy syndrome [32]). The widespread reluctance to use atrial single-chamber pacing is due to concerns about unexpected AV block in patients with AAI(R) pacemakers [33]. Long-term data show the need to upgrade AAI(R) systems to dual-chamber in approximately 1.5-2.0% of patients [31,34] due to symptomatic AV block. In an additional proportion of patients (approximately 0.5–1%), upgrade to dual-chamber mode is performed due to suspected paroxysmal AV block [34]. The need to upgrade AAI(R) pacemaker systems at a rate of 2.5% per year is too high and may, in fact, only represent the tip of the iceberg. Beat-to-beat Holter monitoring in the AAI mode suggests that AV block is more frequent in sinus node disease than previously suggested [35]. Atrial single-chamber pacing may be particularly disadvantageous in the rate responsive or overdrive mode. In this situation, an inappropriately fast atrial pacing rate may cause pacemaker syndrome with atrial contraction synchronized to the T wave (Figure 9.1).

I have come to the conclusion that single-chamber atrial pacing seems to be superior to dual-chamber pacing in preventing heart failure or heart failure progression in sinus node disease. The small but, however, not entirely predictable risk of AV block limits the use of atrial single-chamber pacemaker systems. Implantation of dual-chamber devices and programming to AAI(R) mode may be a more valuable option, with Wenckebach point testing at 6-month intervals and reprogramming to the dual-chamber mode whenever AV conduction fails with atrial rates of 100–120 bpm. However, the lack of a ventricular monitor as a safety feature in case of high-degree AV block still causes concern.

Dual-chamber modes with an AV hysteresis
The AV hysteresis function has been developed specifically to promote intrinsic AV conduction in patients with only intermittent and/or slightly impaired AV conduction. These algorithms prolong the programmed AV delay (e.g. 120 ms) by a certain value (e.g. 40 ms) after a prespecified period (e.g. every 32 cycles).

Whenever this prolongation results in detection of intrinsic AV conduction, the AV delay is maintained at this extended value, otherwise it switches back to the programmed one.

Efficacy of these algorithms in reducing the amount of ventricular pacing has been disappointing. The first algorithm, developed by Vitatron B.V. (Dieren, The Netherlands) reduced the percentage of ventricular pacing in patients with intermittent AV block from 93% to 43% by adding 65 ms to the programmed AV delay of 200 ms [36]. The Search AV® algorithm (Medtronic Inc., Minneapolis, MN) did not prevent 70% ventricular pacing in patients with intact AV conduction, and even in the second generation (Search AV+®), there was still 19% unnecessary ventricular pacing [37]. Similarly, the Autointrinsic Conduction Search® (AICS, St. Jude Medical, Sylmar, CA) reduced ventricular pacing only from 62% to 50% [38]. The INTRINSIC RV trial had to be changed by an amendment because the AV Search Hysteresis® algorithm (Guidant Co., St. Paul, MN) in its original programming was unable to reduce the amount of unnecessary ventricular pacing below 20% [39]. The initial setting (i.e. prolonging the programmed AV delay in a search cycle every 32 beats by 50%) had to be increased to 100% to achieve a mean percentage of ventricular pacing as low as 15%; ventricular pacing for less than 20% of the time was attained in 77% of patients.

Several limitations of AV hysteresis algorithms are responsible for the unsatisfactory reduction of unnecessary ventricular pacing in patients with normal AV conduction:

(i) The maximum value of the programmed AV delay is frequently 300 ms or 350 ms, only few algorithms allow an extension to 450–600 ms.

(ii) AV delay extension is not continuous but in some algorithms rather rare (e.g. every 32nd cycle) and thus not sufficiently sensitive to detect intermittent intrinsic conduction,

(iii) some criteria to prolong the AV delay are too stringent (e.g. if eight out of eight cycles must show intrinsic conduction to switch to a longer AV delay),

(iv) some criteria to switch back to the short AV delay programming are too easily met (e.g. if only 1 out of 8 cycles without intrinsic conduction triggers a switch back to the short AV delay),

(v) repetition of search for AV conduction may be too infrequent (e.g. every 16 hours).

In conclusion, AV hysteresis functions are unsatisfactory in preventing unnecessary ventricular pacing. Other options (AAI mode, permanent long AV delay, dedicated AAI–DDD mode switching) should be preferred.

Dual-chamber modes with a long AV delay

Programming long AV delays represents an effective and simple way to prevent unnecessary ventricular pacing in dual-chamber devices. However, "long"

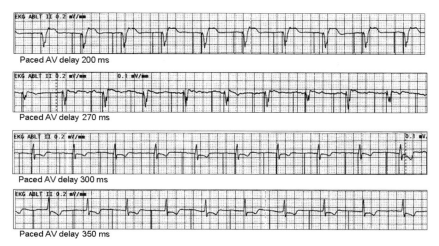

Fig. 9.2 Example of a very long AV delay. In order to prevent unnecessary ventricular pacing in a patient with sinus node syndrome, prolongation to a value of 350 ms is necessary to prevent fusion or pseudofusion.

in this context means that the AV delay has to be programmed to values ≥300 ms (Figure 9.2). This abnormally long AV delay is frequently necessary if atrial leads are implanted in the right atrial appendage or high lateral right atrial wall (Figure 9.3). From these pacing sites, propagation of the atrial stimulus and thus the interval from pacing to intrinsic conduction to the ventricle can be highly prolonged. Data on file suggest that with atrial leads in conventional sites, 87% of patients without AV block require programming of the paced AV delay to a value ≥360 ms to allow intrinsic AV conduction at 90 bpm (David A. Casavant, Medtronic, Inc., personal communication). A study comparing dual-chamber pacing with long versus short AV delay in patients with sinus node disease showed that ventricular pacing was still present for 17% of the time despite programming the "long" AV delay to 300 ms [40].

Programming long AV delays significantly impairs device function (Table 9.1). There are interlocks in most systems that limit the maximum sensor and tracking rate with longer AV delays. Additionally, AV delay is blanked in many devices, allowing no atrial sensing during this period. This may cause "2:1 lock-in" of atrial flutter (i.e. every second atrial flutter potential coincides with the blanking period and is not sensed) [41,42]. In some dual-chamber ICDs, there are interlocks between the detection of slow ventricular tachycardia and atrial blanking periods. This is due to cross-chamber blanking, which can impair the detection of ventricular tachyarrhythmias. In particular, if long AV delays are programmed, ventricular and atrial events

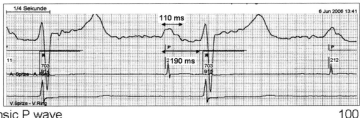

Intrinsic P wave   100 mm/s

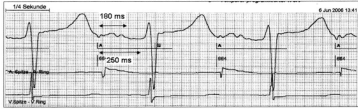

Paced P wave   100 mm/s

Fig. 9.3 Prolongation of the P wave duration and the AV delay by pacing from the right atrial appendage. In this patient with sinus node disease and normal duration of the intrinsic P wave and PQ time, atrial pacing significantly prolongs P wave duration and causes AV block I°.

may be synchronized in a way that prolongs or prevents the detection of ventricular tachyarrhythmia [43].

As soon as long AV delays fail to prevent ventricular pacing, there is an increased risk of retrograde conduction through the AV node. This can cause endless loop tachycardia [44]. Additionally, it can cause a different form of pacemaker mediated tachycardia, termed "rapid non–reentrant VA synchrony" [45] or "AV desynchronizing arrhythmia" [46]. In this arrhythmia, atrial pacing immediately after a blanked or refractory retrograde P wave cannot capture and

Table 9.1 Problems with a long AV delay in dual-chamber devices.

Limited maximum sensor rate
Limited maximum tracking rate
Ventricular tachycardia detection cannot be programmed to slow rates
Underdetection of atrial flutter (and fibrillation)
Underdetection or delayed detection of ventricular tachycardia/fibrillation
Risk of endless loop tachycardia ↑
Risk of repetitive non–reentrant VA synchrony/AV desynchronizing arrhythmia ↑
Risk of induction of ventricular tachycardia in "functional" ventricular
   undersensing ↑

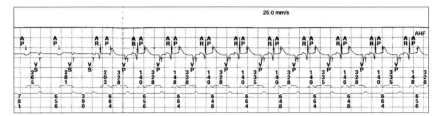

Fig. 9.4 Repetitive Non–Reentrant VA Synchrony. In this atrial electrogram stored upon detection of atrial tachyarrhythmia, a premature ventricular beat (3rd "VS" marker, signifying "ventricular sensing") is followed by a sinus beat, which falls into the refractory period (AR: atrial refractory sense) and does not reset atrial timing. Therefore, ineffective atrial pacing (AP) ensues, followed by asynchronous ventricular pacing (VP) with retrograde VA conduction, followed by ineffective atrial pacing, and so forth.

is thus followed by an asynchronous ventricular stimulus that perpetuates the arrhythmia, causing symptoms of a pacemaker syndrome (Figure 9.4). These arrhythmias have been observed particularly after ventricular premature beats [47]. Finally, cross-chamber blanking occurs in the ventricle during atrial pacing. If a premature ventricular beat occurs exactly at the time of atrial pacing, it may be blanked out and the following ventricular stimulus occurs after expiration of the programmed AV delay (Figure 9.5). The longer the programmed AV delay in this situation, the higher the risk of proarrhythmic ventricular pacing during the ventricular vulnerable phase.

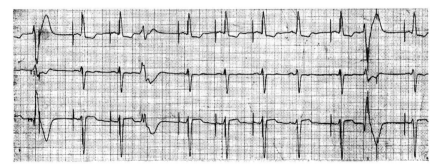

Fig. 9.5 Premature ventricular beats (PVBs) in dual-chamber pacing. The first PVB occurs shortly after atrial pacing and triggers ventricular safety pacing. The second PVB occurs shortly before the atrial stimulus would have occurred but is inhibited. The third PVB is so exactly synchronized with the atrial pace that it is completely blanked and does not trigger ventricular safety pacing. In this case, the ventricular pace occurs 200 ms after atrial pacing. If a longer AV delay would have been programmed, the ventricular pace could have occurred later, in the vulnerable phase of ventricular repolarization. (Reproduced with the kind permission of Bernard Dodinot.)

Dual-chamber pacing with long AV delay is frequently used in the absence of other options, but it can prevent unnecessary ventricular pacing only to some extent, usually only to approximately 20%, and is associated with a number of side effects. The unresolved problem of dual-chamber pacing in this context is the ventricular stimulus that is not prevented (e.g. after a blocked atrial premature beat or ventricular premature beat with retrograde conduction). In this situation, reentrant and non–reentrant arrhythmias can occur and persist.

Dual-chamber mode with mode switching between AAI(R) and DDD(R)

Recent studies demonstrating lack of improvement or even deterioration of patient outcome with dual-chamber compared to single-chamber ventricular devices have renewed efforts to optimize dual-chamber pacing therapy. In 2005, Savouré et al. [48] reported about the AAIsafeR® algorithm (Ela Medical, Montrouge, France), which allows AAI(R) pacing together with monitoring intrinsic AV conduction. It allows block of single atrial events to a prespecified level before it switches to dual-chamber pacing. It is important to note that although the pacemaker works in AAI(R) mode, the AAIsafeR® algorithm does not initiate an AV delay after which ventricular pacing resumes. Therefore, problems associated with DDD pacing and long AV delay, as outlined above, are prevented. The AAIsafeR® algorithm offers a set of criteria to switch to the dual-chamber mode (Figure 9.6): (i) the III° AV block criterion after two consecutive blocked P waves, (ii) the II° AV block criterion if 3 out of 12 P waves are not conducted, (iii) the I° AV block criterion if seven consecutive PR/AR intervals exceed 350 ms (programmable at rest or exercise) and (iv) as a safety feature, ventricular pauses (programmable: 2, 3, or 4 sec). Early results in 43 patients with sinus node disease or paroxysmal AV block showed a reduction of ventricular pacing to 0.2% with appropriate switches in 35% of patients; no adverse events were observed [48]. A ventricular pacing percentage of only 0.2% without any adverse events was confirmed in 123 patients with sinus node disease, bradycardia-tachycardia syndrome or paroxysmal AV block who received dual-chamber pacemakers fitted with the AAIsafeR2® algorithm [49]. In a third study, the AAIsafeR® algorithm was activated in 96 patients with sinus node disease, AV block, or other pacing indications [50]. Over 7 months, the algorithm was deactivated in only 6 patients due to AV block. Again, no adverse events or symptoms with algorithm activity were reported. The percentage of ventricular pacing was reduced from 95% in DDD mode, 87% in DDI mode, and 31% in DDD mode with AV hysteresis to 9% (median: 0%) with AAIsafeR®. As desired, no reentrant or non–reentrant pacemaker mediated arrhythmias occurred.

A second algorithm, Managed Ventricular Pacing® (MVP®, Medtronic Inc., Minneapolis, MN), was developed to prevent unnecessary ventricular pacing in dual-chamber devices. This algorithm provides AAI(R) pacing with ventricular monitoring, too, and switches to dual-chamber pacing if two out of four atrial events are not followed by an intrinsic ventricular event. Working in the

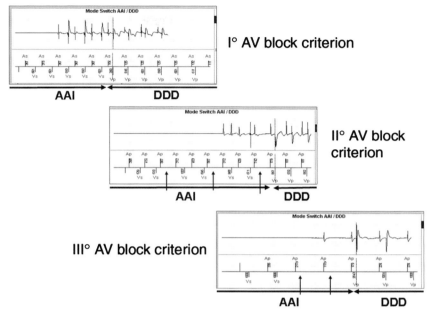

Fig. 9.6 Example of Intervention of AAIsafeR® Mode Switching from AAI(R) to DDD(R) in Response to AV Block. In these stored electrograms (superimposed atrial/ventricular channel), the device switched back to dual-chamber pacing in reaction to different degrees of AV block according to prespecified criteria. AP: Atrial paced event, AS: Atrial sensed event, VP: ventricular paced event, VS: ventricular sensed event, arrows: missing AV conduction in II° and III° AV block, numbers: AV delay (above line) and ventricular cycle length (below line).

dual-chamber mode, the device switches back to AAI to check intrinsic AV conduction after progressively longer time intervals (1 min, 2 min, 4 min, 8 min, etc.). First-degree or second-degree AV block type Wenckebach up to 3:2 will thus not trigger dual-chamber pacing. In a first study, this algorithm was downloaded into dual-chamber ICDs in 30 patients without a history of AV block [51]. Mean spontaneous PR interval was 204 ms, devices were programmed to a sensed AV delay of 170 ms (paced 200 ms). As anticipated, unnecessary ventricular pacing was present during 81% of the time in the DDD mode; it was reduced to 4% after activation of MVP®. Unexpectedly, 10% of these patients with seemingly normal AV conduction had intermittent higher degree AV block with appropriate switch to DDD (mean: nine episodes per day). In a second study, the algorithm was downloaded in 181 unselected patients with a dual-chamber ICD (complete AV block in 5.5%) with a reduced left ventricular function (mean ejection fraction: $36 \pm 14\%$, NYHA Class II–III in 36%, [52]). In this group, with a baseline PR interval of 190 ms, AV intervals in the DDDR mode were programmed to a mean of 216 ms (paced) and 189 ms (sensed). However, ventricular pacing was still present for 74% of the time compared to only 4% with MVP® activated. Again, no adverse events associated with MVP® algorithm function were found. The algorithm was also tested in 129 patients with a conventional indication for permanent pacing [53] where a reduction of ventricular pacing from 90% to 1.4% was found. It is interesting to note that in patients with AV block as an indication for permanent pacemaker therapy, the amount of ventricular pacing could be reduced by 60%. In patients with III° permanent AV block ($n = 13$), ventricular pacing was unchanged at 99% with MVP® activated; no symptoms or adverse events in conjunction with algorithm activity were observed. MVP® provides an excellent way to reduce unnecessary ventricular pacing particularly in the large group of patients with permanent I° AV block and intermittent III° AV block.

In a substudy, an in-depth analysis with 24-hours Holter monitoring with extended telemetry was performed in patients with the MVP® algorithm active [35]. The dedicated Holter system allowed simultaneous recording of surface ECG, marker annotations, and A-V electrograms (Figure 9.7). A total of 682 mode switches from AAI(R) to DDD(R) were recorded, of which 92% were adequately caused by AV block. Surprisingly, two patients without AV block known before implantation required ventricular pacing due to AV block for 71% and 93% of the 24-hour period (Figure 9.8). In two patients, ventricular undersensing and frequent premature beats were responsible for inappropriate

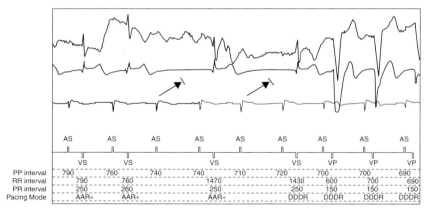

Fig. 9.7 Example of a 24 h Holter ECG with extended telemetry demonstrating MVP® activity. The system offers ventricular electrogram (V-EGM), atrial electrogram (A-ECG), and annotations of markers, cycle lengths (in ms), and pacing mode. In this tracing, 2:1 AV block occurs and triggers switch back to DDDR. AAIR+: DDD with MVP® function active. Paper speed: 25 mm/s.

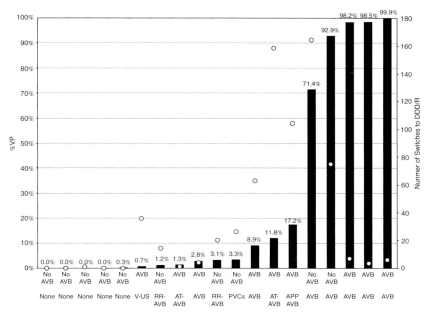

Fig. 9.8 Beat-to-beat analysis of MVP® function in 19 patients. In 5 of 10 patients without AV block ("No AVB") as a pacing indication, ventricular pacing >1% occurred, in two patients due to an unexpected high-degree AV block ("AVB"), in two patients due to AV block during rate responsive pacing ("RR-AVB") and in one patient inappropriately due to ventricular premature beats. In three patients with permanent AV block, ventricular pacing remained >98% with only few attempts of MVP® to change to AAIR. In six out of nine patients with AV block as pacing indication, ventricular pacing was reduced to <20%. AV block occurred only during atrial tachyarrhythmia ("AT-AVB") in two patients, only during atrial overdrive pacing ("APP-AVB") in one patient, and inappropriately due to ventricular undersensing in one patient.

switches to DDD(R) (8% of all switches, 0.2% of total time of Holter recordings). Patients without AV block were effectively paced in the AAIR mode for 93% of the time, and patients with AV block as pacing indication were also paced in AAIR mode for 48% of the time. Importantly, there was no instance where two or more consecutive sinus beats were blocked. There were no concerns about the safety of the algorithm, even in patients with permanent III° AV block, and no symptoms associated with MVP® operation.

Similarly, in 107 unselected, consecutive patients who received a dual-chamber pacemaker with MVP® for sinus node disease or AV block, MVP® operation resulted in ventricular pacing for only 3.9% during a follow-up of 76 days [54]. The median cumulative percentage of ventricular pacing was reduced to 1.4% in patients with sinus node disease and, surprisingly, to 28.8% in patients with AV block as indication for pacing. A cumulative percentage of ventricular pacing ≤ 40% was found in 72% of all patients: in 50% of patients with AV block and in 86% of patients with sinus node disease.

The superiority of an AAI(R)/DDD(R) mode switching algorithm over an AV hysteresis has been recently demonstrated in an analysis of the EnRhythm® and EnPulse® clinical studies [55]. In 322 patients, MVP® operation (used in 129) as compared to the Search AV+® algorithm resulted in a significantly lower median percentage of ventricular pacing in almost all categories of AV conduction: No AV block: 0.3 versus 2.9%, I° AV block: 0.9 versus 80.6%, II° AV block: 37.6% versus 99.3%, intermittent III° AV block: 1.2 versus 42.2%. Only in permanent III° AV block, there was no difference (98.9% vs. 100%). Dedicated AAI(R)/DDD(R) mode switching is much more effective in preventing unnecessary ventricular pacing, particularly in patients with I° AV block where very long AV delays would have to be programmed, so that the programming does not limit other device functions (see above).

The clinical consequences of prevention of unnecessary right ventricular pacing were assessed in a trial [56]. More than 1,000 patients with sinus node disease, intact atrio-ventricular conduction, and a normal QRS interval were randomized to receive dual-chamber pacing alone or together with MVP®. During a follow-up period of 1.7 years, the median percentage of ventricular pacing was much lower in the MVP® treated patients (9% vs. 99%). The primary endpoint–time to persistent atrial fibrillation–was reached by 13% of patients with conventional dual-chamber pacing compared to only 8% in the group assigned to MVP®, which translates into a 40% reduction in the relative risk of developing persistent atrial fibrillation during pacing for sinus node disease.

The safety of AAI(R)/DDD(R) mode switching has been questioned in some case reports, for example, in a patient with AV block where the development of ventricular tachyarrhythmia may have been facilitated by long-short sequences in response to ventricular bigeminy [57]. Also, in patients with a dual AV node physiology, long AV conduction together with short VA intervals may occur [58]. Junctional escape rhythms may also pose a problem for the algorithm [59], but can usually be controlled easily by increasing the lower rate limit. These events seem to be rare and irrelevant compared to the potential benefit of AAI(R)/DDD(R) mode switching, reducing the proportion of ventricular pacing far more effective and with fewer side effects than dual-chamber pacing with long AV delay.

In conclusion, AAI(R)/DDD(R) mode switching seems to be the preferred way to prevent unnecessary right ventricular pacing effectively and without compromising other pacing options. This refers to patients with sinus node disease, first-degree to second-degree AV block, and intermittent III° AV block. Only patients with known permanent III° AV block are not candidates for this option.

I° AV block in patients with heart failure

What is more important in patients with I° AV block and heart failure: prevention of right ventricular pacing or of presystolic mitral regurgitation? This important question is completely unsolved. Although prevention of right ventricular pacing is desirable, long PQ times may be associated with significant presystolic mitral regurgitation. A study of 17 patients suggests that right ventricular pacing at an optimized AV delay may be superior to intrinsic conduction if the latter exceeds 270 ms [60]. However, the ideal pacing mode depended on the echocardiographic parameter used for optimization (transaortic versus transmitral flow) and the paced rate (e.g. 70 bpm or 90 bpm). Additionally, only patients with an ejection fraction ≥50% were included in this single study on that issue.

Although AV delay optimization is being investigated extensively in patients with cardiac resynchronization therapy, there is no sufficient knowledge about this practical issue in patients with heart failure. Some older studies suggest that abolition of diastolic mitral regurgitation by programming a short AV delay may be useful [61–63], while others did not find a significant influence of different AV delay settings on cardiac output in right ventricular pacing and heart failure [64]. It remains to be determined if–as another option–cardiac resynchronization therapy may be beneficial in patients with heart failure, I° AV block and narrow QRS.

Right ventricular pacing sites

In patients with permanent or frequent high-degree AV block, ventricular pacing cannot be avoided. At the time of device implantation, the indication for cardiac resynchronization therapy needs to be considered. However, a considerable proportion of these patients will not receive biventricular devices, either because there is no indication for this treatment (narrow QRS, lack of dyssynchrony) or because of other reasons (inaccessibility of the coronary sinus for pacing, other reasons for failure of implantation of a biventricular device, lack of availability of biventricular pacing, patient's/physician's preference, comorbidity, etc.). In these patients, right ventricular pacing sites other than the apex should be considered. Even though there is no clear evidence, a number of findings suggest that any pacing site other than the right ventricular apex may be at least as good if not better.

Right ventricular outflow tract (RVOT) septum

Although apical right ventricular pacing alters left ventricular hemodynamics and the normal histological appearance of myocardial structures [11,65], these changes were absent or at least attenuated with high septal pacing, which maintains a normal pattern of biventricular activation from basal to apical [22,66–73]. The RVOT is particularly attractive as a pacing position because it is easy to reach and requires only a single ventricular lead in contrast to bifocal right ventricular or biventricular pacing. Additionally, the high septum offers trabeculated myocardium (septoparietal trabeculations, [74]) with favorable lead stability and sensing respectively pacing properties [75].

A number of studies have been performed with right ventricular outflow and/or septal pacing compared to right ventricular apical pacing [22,66,76–91]. Although some of these studies were positive, (i.e. found a beneficial effect of outflow tract septal pacing), almost the same number of studies did not find a clear benefit (Table 9.2). The interpretation of these results is difficult: some studies were regarded as positive only if there was an improvement compared to sinus rhythm (e.g. [92]), while others were regarded as positive if RVOT pacing resulted into significantly better hemodynamics than right ventricular apical pacing (e.g. [93]). Hemodynamic parameters and measurement techniques were significantly different (right ventricular catheterization, thermodilution, echocardiography; systolic or diastolic function, etc.) as were primary endpoints (e.g. hemodynamics vs. quality of life [94]). Importantly, the majority of studies only provided acute data obtained during electrophysiologic study, cardiac surgery, or elective right heart catheterization. Very few studies investigated results from chronically implanted leads, information covering a period >18 months after implant is almost absent.

The potentially most important criticism on previous studies refers to the validation of right ventricular septal lead position. From published fluoroscopy pictures and surface ECGs, it seems that a number of leads have actually been implanted in the anterior aspects or lateral wall of the RVOT, which have not the same electrophysiological properties as the septum, particularly not the same fast conduction to the left ventricular myocardium.

Lieberman et al. [95] proposed a classification of exact RVOT pacing sites (high, low, septal, free wall) based on fluoroscopic and ECG criteria. Mond et al. [72] have elegantly proposed methods how to reach the "sweet spot" in the septal RVOT (Figure 9.9) easily and with almost immediate success in all patients, and how to recognize the exact position of the lead tip from the surface ECG [72–75,96]. The high RVOT septal area can be reached very reliably by manually preshaping the stylet forming three curves (Figure 9.10). To verify if the correct position has been achieved, fluoroscopy in at least two projections, anterior-posterior and left anterior oblique (LAO) 40 degrees, is required (Figures 9.11 and 9.12). As a third projection, a right anterior oblique view (e.g. 30 degrees) may be useful to exclude inadvertent positioning in the coronary sinus. In the surface ECG, positioning in the septal RVOT can be verified by a negative S wave in lead I, positive R waves in leads II and III (Figure 9.6). The QRS is usually free of notches and frequently relatively narrow (<160 ms) for right ventricular pacing. If the lead is positioned in the anterior aspect of the RVOT (see Figure 9.9), lead I is typically isoelectric. If the lead is positioned in the lateral free wall, lead I typically shows a positive R wave, usually together with notches in leads II and

Table 9.2   Studies comparing septal outflow tract with apical pacing in the right ventricle.

Author	Year	n	Indication	A/C	HF	Outcome
			Negative studies			
Buckingham [76]	1997	11	EP study	A	none	No difference in cardiac output
Blanc [92]	1997	27	HF + AV block I°	A	all	No difference from baseline in systolic BP, PCWP, V wave
Alboni [79]	1998	21	SND, AV block	A	none	No difference in echocardiographic or invasive hemodynamic parameters
Buckingham [77]	1998	14	EP study	A	all	Trend toward improved cardiac index, LVEF, LVEDP, dP/dt, time constant of relaxation
Victor [80]	1999	16	AV block III° + AF	C	$n = 6$	After 3 months no difference in NYHA class, LVEF, cardiac output, VO_{2max}
Buckingham [78]	1999	37	Cardiac surgery	A	$n = 27$	No difference in cardiac output
Schwaab [81]	1999	14	AV block III°	A	$n = 3$	No difference in cardiac output
Gold [82]	2000	21	AV block	A	all	No effect on cardiac index, PCWP, right atrial pressure
Bourke [83]	2002	20	AVNA + AF	C	$n = 3$	No difference in LVEF or mean filling rate (dV/dt)
Stambler [94]	2003	10	AF, VVI	C	all	No difference in LVEF or QoL
Lieberman [22]	2006	31	EP study, device implantation	A	$n = 14$	No difference in any hemodynamic parameter
			Positive studies			
Giudici [84]	1997	89	SND, AVNA + AF	A	n. a.	Cardiac index ↑
Le Helloco [85]	1999	15	Dilative CMP	A	all	Cardiac index ↑
Karpawich [66]	1997	22	EP study	A	none	Cardiac index ↑, dP/dt ↑, Vmax ↑, Vpm ↑
De Cock [86]	1998	17	(invasive hemodynamic study)	A	$n = 3$	Cardiac index ↑
Saxon [87]	1998	11	during cardiac surgery	A	all	Fractional area change ↑
Mera [88]	1999	12	AVNA + AF	C	all	FS ↑, LVEF ↑
Kolettis [89]	2000	20	Cardiac catheter	A	none	Isovolumic relaxation time constant ↑
Tse [90]	2002	24	AV block	C	None	Perfusion & LVEF ↑ at 18 months
Victor [93]	2006	28	AVNA + AF	C	$n = 12$	LVEF ↑ after 3 months
Lewicka-Nowak [91]	2006	27	SND, AV block, etc.	C	$n = 3$	LVEF ↑, NT-proBNP↓ after 90 months

A/C: acute, chronic; AF: atrial fibrillation; AVNA: AV node ablation; BP: blood pressure; CMP: cardiomyopathy; CPx: cardiopulmonary exercise testing EP: electrophysiologic; FS: fraction shortening; HF: heart failure; LVEDP: left ventricular enddiastolic pressure; LVEF: left ventricular ejection fraction; n: no. of patients; n.a.: not available; PCWP: pulmonary capillary wedge pressure; QoL: Quality of life; SND: sinus node disease; V_{max}: maximal velocity of fibre shortening; VO_{2max}: maximum oxygen consumption; Vpm: peak measured fiber-shortening velocity.

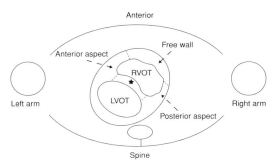

Fig. 9.9 Classification of RVOT segments in a transverse cross-section of the heart. The "sweet spot" is in the septal area (marked by a star), while anterior and lateral aspects of the RVOT in the free wall are not associated with facilitated conduction.

III [72,73]. The high and low septal positions can be distinguished by looking at lead aVF, which is positive in a high and isoelectric in a low septal position [95].

If these criteria to verify and classify the exact RVOT or septal lead position are regarded, future studies may clarify if pacing from this site offers advantages in patients who need ventricular pacing. It may be that a specific spot is ideal in all patients or that other criteria (e.g. QRS duration, [81]) have to be developed to find the individually optimal pacing site within the septal/RVOT area.

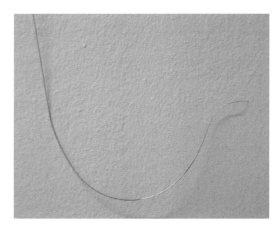

Fig. 9.10 Preshaping the stylet to reach the high septal RVOT. Three curves have to be shaped: A wide C to reach the RVOT, a "swan neck" of approximately 1.5 cm (similar to the shape of an Amplatz catheter for coronary angiography), and within this "swan neck," a gentle curve backward.

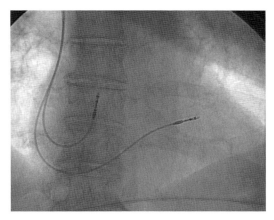

Fig. 9.11 Lead position in the high septal RVOT. In anterior–posterior projection, the lead tip points upward to the right.

His and parahisian pacing

Theoretically, at least in patients without bundle branch block ventricular lead implantation would be ideal at the His bundle. Using the specific His–Purkinje conduction system, the right and left ventricles would be excited in a physiologic way with normal, simultaneous biventricular contraction using the geometric spiral arrangement of ventricular myocardial fibers [66]. Positioning the lead

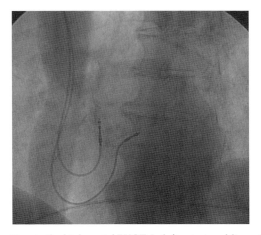

Fig. 9.12 Lead position in the high septal RVOT. In left anterior oblique 40-degree projection, the lead tip points strictly to the right (spine). In this patient with a dual-chamber pacemaker, also the atrial lead has been implanted in the high atrial septum, near the right atrial insertion of Bachmann's bundle.

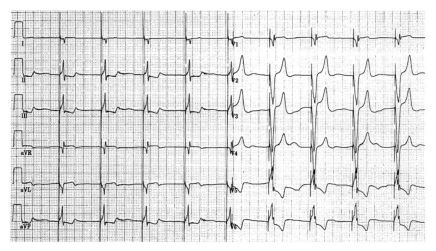

Fig. 9.13 ECG in high septal RVOT pacing. In this patient with permanent AF and AV block III°, a negative S wave in lead I, positive R waves in leads II and III, and the absence of notching in these leads verify positioning in the septal RVOT. In addition, a positive R wave in lead aVF suggests a position in the high septum. The slow increase of R wave voltage after the pacing spike coupled with a much steeper R wave increase later in the ascending limb of the R wave (very similar to a delta wave in Wolf–Parkinson–White syndrome with fusion of accessory pathway and AV conduction) suggests parahisian pacing, which captures normal myocardium first until the His bundle with much faster conduction is excited. Paper speed: 25 mm/s.

as close as possible to the His-Purkinje system avoids conduction through the unspecialized myocardium and thus potentially the disadvantages of artificial ventricular pacing [19,97,98] without the need of more than one single ventricular lead.

Deshmukh et al. [99] reported first results of chronic His-bundle pacing in 18 patients. Although the report about successful His-bundle pacing with a paced QRS almost identical to the intrinsic, narrow QRS was certainly a breakthrough, the study also demonstrated the problems of His-bundle pacing: Lead implantation was only successful in 12 out of 18 selected patients, the mean duration of implantation was almost 4 hours, mean pacing thresholds were as a high as 2.4 V at 0.5 ms acutely, exit block or dislodgement occurred in 2 of 12 patients and thresholds >7 V in another 3 patients. Finally, sensed R waves were below 1.5 mV in 8 of these 12 patients (mean value: 1.7 mV).

A number of studies on His bundle pacing have been published recently. Using a steerable catheter and a 4.1 F lead, Zanon et al. successfully implanted ventricular leads at the His bundle in 24 out of 26 patients (92% success,

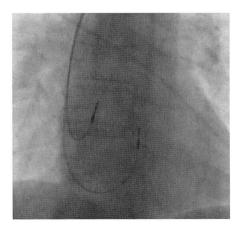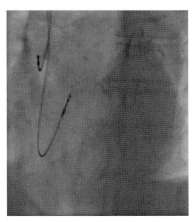

Fig. 9.14 Fluoroscopy of a typical ventricular lead position in permanent direct His-bundle pacing. Anterior-posterior (AP) and left anterior oblique (LAO) 40-degree projection.

[100]). The mean total procedure time including positioning of a diagnostic His-bundle catheter was only 75 min, Mean pacing thresholds were 2.3 V at 0.5 ms impulse duration, and sensed R wave potentials 2.9 mV. No lead dislodgement or exit block occurred during a follow-up period of 3 months, there was undersensing in one patient. Similar results have been reported by a Spanish group [101].

In direct His-bundle pacing, the ventricular lead is typically positioned at the proximal septum (Figure 9.14). Importantly, paced and sensed QRS morphology are identical in all 12 leads (Figure 9.15), which was achieved in studies in >90% of patients [100]. In contrast, parahisian pacing may be attempted. Cantu et al. [102] defined criteria for His-bundle versus parahisian pacing; they demanded for selective His bundle pacing that the intrinsic and paced QRS have to be equal in duration and morphology, the His-ventricular (H-V) interval has to equal the paced-ventricular interval, and at low output, only the His bundle is captured, producing a narrow QRS, while increasing the output results in additional right ventricular capture with widening of the QRS. Conversely, parahisian pacing has been defined as an intrinsic QRS different from the paced one in morphology or duration, and widening of the QRS with output reduction due to loss of His-bundle capture. Occhetta et al. [103] reported results of parahisian pacing in 16 patients with atrial fibrillation and AV node ablation. They used conventional bipolar screw-in leads and a steerable stylet (Locator®, St. Jude Medical, Sylmar, CA) to implant the lead in the high interventricular septum as close as possible to the His potential marked by a diagnostic electrophysiologic catheter. They

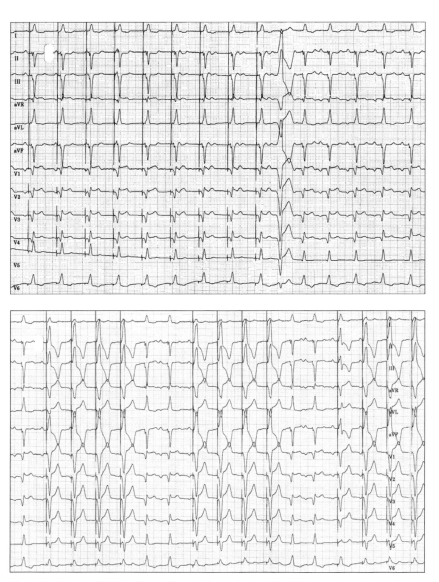

Fig. 9.15 Surface ECG in direct His-bundle pacing. (a) In VVI pacing (which excludes fusion beats) at 1.5 V/0.4 ms, all 12 leads show the QRS complex identical during sensing and pacing. (b) When the pacing output is increased to 2.5 V/0.4 ms, the QRS gets broad and is now similar to RVOT pacing. Paper speed: 25 mm/s.

distinguished direct His-bundle pacing according to the criteria proposed by Deshmukh et al. [104]:

1 QRS morphology identical between native and paced complexes in the 12-lead surface ECG;
2 Interval between His potential and ventricular signal equals ($\pm$20 ms) interval between pacing spike and QRS; and
3 Pacing threshold >2 V.

In contrast, they defined criteria for para-hisian pacing by:

1 Paced QRS at least 50 ms shorter than right ventricular apical paced QRS and always shorter than 130 ms;
2 Paced QRS axis concordant with the electrical axis of the native QRS (discrepancy <30°); and
3 Pacing threshold <1 V. Lead position was only accepted if the sensed R wave was >5 mV and atrial far-field signals were absent (indicating that the lead position was too high).

In their study, Occhetta et al. [103] reported a pacing threshold of only 0.9 V at 0.5 ms and a mean sensed R wave potential of 6.9 mV; only in one patient, no sufficiently stable lead position could be achieved. An animal study confirmed that parahisian pacing can achieve a QRS pattern almost identical to intrinsic conduction together with simpler implantation requirements and better sensing/pacing results [105]. Comparing His-bundle pacing to other alternative right ventricular pacing sites, however, a recent study found no difference in contractility and end systolic pressure [106].

In conclusion, His-bundle and parahisian pacing represent a highly interesting way to pace the right ventricle with a single lead and use the intrinsic His–Purkinje system for a completely normal ventricular activation. Recent progress in lead technology and delivery systems have dramatically facilitated this approach. However, the risks of sensing or pacing failure, lead dislodgement, or infrahisian conduction block unresolved by pacing at the site of the His bundle are not known in the longer (>3 months) term. All studies performed until today therefore used a second "back-up" lead in the right ventricular apex.

Bifocal right ventricular pacing

In 1997, Buckingham et al. [76] reported a moderate improvement in cardiac output for right ventricular outflow tract compared to apical pacing. They also found that if both sites were paced simultaneously, the QRS complex narrowed. In 1999, Pachón et al. [107] used bifocal right ventricular pacing in the RVOT and apex as a method for at least partial resynchronization of the left ventricle, which was easier to achieve than biventricular pacing. In five patients with severe dilated cardiomyopathy, atrial fibrillation, and AV block they found that bifocal right ventricular pacing improved ejection fraction and cardiac output together with a reduction of mitral regurgitation. They repeated this experience in 39 patients with severe heart failure from ischemic and Chagasic cardiomyopathy [108]. Bifocal right ventricular pacing produced a narrow QRS, at the same time improving systolic and diastolic function with better left ventricular ejection fraction, cardiac output, peak filling rate, and transmitral flow. Also mitral regurgitation was significantly reduced. These hemodynamic and echocardiographic findings translated into an impressive improvement in quality of life. Pachón et al. [109] found these improvements much more extensive in bifocal than in septal single-site right ventricular pacing. These results were confirmed in a study with 30 patients suffering from Chagasic cardiomyopathy where bifocal right ventricular pacing was able to improve NYHA functional class and echocardiographic parameters of left ventricular function. However, mortality from ventricular tachyarrhythmias was high in this study using pacemakers and not ICDs, therefore no conclusions concerning the long-term utility of this pacing modality could be drawn.

The BRIGHT study randomized 42 patients with an indication for cardiac resynchronization therapy (NYHA III-IV, left bundle branch block, ejection fraction <35%) to bifocal right ventricular pacing or no pacing (VVI, 40 bpm, [110]). In a cross-over design of two 3-month periods, bifocal right ventricular pacing was associated with a significant increase in left ventricular ejection fraction (from 26% to 36%), decrease of NYHA class (2.8 to 2.3), increase in 6-minute walking distance, and better quality of life as assessed by the Minnesota Living with Heart Failure questionnaire.

In 36 patients with a QRS ≥130 ms, severe left ventricular dysfunction, and NYHA functional Class III–IV, Rocha et al. [111] prospectively compared bifocal right ventricular pacing to biventricular pacing (nonrandomized). No significant differences were found during a follow-up period of 18 months for bifocal pacing compared to 10 months for biventricularly paced patients. Echocardiographic results and clinical response were similar, except for a narrower QRS and a trend toward less hospitalization with biventricular pacing. The improvement compared to baseline was stronger in the biventricular group. Similarly, Bulava et al. [112] report about 50 patients with severe ischemic or non-ischemic cardiomyopathy. Bifocal right ventricular pacing increased left ventricular contractility (dP/dt), particularly if the leads were placed as far from each other as possible. Regional systolic contraction shortened and also interventricular mechanical delay decreased with bifocal right ventricular pacing, leading to longer diastolic filling times. However, all hemodynamic improvements were more pronounced in biventricular pacing. As a confirmation, another acute echocardiographic study showed a stronger effect on interventricular and intra-left ventricular dyssynchrony by biventricular pacing compared to bifocal right ventricular pacing in 21 patients with severe heart failure [113].

In conclusion, bifocal right ventricular pacing may be used as an alternative method of pacing in patients where a left ventricular lead cannot be implanted via the coronary sinus and an epicardial surgical approach via lateral thoracotomy is not an option [114]. Due to the need of a third lead (increased risk for lead fracture/insulation failure and subclavian vein thrombosis), and the lack of sufficient studies (randomized, follow-up >12 months), it should not be considered as an alternative to RVOT single-site pacing in patients with a conventional pacing indication.

Conclusions

There is strong evidence that pacing from the right ventricular apex has deleterious hemodynamic effects, which are most prominent in patients with heart failure. The most efficient way to avoid pacing-induced deterioration of cardiac function is the prevention of unnecessary right ventricular pacing, which is feasible in the majority (approximately 60%) of patients, namely those without AV conduction disturbances and no indication for a biventricular device (Figure 9.16). Study results and published experience strongly advocate the use of dedicated algorithms to switch from AAI to DDD pacing, allowing single P waves to remain nonconducted instead of switching rigorously to ventricular pacing if AV conduction is temporarily impaired. In patients with permanent or frequent

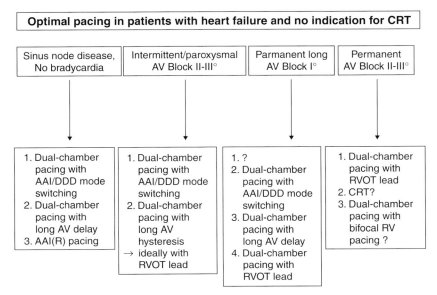

Optimal pacing in patients with heart failure and no indication for CRT

Sinus node disease, No bradycardia	Intermittent/paroxysmal AV Block II-III°	Parmanent long AV Block I°	Permanent AV Block II-III°
1. Dual-chamber pacing with AAI/DDD mode switching 2. Dual-chamber pacing with long AV delay 3. AAI(R) pacing	1. Dual-chamber pacing with AAI/DDD mode switching 2. Dual-chamber pacing with long AV hysteresis → ideally with RVOT lead	1. ? 2. Dual-chamber pacing with AAI/DDD mode switching 3. Dual-chamber pacing with long AV delay 4. Dual-chamber pacing with RVOT lead	1. Dual-chamber pacing with RVOT lead 2. CRT? 3. Dual-chamber pacing with bifocal RV pacing ?

Fig. 9.16 Proposed algorithm for pacing mode and site selection. CRT: Cardiac resynchronization therapy, RVOT: Right ventricular outflow tract.

AV block where ventricular pacing cannot be avoided, theoretical considerations and animal studies suggest that pacing from the high septal RVOT can maintain a normal vector of ventricular activation from basis to apex and may thus prevent unfavorable ventricular remodeling. Clinical studies are less clear and usually show that high septal RVOT pacing is only better than right ventricular apical pacing but inferior to intrinsic ventricular activation if present. Therefore, RVOT pacing may be used as an alternative to right ventricular pacing but not to intrinsic ventricular activation or biventricular pacing if the latter is indicated. A second alternative may be the implantation of the ventricular lead near the His bundle to use the His–Purkinje specialized conduction system for a physiologic ventricular activation. However, feasibility and long-term safety of this technique still has to be delineated in further studies (larger and with longer follow-up) before this technique can be recommended.

In patients with heart failure and AV block where left ventricular lead implantation is not possible due to coronary sinus anatomy and a surgical approach is not feasible, bifocal right ventricular may provide an option, which is at least superior to right ventricular apical pacing.

References

1. Tantengco MVT, Thomas RL, Karpawich PP. Left ventricular dysfunction after long-term right ventricular apical pacing in the young. *J Am Coll Cardiol*. 2001;37: 2093–100.
2. Thambo JB, Bordachar P, Garrigue S, Lafitte S, Sanders P, Reuter S, Girardot R, Crepin D, Reant P, Roudaut R, Jaïs P, Haïssaguerre M, Clementy J, Jimenez M. Detrimental ventricular remodeling in patients with congenital complete heart block and chronic right ventricular apical pacing. *Circulation*. 2004;110:3766–72.
3. Freudenberger RS,Wilson AC, Lawrence-Nelson J, Hare JM, Kostis JB. Myocardial Infarction Data Acquisition System Study Group (MIDAS 9). Permanent pacing is a risk factor for the development of heart failure. *Am J Cardiol*. 2005;95:671–4.
4. O'Keefe JH Jr, Abuissa H, Jones PG, Thompson RC, Bateman TN, McGhie AI, Ramza BM, Steinhaus DM. Effect of chronic right ventricular apical pacing on left ventricular function. *Am J Cardiol*. 2005;95:771–3.
5. Barold SS, Lau CP. Primary prevention of heart failure in cardiac pacing. *Pacing Clin Electrophysiol*. 2006;29:217–219.
6. Ellenbogen KA, Wood MA. Pacemaker selection—the changing definition of physiologic pacing. *N Engl J Med*. 2005;353:202–4.
7. Sweeney MO, Hellkamp AS, Ellenbogen KA, et al. Adverse effect of ventricular pacing on heart failure and atrial fibrillation among patients with normal baseline QRS duration in a clinical trial of pacemaker therapy for sinus node dysfunction. *Circulation*. 2003;23:2932–7.
8. Wilkoff BL, Cook JR, Epstein AE, Greene L, Hallstrom AP, Hsia H, Kutalek SP, Sharma A. Dual-chamber pacing or ventricular backup pacing in patients with an implantable defibrillator: the Dual Chamber and VVI Implantable Defibrillator (DAVID) Trial. *JAMA*. 2002;288:3115–23.

9. Gilmore JP, Sarnoff SJ, Mitchell JH, et al. Synchrony of ventricular contraction: Obser-vationscomparing hemodynamic effects of atrial and ventricular pacing. *Br Heart J.* 1963;25:299–307.

10. Prinzen FW. Augustijn CH, Arts T, et al. Redistribution of myocardial fiber strain and blood flow by asynchronous activation. *Am J Physiol.* 1990;259:H300–H308.

11. Karpawich PP, Justice CD, Cavit DL. et al. Developmental sequelae of fixed-rate, ven-tricular pacing in the immature canine heart: An electrophysiologic, hemodynamic and histopathologic evaluation. *Am Heart J.* 1990; 119:1077–83.

12. Adomian CE, Boazoll J. Myofibrillar disarray produced in normal hearts by chronic electrical pacing. *Am Heart J.* 1986;112:79–83.

13. Karpawich PP, Rabah R, Haas JE. Altered cardiac histology following apical right ventricular pacing in patients with congenital atrioventricular block. *Pacing Clin Electrophysiol.* 1999;22:1372–7.

14. Moak JP, Barron KS, Hougen TJ, Wiles HB, Balaji S, Sreeram N, Cohen MH, Nor-denberg A, Van Hare GF, Friedman RA, Perez M, Cecchin F, Schneider DS, Nehgme RA, Buyon JP. Congenital heart block: development of late-onset cardiomyopathy, a previously underappreciated sequela. *J Am Coll Cardiol.* 2001;37:238–42.

15. Ichiki H, Oketani N, Hamasaki S, Ishida S, Kataoka T, Ogawa M, Saihara K, Okui H, Fukudome T, Shinasato T, Kubozono T, Ninomiya Y, Matsushita T, Otsuji Y, Tei C. Effect of right ventricular apex pacing on the Tei index and brain natriuretic pep-tide in patients with a dual-chamber pacemaker. *Pacing Clin Electrophysiol.* 2006;29: 985–90

16. Simantirakis EN, Prassopoulos VK, Chrysostomakis SI, Kochiadakis GE, Koukouraki SI, Lekakis JP, Karkavitsas NS, Vardas PE. Effects of asynchronous ventricular activa-tion on myocardial adrenergic innervation in patients with permanent dual-chamber pacemakers. *Eur Heart J.* 2001;22:323–33

17. Al-Hesayen A, Parker JD. Adverse effects of atrioventricular synchronous right ven-tricular pacing on left ventricular sympathetic activity, efficiency, and hemodynamic status. *Am J Physiol Heart Circ Physiol.* 2006;291:2377–9.

18. Askenazi J, Alexander JH, Koenigsberg DI, Belic N, Lesch M. Alteration of left ven-tricular performance by left bundle branch block simulated with atrioventricular sequential pacing. *Am J Cardiol.* 1984;53:99–104.

19. Bedotto JB, Grayburn PA, Black WH, Raya TE, McBride W, Hsia HH, Eichhorn EJ. Alterations in left ventricular relaxation during atrioventricular pacing in humans. *J Am Coll Cardiol.* 1990;15:658–64.

20. Zile MR, Blaustein AS, Shimizu G, Gaasch WH. Right ventricular pacing reduces the rate of left ventricular relaxation and filling. *J Am Coll Cardiol.* 1987;10:702–9.

21. Leclercq C, Gras D, Le Helloco A, Nicol L, Mabo P, Daubert C. Hemodynamic impor-tance of preserving the normal sequence of ventricular activation in permanent car-diac pacing. *Am Heart J.* 1995;129:1133–41.

22. Lieberman R, Padeletti L, Schreuder J, Jackson K, Michelucci A, Colella A, Eastman W, Valsecchi S, Hettrick DA. Ventricular pacing lead location alters systemic hemo-dynamics and left ventricular function in patients with and without reduced ejection fraction. *J Am Coll Cardiol.* 2006;48:1634–41.

23. Nahlawi M, Waligora M, Spies SM, Bonow RO, Kadish AH, Goldberger JJ. Left ventricular function during and after right ventricular pacing. *J Am Coll Cardiol.* 2004;44:1883–8.

24. Schmidt M, Brömsen J, Herholz C, Adler K, Neff F, Kopf C, Block M. Evidence of left ventricular dyssynchrony resulting from right ventricular pacing in patients with severely depressed left ventricular ejection fraction. *Europace.* 2007;9:34–40.

25. Sharma AD, Rizo-Patron C, Hallstrom AP, O'Neill GP, Rothbart S, Martins JB, Roelke M, Steinberg JS, Greene HL. Percent right ventricular pacing predicts outcomes in the DAVID trial. *Heart Rhythm.* 2005;2:830–4.

26. Steinberg JS, Fischer A, Wang P, Schuger C, Daubert J, McNitt S, Andrews M, Brown M, Hall WJ, Zareba W, Moss AS. The clinical implications of cumulative right ventricular pacing in the Multicenter Automatic Defibrillator Trial II. *J Cardiovasc Electrophysiol.* 2005;16:359–65.

27. Sweeney MO, Hellkamp AS. Heart failure during cardiac pacing. *Circulation.* 2006;113:2082–8.

28. Wilkoff BL. The dual chamber and VVI implantable defibrillator trial (DAVID) II. Presented at the late breaking trials session, Heart Rhythm 2007, San Francisco, May 10, 2007.

29. Andersen HR, Nielsen JC, Thomsen PE, Thuesen L, Mortensen PT, Vesterlund T, Pedersen AK. Long-term follow-up of patients from a randomised trial of atrial versus ventricular pacing for sick-sinus syndrome. *Lancet.* 1997;350:1210–6.

30. Andersen HR, Nielsen JC, Thomsen PE, Thuesen L, Vesterlund T, Pedersen AK, Mortensen PT. Atrioventricular conduction during long-term follow-up of patients with sick sinus syndrome. *Circulation.* 1998;98:1315–21.

31. Brandt J, Anderson H, Fåhraeus T, Schüller H. Natural history of sinus node disease treated with atrial pacing in 213 patients: implications for selection of stimulation mode. *J Am Coll Cardiol.* 1992;20:633–9.

32. Markewitz A. Yearly report of the German pacemaker registry. *Herzschrittm Elektrophys.* 2007;18:166–93.

33. Barold SS. Permanent single chamber atrial pacing is obsolete. *Pacing Clin Electrophysiol.* 2001;24:271–5.

34. Kristensen L, Nielsen JC, Pedersen AK, Mortensen PT, Andersen HR. AV block and changes in pacing mode during long-term follow-up of 399 consecutive patients with sick sinus syndrome treated with an AAI/AAIR pacemaker. *Pacing Clin Electrophysiol.* 2001;24:358–65.

35. Israel CW, Boriani G, Brandt J, Gillis AM, Demas M, Sheldon T, Pürerfellner H, Hohnloser SH. Automatic mode change from an atrial to dual-chamber pacing mode to avoid unnecessary ventricular pacing: Holter analysis of a new pacing mode. *Heart Rhythm.* 2006;3 Suppl 1:S130 (abstract).

36. Stierle U, Krüger D, Vincent AM, Mitusch R, Giannitsis E, Wiegand U, Potratz J. An optimized AV delay algorithm for patients with intermittent atrioventricular conduction. *Pacing Clin Electrophysiol.* 1998;21:1035–43.

37. Melzer C, Sowelam S, Sheldon TJ, Bondke HJ, Baumann G, Combs B, Theres H. Reduction of right ventricular pacing in patients with sinus node dysfunction using an enhanced search AV algorithm. *Pacing Clin Electrophysiol.* 2005;28:521–7.

38. Deering TF, Wilensky M, Tondato F, Dan D, Tyler J. Auto intrinsic conduction search algorithm: a prospective analysis. *Pacing Clin Electrophysiol.* 2003;26:1080 (abstract).

39. Olshansky B, Day J, McGuire M, Hahn S, Brown S, Lerew DR. Reduction of right ventricular pacing in patients with dual-chamber ICDs. *Pacing Clin Electrophysiol.* 2006;29:237–43.

40. Nielsen JC, Kristensen L, Andersen HR, Mortensen PT, Pedersen OL, Pedersen AK. A randomized comparison of atrial and dual-chamber pacing in 177 consecutive patients with sick sinus syndrome: echocardiographic and clinical outcome. *J Am Coll Cardiol.* 2003;42:614–23.

41. Goethals M, Timmermans W, Geelen P, Backers J, Brugada P. Mode switching failure during atrial flutter: the "2:1 lock-in" phenomenon. *Europace.* 2003;5:95–102.

42. Pajitnev D, Israel CW, Hohnloser SH, Barold SS. The "inverse 2:1 lock-in" response to atrial flutter. *Pacing Clin Electrophysiol.* 2005; Sep;28(9):982–4.

43. Shivkumar K, Feliciano Z, Boyle NG, Weiner I. Intradevice interaction in a dual chamber implantable cardioverter defibrillator preventing ventricular tachyarrhythmia detection. *J Cardiovasc Electrophysiol.* 2000;11:1285–1288.

44. Dennis MJ, Sparks PB. Pacemaker mediated tachycardia as a complication of the autointrinsic conduction search function. *Pacing Clin Electrophysiol.* 2004;27:824–6.

45. Barold SS, Levine PA. Pacemaker repetitive nonreentrant ventriculoatrial synchronous rhythm. A review. *J Interv Card Electrophysiol.* 2001;5:45–58.

46. Sweeney MO. Novel cause of spurious mode switching in dual-chamber pacemakers: atrioventricular desynchronization arrhythmia. *J Cardiovasc Electrophysiol.* 2002;13:616–619.

47. Nielsen JC, Pedersen AK, Mortensen PT, Andersen HR. Programming a fixed long atrioventricular delay is not effective in preventing ventricular pacing in patients with sick sinus syndrome. *Europace.* 1999;1:113–20.

48. Savouré A, Fröhlig G, Galley D, Defaye P, Reuter S, Mabo P, Sadoul N, Amblard A, Limousin M, Anselme F. A new dual-chamber pacing mode to minimize ventricular pacing. *Pacing Clin Electrophysiol.* 2005;28 Suppl 1:S43–S46.

49. Fröhlig G, Gras D, Victor J, Mabo P, Galley D, Savouré A, Jauvert G, Defaye P, Ducloux P, Amblard A. Use of a new cardiac pacing mode designed to eliminate unnecessary ventricular pacing. *Europace.* 2006;8:96–101.

50. Pioger G, Leny G, Nitzsché R, Ripart A. AAIsafeR limits ventricular pacing in unselected patients. *Pacing Clin Electrophysiol.* 2007;30 Suppl 1:S66–S70.

51. Sweeney MO, Shea JB, Fox V, Adler S, Nelson L, Mullen TJ, Belk P, Casavant D, Sheldon T. Randomized pilot study of a new atrial-based minimal ventricular pacing mode in dual-chamber implantable cardioverter-defibrillators. *Heart Rhythm.* 2004;1:160–7

52. Sweeney MO, Ellenbogen KA, Casavant D, Betzold R, Sheldon T, Tang F, Mueller M, Lingle J; The Marquis MVP Download Investigators. Multicenter, prospective, randomized safety and efficacy study of a new atrial-based managed ventricular pacing mode (MVP) in dual chamber ICDs. *J Cardiovasc Electrophysiol.* 2005;16: 811–7.

53. Gillis AM, Pürerfellner H, Israel CW, Sunthorn H, Kacet S, Anelli-Monti M, Tang F, Young M, Boriani G; Medtronic Enrhythm Clinical Study Investigators. Reducing unnecessary right ventricular pacing with the managed ventricular pacing mode in patients with sinus node disease and AV block. *Pacing Clin Electrophysiol.* 2006;29:697–705.

54. Milasinovic G, Tscheliessnigg K, Boehmer A, Vancura V, Schuchert A, Brandt J, Wiggenhorn C, Hofman M, Sperzel J. Percent ventricular pacing with managed ventricular pacing mode in standard pacemaker population. *Europace.* 2008;10: 151–5.

55. Pürerfellner H, Brandt J, Israel C, Sheldon T, Johnson J, Tscheliessnigg K, Sperzel J, Boriani G, Puglisi A, Milasinovic G. Comparison of two strategies to reduce ventricular pacing in pacemaker patients. *Pacing Clin Electrophysiol.* 2008;31:167–76.

56. Sweeney MO, Bank AJ, Nsah E, Koullick M, Zeng QC, Hettrick D, Sheldon T, Lamas GA; Search AV Extension and Managed Ventricular Pacing for Promoting Atrioventricular Conduction (SAVE PACe) Trial.Minimizing ventricular pacing to reduce atrial fibrillation in sinus-node disease. *N Engl J Med.* 2007;357:1000–8.

57. Mechelen R van, Schoonderwoerd R. Risk of managed ventricular pacing in a patient with heart block. *Heart Rhythm.* 2006;3:1384–5.

58. Chalfoun N, Kuhne M, Boonyapisit W, Jongnarangsin K. Managed ventricular pacing with a short VA interval: what is the mechanism? *Heart Rhythm.* 2007;4:1100–1.

59. Mansour F, Talajic M, Thibault B, Khairy P. Pacemaker troubleshooting: When MVP is not the most valuable parameter. *Heart Rhythm.* 2006;3:612–4.

60. Iliev II, Yamachika S, Muta K, Hayano M, Ishimatsu T, Nakao K, Komiya N, Hirata T, Ueyama C, Yano K. Preserving normal ventricular activation versus atrioventricular delay optimization during pacing: the role of intrinsic atrioventricular conduction and pacing rate. *Pacing Clin Electrophysiol.* 2000;23:74–83.

61. Auricchio A, Sommariva L, Salo RW, Scafuri A, Chiariello L. Improvement of cardiac function in patients with severe congestive heart failure and coronary artery disease by dual chamber pacing with shortened AV delay. *Pacing Clin Electrophysiol.* 1993; Oct;16(10):2034–43.

62. Brecker SJ, Xiao HB, Sparrow J, Gibson DG. Effects of dual-chamber pacing with short atrioventricular delay in dilated cardiomyopathy. *Lancet.* 1992;340:1308–12.

63. Hochleitner M, Hörtnagl H, Ng CK, Hörtnagl H, Gschnitzer F, Zechmann W. Usefulness of physiologic dual-chamber pacing in drug-resistant idiopathic dilated cardiomyopathy. *Am J Cardiol.* 1990; Jul 15;66(2):198–202.

64. Shinbane JS, Chu E, DeMarco T, Sobol Y, Fitzpatrick AP, Lau DM, Klinski C, Schiller NB, Griffin JC, Chatterjee K. Evaluation of acute dual-chamber pacing with a range of atrioventricular delays on cardiac performance in refractory heart failure. *J Am Coll Cardiol.* 1997;30:1295–300.

65. Karpawich PP, Justice CD, Chang CH, el al. Septal ventricular pacing in the immature canine heart: A new perspective. *Am Heart J.* 1991; 121:827–33.

66. Karpawich PP. Mital SR. Comparative left ventricular function following atrial, septal and apical single chamber heart pacing in the young. *PACE.* 1997; 20:1983–8.

67. Prinzen FW, Peschar M. Relationship between the pacing induced sequence of activation and left ventricular pump function in animals. *Pacing Clin Electrophysiol.* 2002; 25:484–98.

68. Sweeney MO, Prinzen FW. A new paradigm for physiologic ventricular pacing. *J Am Coll Cardiol.* 2006; 47:282–8.

69. Barin ES, Jones SM, Ward DE, et al. The right ventricular outflow tract as an alternative permanent pacing site; Long-term follow-up. *PACE.* 1991;14:3–6

70. Brady PA, Hammill SC. Ventricular-based pacing: One site fits all? *J Cardiovasc Electrophysiol.* 2003; 14:1187–8.

71. Lev M. The conduction system. In: SE Gould ed., *Pathology of the heart and blood vessels,* 3rd edition. Springfield, IL, Charles C. Thomas Pub., 1968:199–209.

72. Mond HG, Hillock RJ, Stevenson IH, McGavigan AD. The right ventricular outflow tract: the road to septal pacing. *Pacing Clin Electrophysiol.* 2007;30:482–91.

73. McGavigan AD, Roberts-Thomson KC, Hillock RJ, Stevenson IH, Mond HG. Right ventricular outflow tract pacing: radiographic and electrocardiographic correlates of lead position. *Pacing Clin Electrophysiol.* 2006;29:1063–8.

74. Anderson RH, Razavi R, Taylor AM. Cardiac anatomy revisited. *J Anat.* 2004;205:159–77.

75. Vlay SC. Right ventricular outflow tract pacing: practical and beneficial. A 9-year experience of 460 consecutive implants. *Pacing Clin Electrophysiol.* 2006;29:1055–62.

76. Buckingham TA, Candinas R, Schläpfer J, Aebischer N, Jeanrenaud X, Landolt J, Kappenberger L. Acute hemodynamic effects of atrioventricular pacing at differing sites in the right ventricle individually and simultaneously. *Pacing Clin Electrophysiol.* 1997;20:909–15.

77. Buckingham TA, Candinas R, Attenhofer C, Van Hoeven H, Hug R, Hess O, Jenni R, Amann FW. Systolic and diastolic function with alternate and combined site pacing in the right ventricle. *Pacing Clin Electrophysiol.* 1998;21:1077–84.

78. Buckingham TA, Candinas R, Duru F, Pagotto E, Schönbeck M, Amann FW, Turina M, Schmid ER. Acute hemodynamic effects of alternate and combined site pacing in patients after cardiac surgery. *Pacing Clin Electrophysiol.* 1999;22:887–93.

79. Alboni P, Scarfò S, Fucà G, Mele D, Dinelli M, Paparella N. Short-term hemodynamic effects of DDD pacing from ventricular apex, right ventricular outflow tract and proximal septum. *G Ital Cardiol.* 1998;28:237–41.

80. Victor F, Leclercq C, Mabo P, Pavin D, Deviller A, de Place C, Pezard P, Victor J, Daubert C. Optimal right ventricular pacing site in chronically implanted patients: a prospective randomized crossover comparison of apical and outflow tract pacing. *J Am Coll Cardiol.* 1999;33:311–6.

81. Schwaab B, Fröhlig G, Alexander C, Kindermann M, Hellwig N, Schwerdt H, Kirsch CM, Schieffer H. Influence of right ventricular stimulation site on left ventricular function in atrial synchronous ventricular pacing. *J Am Coll Cardiol.* 1999;33: 317–23.

82. Gold MR, Brockman R, Peters RW, Olsovsky MR, Shorofsky SR. Acute hemodynamic effects of right ventricular pacing site and pacing mode in patients with congestive heart failure secondary to either ischemic or idiopathic dilated cardiomyopathy. *Am J Cardiol.* 2000;85:1106–9.

83. Bourke JP, Hawkins T, Keavey P, Tynan M, Jamieson S, Behulova R, Furniss SS. Evolution of ventricular function during permanent pacing from either right ventricular apex or outflow tract following AV-junctional ablation for atrial fibrillation. *Europace.* 2002;4:219–28.

84. Giudici MC, Thornburg GA, Buck DL, Coyne EP, Walton MC, Paul DL, Sutton J. Comparison of right ventricular outflow tract and apical lead permanent pacing on cardiac output. *Am J Cardiol.* 1997;79:209–12.

85. Le Helloco A, Hacot JP, Lelong B, Schleich JM, Laurent M, Almange C. Comparison of apical and infundibular pacing in patients with primary dilated or ischemic cardiomyopathy. *Arch Mal Coeur Vaiss.* 1999;92:19–26.

86. de Cock CC, Meyer A, Kamp O, Visser CA. Hemodynamic benefits of right ventricular outflow tract pacing: comparison with right ventricular apex pacing. *Pacing Clin Electrophysiol.* 1998;21:536–41.

87. Saxon LA, Kerwin WF, Cahalan MK, Kalman JM, Olgin JE, Foster E, Schiller NB, Shinbane JS, Lesh MD, Merrick SH. Acute effects of intraoperative multisite ventricular

pacing on left ventricular function and activation/contraction sequence in patients with depressed ventricular function. *J Cardiovasc Electrophysiol.* 1998;9:13–21.

88. Mera F, DeLurgio DB, Patterson RE, Merlino JD, Wade ME, León AR. A comparison of ventricular function during high right ventricular septal and apical pacing after His-bundle ablation for refractory atrial fibrillation. *Pacing Clin Electrophysiol.* 1999;22:1234–9.

89. Kolettis TM, Kyriakides ZS, Tsiapras D, Popov T, Paraskevaides IA, Kremastinos DT. Improved left ventricular relaxation during short-term right ventricular outflow tract compared to apical pacing. *Chest.* 2000;117:60–4.

90. Tse HF, Yu C, Wong KK, Tsang V, Leung YL, Ho WY, Lau CP. Functional abnormalities in patients with permanent right ventricular pacing: the effect of sites of electrical stimulation. *J Am Coll Cardiol.* 2002;40:1451–8.

91. Lewicka-Nowak E, Dabrowska-Kugacka A, Tybura S, KrzymiÒska-Stasiuk E, Wilczek R, Staniewicz J, Swiatecka G, Raczek G. Right ventricular apex versus right ventricular outflow tract pacing: prospective, randomised, long-term clinical and echocardiographic evaluation. *Kardiol Pol.* 2006;64:1082–91.

92. Blanc JJ, Etienne Y, Gilard M, Mansourati J, Munier S, Boschat J, Benditt DG, Lurie KG. Evaluation of different ventricular pacing sites in patients with severe heart failure: results of an acute hemodynamic study. *Circulation.* 1997;96:3273–7.

93. Victor F, Mabo P, Mansour H, Pavin D, Kabalu G, de Place C, Leclercq C, Daubert JC. A randomized comparison of permanent septal versus apical right ventricular pacing: short-term results. *J Cardiovasc Electrophysiol.* 2006;17:238–42.

94. Stambler BS, Ellenbogen K, Zhang X, Porter TR, Xie F, Malik R, Small R, Burke M, Kaplan A, Nair L, Belz M, Fuenzalida C, Gold M, Love C, Sharma A, Silverman R, Sogade F, Van Natta B, Wilkoff BL; ROVA Investigators. Right ventricular outflow versus apical pacing in pacemaker patients with congestive heart failure and atrial fibrillation. *J Cardiovasc Electrophysiol.* 2003;14:1180–6.

95. Lieberman R, Grenz D, Mond HG, Gammage MD. Selective site pacing: defining and reaching the selected site. *Pacing Clin Electrophysiol.* 2004;27:883–6.

96. Hillock RJ, Stevenson IH, Mond HG. The right ventricular outflow tract: a comparative study of septal, anterior wall, and free wall pacing. *Pacing Clin Electrophysiol.* 2007;30:942–7.

97. Burkoff D, Oikawa RY, Sagawa K. Influence of pacing site on canine left ventricular contraction. *Am J Physiol.* 1986; 251:H428–H435.

98. Heydrickx GR. Vilaine JP, Knight DR, et al. Effects of altered site of electrical activation on myocardial performance during inotropic stimulation. *Circulation.* 1985; 71:1010–16.

99. Deshmukh P, Casavant DA, Romanyshyn M, Anderson K. Permanent, direct His-bundle pacing. A novel approach to cardiac pacing in patients with normal His-Purkinje activation. *Circulation.* 2000;101:869–877.

100. Zanon F, Baracca E, Aggio S, Pastore G, Boaretto G, Cardano P, Marotta T, Rigatelli G, Galasso M, Carraro M, Zonzin P. A feasible approach for direct His-bundle pacing using a new steerable catheter to facilitate precise lead placement. *J Cardiovasc Electrophysiol.* 2006;17:29–33.

101. Barba-Pichardo R, Moriña-Vázquez P, Venegas-Gamero J, Maroto-Monserrat F, Cid-Cumplido M, Herrera-Carranza M. Permanent His-bundle pacing in patients with infra-Hisian atrioventricular block. *Rev Esp Cardiol.* 2006;59:553–8.

102. Cantù F, De Filippo P, Cardano P, De Luca A, Gavazzi A. Validation of criteria for selective His bundle and para-Hisian permanent pacing. *Pacing Clin Electrophysiol.* 2006;29:1326–33.
103. Occhetta E, Bortnik M, Magnani A, Francalacci G, Piccinino C, Plebani L, Marino P. Prevention of ventricular desynchronization by permanent para-Hisian pacing after atrioventricular node ablation in chronic atrial fibrillation: a crossover, blinded, randomized study versus apical right ventricular pacing. *J Am Coll Cardiol.* 2006;47:1938–45.
104. Deshmukh P, Romanyshyn M. Direct His-bundle pacing: present and future. *Pacing Clin Electrophysiol.* 2004;27:862–70.
105. Laske TG, Skadsberg ND, Hill AJ, Klein GJ, Iaizzo PA. Excitation of the intrinsic conduction system through His and interventricular septal pacing. *Pacing Clin Electrophysiol.* 2006;29:397–405.
106. Padeletti L, Lieberman R, Schreuder J, Michelucci A, Collella A, Pieragnoli P, Ricciardi G, Eastman W, Valsecchi S, Hettrick DA. Acute effects of His bundle pacing versus left ventricular and right ventricular pacing on left ventricular function. *Am J Cardiol.* 2007;100:1556–60.
107. Pachón Mateos JC, Albornoz RN, Pachón Mateos EI, Gimenez VM, Pachón MZ, Santos Filho ER, Medeiros P, Silva MA, Paulista PP, Sousa JE, Jatene AD. Right ventricular bifocal stimulation in the treatment of dilated cardiomyopathy with heart failure. *Arq Bras Cardiol.* 1999;73:485–98.
108. Pachón JC, Pachón EI, Albornoz RN, Pachón JC, Kormann DS, Gimenes VM, Medeiros PT, Silva MA, Sousa JE, Paulista PP, Souza LC, Jatene AD. Ventricular endocardial right bifocal stimulation in the treatment of severe dilated cardiomyopathy heart failure with wide QRS. *Pacing Clin Electrophysiol.* 2001;24:1369–76.
109. Da Silva Menezes A. Outcome of right ventricular bifocal pacing in patients with permanent atrial fibrillation and severe dilated cardiomiopathy due to Chagas disease: three years of follow-up. *J Interv Card Electrophysiol.* 2004;11:193–8.
110. Res JC, Bokern MJ, de Cock CC, van Loenhout T, Bronzwaer PN, Spierenburg HA; BRIGHT Investigators. The BRIGHT study: bifocal right ventricular resynchronization therapy: a randomized study. *Europace.* 2007;9:857–61.
111. Rocha EA, Gondim TP, Abreu S, Farias R, Marques V, Rocha A, Ribeiro D, Pereira R, Negreiros P, Rodrigues CR, Paes JN, Jr. Ventricular resynchronization: comparing biventricular and bifocal right ventricular pacemakers. *Arq Bras Cardiol.* 2007;88:674–82.
112. Bulava A, Lukl J. Usefulness of bifocal pacing in patients with heart failure and intraventricular conduction delay. *Eur J Heart Fail.* 2007;9:300–5.
113. Lane RE, Mayet J, Peters NS, Davies DW, Chow AW. Comparison of temporary bifocal right ventricular pacing and biventricular pacing for heart failure: evaluation by tissue Doppler imaging. *Heart.* 2008;94:53–8.
114. Barold SS, Herweg B. Pacing in heart failure: how many leads and where? *Heart.* 2008;94:10–2.

Chapter 10

Non-CRT pacing in the failing heart: Cardiac contractility modulation (CCM)

Daniel Burkhoff, Martin Borggrefe, and Christian Butter

Key Points

1. Cardiac Resynchronization Therapy (CRT) is an important therapy for patients with symptomatic heart failure, ejection fraction less than 35% and prolonged QRS duration.
2. However, 50% or more of heart failure patients with ejection fraction have a normal QRS duration.
3. Cardiac Contractility Modulation (CCM) signals are relatively high electric currents delivered during the absolute refractory period that impact on the physiology of the myocyte.
4. In isolated muscles, CCM signals rapidly increase contractile strength, likely due to an enhancement of the peak of the calcium transient.
5. However, in intact animals and patients with heart failure, where CCM signals are applied in one region of the heart, the time course of increase of global strength is more gradual, suggesting that different mechanisms may be dominant.
6. Studies in animal models of heart failure have shown that expression of malexpressed genes become more normal within 4 hours of CCM signal application in the region where the signal are applied, but not in remote areas.
7. These studies also show that following 3 months of CCM treatment, gene expression is improved in all regions of the heart.
8. Similarly, gene expression is improved in patients following 3 months of CCM treatment and the improvement in exercise tolerance correlated with the improvement in gene expression.

Pacing to Support the Failing Heart, 1st edition. Edited by K. Ellenbogen and A. Auricchio.
© 2008 American Heart Association, ISBN: 978-1-4051-7534-0

9. Results of one randomized, blinded clinical trial conducted in patients with ejection fraction less than 35%, NYHA II or III symptoms despite optimal medical therapy, not eligible for CRT showed that CCM provides significant improvement in exercise tolerance and quality of life, on the order of that observed with CRT in patients with prolonged QRS duration.

10. Results of other ongoing studies will help further define the safety and efficacy of CCM for these patients with no other therapeutic option.

Introduction

Clinical studies have shown that cardiac resynchronization therapy (CRT) improves patient symptoms, quality of life, and exercise tolerance and reduces hospitalizations in patients with advanced heart failure and prolonged QRS duration [1–3]. However, because roughly 70% of patients with heart failure have a normal QRS duration [4], development of a device-based treatment for such patients with persistent symptoms despite optimal medical therapy would have an important impact. New treatments are required to fill this significant unmet clinical need. It is possible to make a rough estimate of the number of heart failure patients with NYHA Class III or Class IV symptoms in the United States who are not eligible for CRT. Of the approximately 5.5 million patients who suffer from symptomatic heart failure [5], roughly one-half have an ejection fraction (EF) $\leq$35%, of which approximately 30% have NYHA Class III or Class IV symptoms, and of which approximately 70% have a QRS duration $\leq$120 ms [4,6]. From these conservative numbers, it is estimated that there are almost 600,000 patients in the United States with EF $\leq$35%, with QRS duration $\leq$120ms with NYHA Class III or Class IV symptoms who do not meet current indications for CRT.

Cardiac contractility modulating (CCM) signals are nonexcitatory signals applied during the absolute refractory period that have been shown to enhance the strength of left ventricular contraction in studies carried out in animals and humans with heart failure. Because the signals have an impact on cell function without any impact on activation sequence, the effects are independent of QRS duration and additive to those of CRT in patients with prolonged QRS [7,8]. We will review the rationale and available clinical results concerning the evaluation of CCM as a treatment for heart failure. Reviews of early findings have appeared in previous papers [9,10].

Pathology of calcium handling in heart failure and rationale for CCM

One cellular defect that underlies myocardial contractile dysfunction in heart failure is reduction in the peak and broadening of the time course of the intracellular calcium transient [11]. Such abnormalities reflect heart failure-associated changes in expression of genes encoding calcium-handling proteins and post-translational modification of their associated proteins. Several of the commonly discussed abnormalities include down-regulation of genes encoding for the sarcoplasmic reticular ATPase-dependent calcium pump (SERCA2a) [12–15], changes in the expression and the hypophosphorylation of phopholamban [14–19], altered regulation of the sodium-calcium exchanger [15,20,21], and the hyperphosphorylation of the ryanodine release channel [22–24]. Accordingly, it has been proposed that treatments aimed at improving the calcium transient in heart failure could be therapeutic [25].

Although the early studies of the mechanisms by which CCM signal have an impact on myocardial contractile force focused on their immediate and direct effects on calcium handling, the most recent studies of the mechanisms by which CCM signal enhance contractile strength have been motivated by prior literature showing that electromagnetic fields can impact on protein–protein interaction and gene expression [26]. Based on these findings, it was hypothesized that CCM signals may have a direct impact on cellular physiology. Accordingly, myocardial samples were obtained for molecular and biochemical analysis from normal canine myocardium, failing canine myocardium, and failing canine myocardium following 3 months of CCM signal application [27,28]. Myocardial biopsies were also obtained from patients prior to and following 3 months of CCM therapy [29]. In the studies in canine hearts, it was shown that CCM signals have a relatively rapid beneficial impact on gene expression in the region where they are applied, but not in remote regions. Among the genes examined in these studies were SERCA2a, ANP, BNP and α-myosin heavy chain. The relatively rapid and local impact of CCM on gene expression implies a direct effect of the signals. In the chronic setting, however, improved expression of these genes was present both in local and remote of signal delivery regions. These later findings imply indirect beneficial effects of the CCM signals on myocardial gene expression; it has been hypothesized that sustained hemodynamic benefits of long-term CCM signal application result in reverse remodeling even in areas remote from where the signals are applied. In addition to the findings concerning gene expression, similar improvements were seen at the protein level for most of the proteins examined. Interestingly, phospholamban (PLB) was one protein whose total expression was not changed significantly by CCM. However, it was found that the ratio of total-to-phosporylated PLB improved in a manner that would result in improved SR calcium handling [28]. These findings related to the impact on gene expression obtained in failing canine myocardium were recapitulated in right ventricular myocardial biopsies obtained after 3 months of CCM treatment [29]. Thus, the mechanisms by which CCM signals have an impact on myocardial properties appears to go far beyond the original hypotheses related to acute augmentation of calcium handling [10].

Clinical evidence

The initial clinical study of CCM signals involved short-term (10–30 min) CCM signal application, which showed the feasibility of delivering CCM signals in humans and demonstrating that contractile performance could be enhanced [7]. The initial study of chronic CCM signals delivery commenced when an implantable pulse generator (IPG) was developed (Figure 10.1) [30,31]. The device [30,31], does not have pacing or antitachycardia therapy capabilities but is designed to work in concert with pacemakers (including CRT devices) and implantable cardioverter defibrillators (ICDs). The IPG has a rechargeable battery that the patients recharge at home once per week via a transcutaneous energy transfer (TET) charging unit. The implant procedure is also similar to that of a standard dual chamber pacemaker and has been described in detail previously, along with a detailed description of the system [9]. In addition, the system includes an acute monitoring system used to measure hemodynamic responses during the system implant and the system programmer. The hemodynamic evaluation primarily relies on assessment of changes of peak rate of left ventricular rise (dP/dt); for this evaluation, left ventricular pressure (LVP) is measured with a Millar catheter inserted into the left ventricle under fluoroscopic guidance via a femoral artery. In all prior clinical studies, CCM signals are applied after initial lead placement and a $\geq 5\%$ increase in dP/dt within 5–10 minutes is taken as evidence that the leads are in an appropriate position, as shown in Figure 10.2. If such a response is not observed, the leads are repositioned and another test application of CCM is performed. If, after several attempts, an acute hemodynamic response is not able to be elicited, patients have been considered to be ineligible and the IPG is not implanted. The current rate of failure to achieve such an acute hemodynamic response is approximately 2% of attempted implants.

The initial study of chronic CCM signal delivery (called the FIX-HF-3 study [30,31]) was performed in 23 patients with NYHA Class III symptoms and QRS duration ≤ 120 ms. This was a multicenter, unblinded, uncontrolled, treatment only, feasibility study designed mainly to test the functionality of the device over an 8-week period in Europe. The average age of the patients was 62 ± 9 years, they were primarily male (92%) and were split between idiopathic and ischemic cardiomyopathy (41% and 59%, respectively). Baseline ejection fraction averaged $22 \pm 7\%$ and Minnesota Living with Heart Failure Questionnaire (MLWHFQ) score averaged 43 ± 22. The study revealed that the device operated as intended, there was no change in ambient ectopy observed between baseline and 8 weeks of treatment and no overt safety concerns were revealed. At the end of the 8 week study period, heart failure symptoms improved significantly from NYHA Class III to Class II in 15 patients and to Class I in 4 patients, left ventricular ejection fraction improved from $22 \pm 7\%$ to $28 \pm 8\%$, and the MLWHFQ improved from 43 ± 22 to 25 ± 18. The 6-minute walk test increased from 411 ± 86 to 465 ± 81 m. These findings were sufficient to support further clinical evaluation of CCM.

The next study was carried out in the United States (the FIX-HF-5 Phase I study) [32]. Forty-nine subjects with EF$\leq 35\%$, normal QRS duration (105 $\pm$

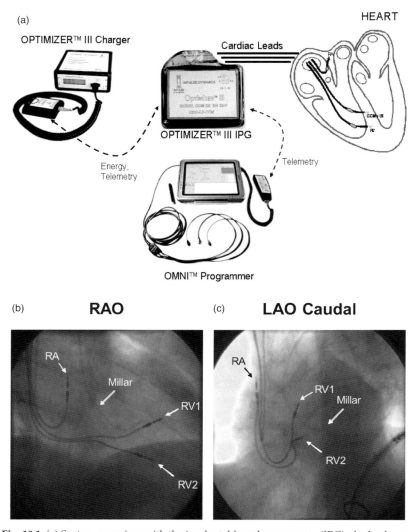

Fig. 10.1 (a) System overview with the implantable pulse generator (IPG), the leads connecting to the heart, the charger and charging wand, the acute hemodynamic monitoring system used to measure hemodynamic responses during the system implant, and the programmer. (b and c) Right anterior oblique (RAO) and left lateral oblique (LAO) fluoroscopic images of electrode placement during OPTIMIZER System implant. One lead is placed in the right atrium (RA) and two leads are placed on the right ventricular septum (RV1, RV2) approximately midway between the base and the apex, one near the anterior, and one near the posterior interventricular groove. (c) The LAO caudal view shows the electrode tips point toward the patient left, into the septum. A micromanometer (Millar) is placed temporarily to measure physiologic response to acute CCM signal application.

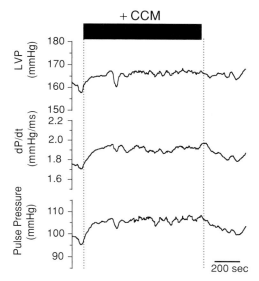

Fig. 10.2 An example of hemodynamic responses to acute CCM signal application. LVP, left ventricular pressure; dP/dt, peak rate of rise of LVP; Pulse Pressure is difference between systolic and diastolic arterial pressure. LVP and dP/dt are measured with a Millar catheter placed under fluoroscopic guidance via the femoral artery.

15 ms) and NYHA Class III or IV despite medical therapy received a CCM pulse generator. Two weeks after implantation, patients were randomized to a treatment group in which their devices were programmed to deliver CCM signals for 5 hours per day ($n = 25$) or to a control group in which the device remained off ($n = 24$). All patients were followed for 6 months; both patients and investigators were blinded to treatment group. Evaluations included NYHA, 6-minute walk (6MW), cardiopulmonary stress test, Minnesota Living with Heart Failure Questionnaire (MLWHFQ) and Holter. Although most baseline features were balanced between groups, EF (31.4 ± 7.4 vs. $24.9 \pm 6.5\%$, $p = 0.003$), end-diastolic dimension (52.1 ± 21.4 vs. 62.5 ± 6.2 mm, $p = 0.01$), peak VO$_2$ (16.0 ± 2.9 vs. 14.3 ± 2.8 ml O$_2$/kg/min, $p = 0.02$) and anaerobic threshold (12.3 ± 2.5 vs. 10.6 ± 2.4 ml O$_2$/kg/min, $p = 0.01$) were all worse in the treatment group as compared to the control. Nevertheless, there was 1 death in control and more treatment patients were free of hospitalization for any cause at 6 months (84% vs. 62%, Figure 10.3, (b)). Compared to baseline, changes in 6MW (13.4 m), peak VO$_2$ (0.2 ml O$_2$/kg/min) and anaerobic threshold (~0.8 ml O$_2$/kg/min, Figure 10.3, (a)) were more positive in the Treatment group than in the Control group. None of these differences was statistically significant because of the small sample size. Nevertheless, despite a distinctly sicker population in the Treatment group, no safety concerns emerged with chronic CCM signal administration and

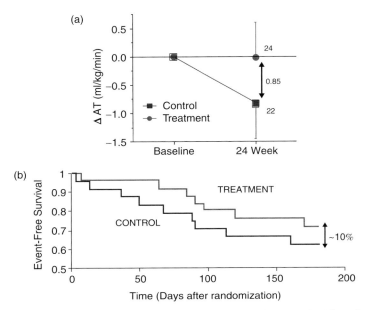

Fig. 10.3 Key findings from the US feasibility study (called the FIX-HF-5 Phase I study) of CCM. In this prospective, double blind study in which all 49 patients were implanted with an OPTIMIZER System, average anaerobic threshold (measured on cardiopulmonary stress testing) decreased by 0.85 ml O2/kg/min in the sham control group and remained constant in the active treatment group (a). The event-free survival (i.e. the proportion of patients alive without being hospitalized) also trended better in the treatment group (b). With the small number of patients, the differences between the groups were not statistically significant in either panel [32].

there were trends toward better outcomes and improved symptoms in response to CCM treatment.

These feasibility studies were followed by a multicenter randomized, double-blind, double-crossover study of CCM in heart failure patients with NYHA Class II or Class III symptoms despite optimal medical therapy (the FIX-HF-4 study) [33]. One hundred and sixty-four subjects with EF <35% and NYHA Class II (24%) or Class III (76%) symptoms received a CCM pulse generator. Patients were randomly assigned to Group 1 ($n = 80$, CCM treatment for the first 3 months, sham treatment for the second 3 months) or Group 2 ($n = 84$, sham treatment for the first 3 months, CCM treatment for the second 3 months). The coprimary endpoints were changes in peak oxygen consumption (peak VO$_2$) and Minnesota Living with Heart Failure Questionnaire (MLWHFQ). Baseline EF ($29.3 \pm 6.69\%$ vs. $29.8 \pm 7.8\%$), peak VO$_2$ (14.1 ± 3.0 vs. 13.6 ± 2.7 ml/kg/min) and MLWHFQ (38.9 ± 27.4 vs. 36.5 ± 27.1) were similar between groups. VO$_{2,peak}$ increased similarly in both groups during the first 3 months (0.40 ± 3.0 vs. $0.37 \pm$

3.3 ml/kg/min) (Figure 10.4a). This was interpreted as evidence of a prominent placebo effect. During the next 3 months, however, $VO_{2,peak}$ decreased in the group switched to sham (-0.86 ± 3.06 ml/kg/min) and increased in patients switched to active treatment (0.16 ± 2.50 ml/kg/min). At the end of the second phase of the study, the difference in peak VO_2 between groups was approximately 1 ml/kg/min. MLWHFQ behaved similarly, trending only slightly better with treatment (-12.06 ± 15.33 vs. -9.70 ± 16.71) during the first 3 months (again, consistent with a large placebo effect) (Figure 10.4b). During the second 3 months, MLWHFQ increased in the group switched to sham ($+4.70 \pm 16.57$) and decreased further in patients switched to active treatment (-0.70 ± 15.13). Serious cardiovascular adverse events were tracked carefully in both groups. The most frequently reported events were episodes of decompensated heart failure, atrial fibrillation, bleeding at the OPTMIZER System implant site and pneumonia. Importantly, there were no significant differences between ON and OFF phases in the number or types of adverse events.

Hospitalizations and mortality were compared for the first period of the study (because these will be difficult to interpret following crossover). In all, there were 14 hospitalizations in Group 1 patients (CCM ON phase) compared to 20 hospitalizations in Group 2 patients (CCM OFF phase). In addition there was 1 death in a Group 2 patient versus no deaths in Group 1 patients. With the relatively small sample size the overall event-free survival (Figure 10.4c) did not reach statistical significance ($p = 0.31$) but showed trends of magnitude that were similar to those reported for CRT [1].

In order to put the results of the FIX-HF-4 study into perspective, it was considered to be relevant to compare these results obtained with CCM in patients with more normal QRS duration to those obtained in patients with more prolonged QRS duration in response to CRT as observed in the MUSTIC study [34]. Such a comparison is interesting in view of the fact that the FIX-HF-4 study design mimicked that of the MUSTIC study of CRT. The MLWHFQ results of the two studies are compared in Figure 10.5; (a) shows results from Group 1 patients (device "ON" first, then "OFF") whereas (b) shows results from Group 2 (device "OFF" first, then "ON"). As seen, results in Group 1 patients are nearly identical in both studies for both "ON" and "OFF" phases. In Group 2 patients, results are similar, but the placebo effect is much more prominent in the present CCM study; that is, patients with device "OFF" first showed little improvement in the MUSTIC study. Thus, the main difference in findings between the studies is explained by the lack of a placebo effect in the MUSTIC study. These findings are similar to those obtained with the 6MW test as shown in (c) and (d). Although this compares results to just a single study of CRT, comparison to the MUSTIC study results is most pertinent and straightforward because the study designs (including duration of treatment) are essentially identical.

In aggregate, the data from the feasibility and larger randomized FIX-HF-4 study show that in patients with heart failure and left ventricular dysfunction,

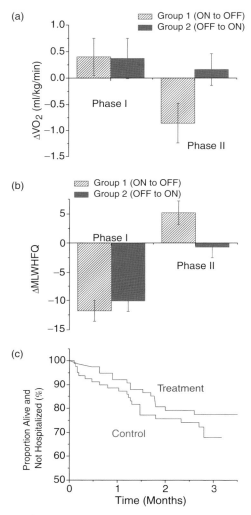

Fig. 10.4 Key results of the FIX-HF-4 study [33]. (a) changes in peak VO$_2$ between the baseline and the end of Phase I (labeled "Phase I") and changes between the end of Phase I and the end of Phase II (labeled "Phase II"). (b) changes in Minnesota Living with Heart Failure Questionnaire (MLWHFQ) with the same format as in the top of this figure. For both parameters, differences were significant but similar during the study Phase I, which was attributed to a placebo effect. Clinically significant and statistically significant differences emerged between the groups during the second phase of the study that revealed treatment benefits. (c) Kaplan–Meier analysis of the proportion of patients surviving without being hospitalized during the first Phase of the study between the baseline and the end of Phase I (labeled "Phase I"). With the relatively small number of patients, the differences were not statistically significant.

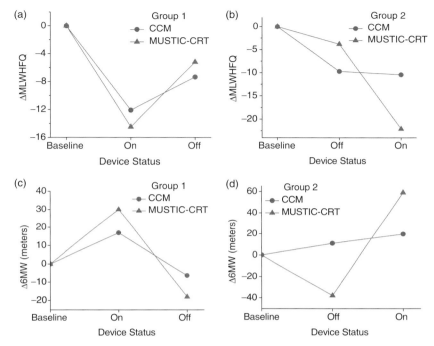

Fig. 10.5 Results of the FIX-HF-4 study of CCM are compared to those of the MUSTIC study [34] of cardiac resynchronization therapy. Although this compares results to just a single study of CRT, comparison to the MUSTIC study results is most pertinent and straightforward because the study designs (including duration of treatment) are essentially identical. Panels (a) and (c) show MLWHFQ and 6MW results from study subjects in which the respective device was "ON" for the first 3 months and "OFF" for the second three months. Panels (b) and (d) show results for same parameters from study subjects in which the respective device was "OFF" for the first 3 months and "ON" for the second 3 months. The main difference in the results of the two studies for both parameters is in Study Group 2, first study phase; subjects in the FIX-HF-4 study of CCM showed a significant placebo effect, which is absent from the MUSTIC study. (For example. (b) and (d), time point labeled "Off").

CCM signals appear to be safe and improve exercise tolerance and quality of life. Currently, a prospective, randomized, 12-month, study in 428 patients with NYHA Class III or Class IV despite optimal medical therapy is underway at 50 centers in the United States (the FIX-HF-5 Phase II study).

Combining CCM with CRT
CCM signals applied in the acute setting to heart failure patients simultaneously receiving CRT were shown to provide additive effects on LV contractility

indexed by dP/dt_{max} [7]. This is expected because of the distinctly different mechanisms of action of CRT and CCM. In view of the fact that symptoms persist in more approximately 30% of patients with prolonged QRS duration receiving CRT, it has been postulated that addition of CCM treatment may provide an option for these patients. We have previously reported on the initial experience of adding CCM treatment in a CRT nonresponder [8]. It was demonstrated that the implantation procedure is technically feasible, that the OPTIMIZER and CRT-D devices can coexist without interference and that acute hemodynamic and clinical improvements can be observed. These preliminary results have provided the impetus for initiation of a prospective study that is now planned to systematically investigate the effects of CCM in CRT nonresponders.

Summary and Conclusions

Studies of CCM signals performed in isolated muscle strips and in intact hearts of animals with CHF have suggested that these signals can enhance myocardial contractile strength. CCM signal delivery with a pacemaker-like device connected to the heart with standard pacing leads has been shown to be straight forward to implement clinically. More recent basic research has demonstrated that CCM signals effect significant changes in myocardial gene expression, improved expression and phosphorylation of key proteins involved in calcium metabolism [28,29]. These findings point toward novel mechanisms of action of this electrical form of treatment. Results obtained in patients with symptomatic heart failure with reduced ejection fraction have been encouraging and support both safety and efficacy. A large, randomized, controlled clinical trial is underway in the United States. Future studies could also evaluate whether CCM is effective in patients with wide QRS who are nonresponsive to CRT [8] or if combining CRT with CCM is more effective than CRT alone. Testing of these hypotheses would be facilitated by development of a single device that incorporates pacing, antitachycardis therapies and CCM.

Acknowledgments

The research presented in this study was supported by grants from IMPULSE Dynamics, Inc., Orangeburg, NY. Daniel Burkhoff is an employee of IMPULSE Dynamics.

References

1. Abraham WT, Fisher WG, Smith AL, et al. Cardiac resynchronization in chronic heart failure. *N Engl J Med.* 2002;346:1845–53.
2. Bristow MR, Saxon LA, Boehmer J, et al. Cardiac-resynchronization therapy with or without an implantable defibrillator in advanced chronic heart failure. *N Engl J Med.* 2004;350:2140–50.

3. Beshai JF, Grimm RA, Nagueh SF, et al. Cardiac-Resynchronization Therapy in Heart Failure with Narrow QRS Complexes. *N Engl J Med*. 2007; Dec 13;357(24): 246–71.

4. Shenkman HJ, Pampati V, Khandelwal AK, et al. Congestive heart failure and QRS duration: establishing prognosis study. *Chest*. 2002;122:528–34.

5. American Heart Association. Heart disease and stroke statistics—2005 update. Pamphlet. American Heart Association, Dallas, TX, 2005.

6. Sandhu R, Bahler RC. Prevalence of QRS prolongation in a community hospital cohort of patients with heart failure and its relation to left ventricular systolic dysfunction. *Am J Cardiol*. 2004;93:244–6.

7. Pappone C, Rosanio S, Burkhoff D, et al. Cardiac contractility modulation by electric currents applied during the refractory period in patients with heart failure secondary to ischemic or idiopathic dilated cardiomyopathy. *Am J Cardiol*. 2002;90: 1307–13.

8. Butter C, Meyhofer J, Seifert M, Neuss M, Minden HH. First use of cardiac contractility modulation (CCM) in a patient failing CRT therapy: Clinical and technical aspects of combined therapies. *Eur J Heart Fail*. 2007;9:955–8.

9. Lawo T, Borggrefe M, Butter C, et al. Electrical signals applied during the absolute refractory period: an investigational treatment for advanced heart failure in patients with normal QRS duration. *J Am Coll Cardiol*. 2005;46:2229–36.

10. Burkhoff D, Ben Haim SA. Nonexcitatory electrical signals for enhancing ventricular contractility: rationale and initial investigations of an experimental treatment for heart failure. *Am J Physiol Heart Circ Physiol*. 2005;288:H2550–H2556.

11. Gomez AM, Valdivia HH, Cheng H, et al. Defective excitation–contraction coupling in experimental heart failure. *Science*. 1997; 276:800–6.

12. Hasenfuss G, Reinecke H, Studer R, et al. Relation between myocardial function and expression of sarcoplasmic reticulum Ca2+-ATPase in failing and nonfailing human myocardium. *Circ Res*. 1994;75:434–42.

13. Frank KF, Bolck B, Brixius K, Kranias EG, Schwinger RH. Modulation of SERCA: implications for the failing human heart. *Basic Res Cardiol*. 2002;97 Suppl 1:I72–I78.

14. Mishra S, Gupta RC, Tiwari N, Sharov VG, Sabbah HN. Molecular mechanisms of reduced sarcoplasmic reticulum Ca(2+) uptake in human failing left ventricular myocardium. *J Heart Lung Transplant*. 2002;21:366–73.

15. O'rourke B, Kass DA, Tomaselli GF, et al. Mechanisms of altered excitation-contraction coupling in canine tachycardia-induced heart failure, I: experimental studies. *Circ Res*. 1999;84:562–70.

16. Haghighi K, Gregory KN, Kranias EG. Sarcoplasmic reticulum Ca-ATPase-phospholamban interactions and dilated cardiomyopathy. *Biochem Biophys Res Commun*. 2004;322:1214–22.

17. Frank K, Kranias EG. Phospholamban and cardiac contractility. *Ann Med*. 2000;32:572–8.

18. Schmidt U, Hajjar RJ, Kim CS, et al. Human heart failure: CAMP stimulation of SR Ca(2+)-ATPase activity and phosphorylation level of phospholamban. *Am J Physiol*. 1999;277:H474–H480.

19. Schwinger RH, Munch G, Bolck B, et al. Reduced Ca(2+)-sensitivity of SERCA 2a in failing human myocardium due to reduced serin-16 phospholamban phosphorylation. *J Mol Cell Cardiol*. 1999;31:479–91.

20. Studer R, Reinecke H, Bilger J, et al. Gene expression of the cardiac Na+-Ca2+ exchanger in end-stage human heart failure. *Circ Res.* 1994;75:443–53.

21. Heerdt PM, Holmes JW, Cai B, et al. Chronic unloading by left ventricular assist device reverses contractile dysfunction and alters gene expression in end-stage heart failure. *Circulation.* 2000;102:2713–19.

22. Marx SO, Reiken S, Hisamatsu Y, et al. PKA phosphorylation dissociates FKBP12.6 from the calcium release channel (ryanodine receptor): defective regulation in failing hearts. *Cell.* 2000;101:365–76.

23. Wehrens XH, Lehnart SE, Marks AR. Intracellular calcium release channels and cardiac disease. *Annu Rev Physiol.* 2004.

24. Li Y, Kranias EG, Mignery GA, Bers DM. Protein kinase A phosphorylation of the ryanodine receptor does not affect calcium sparks in mouse ventricular myocytes. *Circ Res.* 2002;90:309–16.

25. Dorn GW, Molkentin JD. Manipulating cardiac contractility in heart failure: data from mice and men. *Circulation.* 2004;109:150–8.

26. Blank M, Goodman R. Initial interactions in electromagnetic field-induced biosynthesis. *J Cell Physiol.* 2004;199:359–63.

27. Morita H, Suzuki G, Haddad W, et al. Cardiac contractility modulation with nonexcitatory electric signals improves left ventricular function in dogs with chronic heart failure. *J Card Fail.* 2003;9:69–75.

28. Imai M, Rastogi S, Gupta RC, et al. Therapy with cardiac contractility modulation electrical signals improves left ventricular function and remodeling in dogs with chronic heart failure. *J Am Coll Cardiol.* 2007;49:2120–8.

29. Butter C, Rastogi S, Minden HH, et al. Cardiac contractility modulation electrical signals improve myocardial gene expression in patients with heart failure. *J Am Coll Cardial.* 2008; 51:1784-9. 2008; in press.

30. Pappone C, Augello G, Rosanio S, et al. First human chronic experience with cardiac contractility modulation by nonexcitatory electrical currents for treating systolic heart failure: mid-term safety and efficacy results from a multicenter study. *J Cardiovasc Electrophysiol.* 2004;15:418–27.

31. Stix G, Borggrefe M, Wolpert C, et al. Chronic electrical stimulation during the absolute refractory period of the myocardium improves severe heart failure. *Eur Heart J.* 2004;25:650–5.

32. Neelagaru SB, Sanchez JE, Lau SK, et al. Nonexcitatory, cardiac contractility modulation electrical impulses: Feasibility study for advanced heart failure in patients with normal QRS duration. *Heart Rhythm.* 2006;3:1140–7.

33. Borggrefe M, Lawo T, Butter C, et al. Randomized, double blind study of nonexcitatory, cardiac contractility modulation (CCM) electrical impulses for symptomatic heart failure. *Eur Heart J.* 2008; in press.

34. Cazeau S, Leclercq C, Lavergne T, et al. Effects of multisite biventricular pacing in patients with heart failure and intraventricular conduction delay. *N Engl J Med.* 2001;344:873–80.

Chapter 11

Clinical outcomes and chronic management of device patients

Patrick W. Fisher, A. G. Kfoury, and Dale G. Renlund

Key Points

1. Economic and social impact of the increased incidence and prevalence of the chronic heart failure is alarming.
2. Outcomes for patients with chronic heart failure are improved with disease-based management systems in the outpatient setting.
3. Novel technology that incorporates remote wireless implantable sensors in current CRT-D and ICD devices allow monitoring of the outpatient with heart failure using multiple physiological parameters.
4. Remote wireless monitoring is an important milestone in the outpatient management of heart failure patients.
5. The CardioMEMS implantable pressure sensor is a novel tool that uses remote wireless monitoring of directly measured pulmonary artery pressures and hemodynamics. This is a separate modality from the current implantable sensors that measure intrathoracic impedance such as the Optiviol Requires appropriate Mark (e.g. TM or (R)) monitoring system from Medtronic Requires appropriate Mark (e.g. TM or (R)).
6. Improved patient outcomes in the chronic heart failure population depend on the successful collaboration among device (CRT-D, ICD, implantable direct pressure sensors) companies, electrophysiologists, and heart failure specialists or other pertinent clinicians involved in managing these patients.
7. CareLink Network Requires appropriate Mark (e.g. TM or (R)) by Medtronic Requires appropriate Mark (e.g. TM or (R)) provides remote monitoring of arrhythmia and device-related management. Additionally, monitoring of

Pacing to Support the Failing Heart, 1st edition. Edited by K. Ellenbogen and A. Auricchio.
© 2008 American Heart Association, ISBN: 978-1-4051-7534-0

intrathoracic impedance, an indirect measure of right heart pressures is a key feature of this system.

8. LATITUDE Requires appropriate Mark (e.g. TM or (R)) by Boston Scientific Requires appropriate Mark (e.g. TM or (R)) incorporates arrhythmia monitoring and heart rate variability trends with the addition of patient weight, vital sign evaluation, and subjective symptom reporting via wireless transmission.

9. LATITUDE Requires appropriate Mark (e.g. TM or (R)) disperses incoming patient-initiated data alerts to the appropriate clinician. Heart failure-related data useful in clinical management is directed toward the Health Following Physician, whereas all device, and most arrhythmia data alerts are sent directly to the Device Implant Managing Physician.

10. CareLink Network Requires appropriate Mark (e.g. TM or (R)) sends remote received patient data to the electrophysiologist, thus making the applicability in the outpatient management of the heart failure patient limited.

Introduction

Heart failure afflicts more than 5 million Americans, and 500,000 more are diagnosed each year. In fact, heart failure is responsible for 12–15 million office visits and 6.5 million hospital days each year [1,2]. During the last ten years, the annual number of hospitalizations has increased from approximately 550,000 to nearly 900,000 more than one million in 2005, an increase of 171%. Moreover, hospitalization rates for heart failure as a primary or secondary diagnosis rose from 1.7 to 2.6 million [3]. In the United States, the total inpatient and outpatient costs for heart failure in 1991 were approximately $38.1 billion, which was approximately 5.4% of the healthcare budget that year [1]. About $500 million annually is spent on drugs for the treatment of heart failure [2,3]. Accordingly, the increased incidence and prevalence of heart failure remains primarily a disease of the elderly resulting mostly from the improved medical therapy in the treatment of both ischemic and nonischemic dilated cardiomyopathies [4]. Approximately 10 in 1000 Americans older than 65 years have heart failure [3], and approximately 80% of patients hospitalized with heart failure are more than 65 years old [1]. Heart failure is the most common Medicare diagnosis-related group, and more Medicare dollars are spent for the diagnosis and treatment of heart failure than for any other diagnosis [6]. For example, the readmission rates for heart failure are high, approaching 50% at 6 months. With an estimated 700,000 Medicare recipients discharged annually with heart failure coupled with an average cost of $7,000 per readmission, the economic burden is astounding [7]. Indeed, heart failure currently costs US taxpayers approximately $50 billion per year [1,3].

A comprehensive and systematic review of randomized trials demonstrated that the benefits and the cost-effectiveness of heart failure programs compare favorably with established drug treatments for heart failure. McAlister et al. [8,9] found that follow-up monitoring by specially trained staff and/or heart failure clinics are associated with a 27% reduction in heart failure hospitalization rates (NNT = 11), a 43% reduction in total number of heart failure hospitalizations, a 25% reduction in all-cause mortality (NNT = 17), and a 20% reduction in all-cause hospitalizations (NNT = 10). In contrast, the use of angiotensin converting enzyme-inhibitors reduced mortality by 20% (NNT = 19) and reduced heart failure hospitalization rates by 33% (NNT = 16) in similar patient populations.

Moreover, several studies have demonstrated that heart failure patients who are managed by a highly qualified multidisciplinary heart failure team experience fewer hospital readmissions and a smaller economic burden [10]. Coordinating both inpatient and outpatient care with an emphasis on intensive discharge planning as well as patient education significantly reduces costs and readmission rates for heart failure, in addition to improving patient outcomes [8]. Empowering the patient in the care of his or her disease process through intensive patient education and multidisciplinary support likewise improves patient outcomes [8–10]. Furthermore, much of the success in the treatment of heart failure patients can be attributed directly to better patient and family education and heart failure team support, resulting in improved compliance with diet, exercise, medications, and risk factor modification [8]. In contrast, inadequate patient education, support, and follow-up care have been clearly linked as major contributing factors to increased rates of heart failure exacerbation and hospital readmissions. Inadequate education and support lead to poor compliance with diet and daily weight monitoring, patients' lack of insight into their complex medical regimen, and the inability to identify early signs and symptoms of worsening heart failure [9–12].

In the past decade, there have been significant advances in heart failure disease management. One example of a therapy that has made a profound impact on the treatment of patients with advanced heart failure includes implantable devices. In fact, device therapy has emerged as an important modality of therapy for patients with refractory chronic heart failure and severe left ventricular dysfunction. Based on current guidelines and recommendations from the AHA/ACC on devices and heart failure, an expected rise in the number of patients implanted is anticipated [1]. Consequently, technologic advances extending beyond current device-based therapy (e.g. chronic resynchronization therapy (CRT or CRT-D) and implantable cardiac defibrillators (ICD) hold promise for future success in outpatient management.

Remote monitoring

Integration of novel sensor technology coupled with current CRT-D and ICD devices offer improved diagnostic data collection via intrinsic monitoring of a variety of physiologic variables over time (Table 11.1). For example, the opportunity to remotely monitor intrathoracic impedance or other indirect measurements of fluid status in the outpatient population with heart failure is encouraging. Accordingly, device-based monitoring has the potential to improve patient

Table 11.1 Parameters measured by device and Disease Management Programs for Heart Failure

	Mechanism of Reporting	Recommended by Guidelines?	Outcomes Effect Supported by Conclusive Evidence Base?	Ease of Implementation
Daily weights	Telephone (Patient initiated)	Yes	Yes	Easy
Signs/Symptoms of worsening heart failure	Telephone (Patient initiated)	Yes	Yes	Easy
Daily weight & heart failure symptoms	Electronically	Yes	Yes	Moderately difficult
Physiologic parameters (e.g. heart rate variability, activity level, night time heart rate trends)	Yes	No	No	Moderately
Surrogates for excess lung water, (i.e. intrathoracic impedance)	Yes	No	No	Moderately
Hemodynamic pressures via implanted pressure monitors with radiofrequency transmission of the data	Implanted pressure monitors with radio frequency wireless data transmission	No	+/–	Easy

management by providing early warning of imminent decompensated heart failure, prevent recurrent hospitalization for acute decompensation, and ultimately improve patient quality of life. To integrate such diagnostic information into routine clinical practice, the remote monitoring technology and system must be implemented appropriately. This requires a close collaboration between heart failure and electrophysiology subspecialties and improved coordination and efficiency in heart failure outpatient care.

The concept of remote monitoring in patients with resynchronization devices is the next step in bridging technology with actual clinical care of the heart failure patient. The ability to remotely track specific physiological parameters in heart failure patients holds promise for improving patient outcomes and preventing recurrent hospitalizations for acute decompensation, ultimately improving patient quality of life.

Use of diagnostic capabilities inherent in implantable devices (e.g. CRT-D and ICD) coupled with the integration of wireless and remote monitoring capabilities will potentially allow expeditious data transmission from patient to provider, thus adding an additional element to the present disease management systems.

Advanced sensors in device therapy for heart failure

Sensors that measure intrathoracic impedance or direct right heart pressures using remote monitoring technology are exciting. How successful the incorporation and implementation of these sensors and data derived from interrogation into clinical practice is unknown. However, recent focus and effort in implementing novel monitoring systems linked to implantable device therapy is encouraging.

Thoracic impedance monitoring

Thoracic bio-impedance monitoring is not a new concept. In fact, the first studies, albeit small and mostly in large animal models were first performed in the 1960s [13]. Initial studies demonstrated the utility and potential of intrathoracic impedance monitoring in the determination of fluid status. Early research involved external impedance monitoring systems that were neither predictable nor reliably accurate, given the variability introduced by external measurement [14]. Today, the mechanism for measuring intrathoracic impedance assumes that the electrical impedance detected between the right ventricular lead and the pacemaker can is reflective of the true volume or fluid status in the right heart and pulmonary artery (Figures 11.1 and 11.2). Consequently, a drop in intrathoracic impedance is indicative of increased volume status suggesting the presence of progressive subclinical heart failure (Figure 11.2) [15].

The Mid–Heft trial [16] was initiated with the aim of determining feasibility of intrathoracic volume monitoring in a relatively small sample size of heart failure patients. Results, from this small-scale study, showed an inverse relationship between pulmonary capillary wedge pressure and intrathoracic impedance. In addition, a drop in impedance was detected as early as 18 days prior to hospitalization for acute decompensation. On average, signs of progressive heart failure were clinically evident 15 days prior to hospitalization for acute decomposition [16].

A mathematically derived algorithm for fluid determination via intrathoracic impedance values detected subsequent decompensated heart failure events with a sensitivity of 77%. However, the modest sensitivity to increased volume

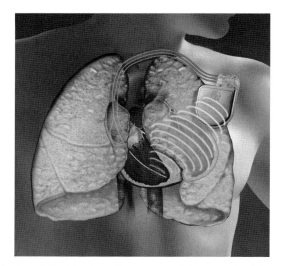

Fig. 11.1 Illustration of electrical impedance detected between the right ventricular lead and the pacemaker in determination of volume status.

status in these patients was accompanied by a false positive rate of 1.5 episodes per patient per year. Preliminary studies have shown that each crossing of the intrathoracic impedance across a threshold alert value was associated with a 51% of heart failure hospitalization and a 47% chance of an increased risk of a clinically relevant heart failure event.

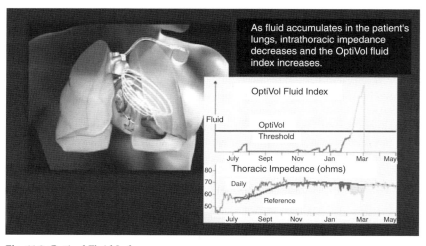

Fig. 11.2 Optivol Fluid Index.

Direct right heart pressure measurement and remote monitoring

More recently, the Chronicle implantable hemodynamic monitor was evaluated in a controlled clinical trial (COMPASS-HF) with 274 enrolled patients [17]. Although the COMPASS-HF study results tout a 22% overall reduction in hospitalizations for heart failure exacerbation, this reduction was not statistically significant and therefore necessitates careful interpretation. One interpretation of this study is that the "hyper" management of the control group made it exceedingly difficult to demonstrate a benefit from invasive hemodynamic monitoring. This was reflected by a frequency of heart failure related events (e.g. hospitalizations, emergency room visits, or urgent clinic visits) of less than 1 in 6 months in patients with NYHA Class III or Class IV heart failure.

Cardiomems implantable hemodynamic sensor

Currently under clinical investigation in the United States, the CardioMEMS radio frequency-based wireless pressure sensor is another novel remote wireless modality for outpatient monitoring of chronic heart failure patients. Recently, in a small-scale study of 12 patients with heart failure (NYHA Class II–IV), the CardioMEMS sensor system demonstrated the accuracy and feasibility in measuring continuous pulmonary artery pressures in the outpatient setting [18,19]. Although controversy exists in the utility and applicability in continuous invasive hemodynamic monitoring in patients hospitalized with acute decompensated heart failure using a PA-catheter [20], the ability to monitor the hemodynamic status in outpatients is propitious. The CardioMEMS sensor is a relatively small radiofrequency sensor that is technically easy to implant. The procedure involves a right heart cardiac catheterization using a catheter-based delivery system with Swan–Ganz catheter guidance (Figure 11.3a). The preferable position of sensor deployment is the distal posterior branch of the left pulmonary artery using the Swan-inflated balloon for optimal determination of vessel diameter (Figure 11.3b). Because it directly and accurately measures pulmonary artery pressures, the CardioMEMS implantable sensor device may provide an alternative to more frequent outpatient hemodynamic monitoring using invasive right heart cardiac catheterization, especially in those patients with secondary pulmonary hypertension or who are awaiting orthotopic heart transplantation.

Moreover, this unique remote monitoring sensor allows the alert threshold to be set individually, decreasing unnecessary false positives. It can therefore be incorporated into the busy outpatient clinical heart failure setting with relative ease and efficiency. Future results from ongoing multicenter clinical trials in the United States should elucidate the clinical applicability of this monitoring system.

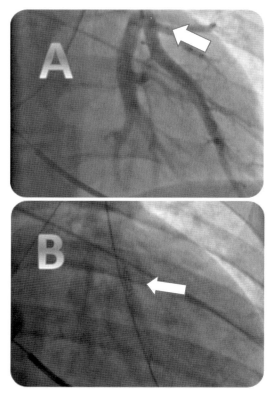

Fig. 11.3 A. Left pulmonary artery angiography demonstrating the tip of a Swan-Ganz catheter to determine appropriate site for deployment of sensor (arrow). B. Sensor deployment (arrow) in the distal posterior branch of the left pulmonary artery prior to removal of guide wire.

HeartPOD implantable hemodynamic sensor

Similar to the CardioMEMS sensor, the HeartPOD direct left atrial pressure (LAP) implantable sensor is currently under clinical investigation. The Heart-POD sensor is another novel implantable monitoring modality for optimizing the outpatient care of chronic heart failure patients. In contrast to the CardioMEMS implantable sensor, the HeartPOD is a direct left atrial pressure (LAP) sensor that transmits LAP measurements via RF wireless transmission to a patient monitor similar in shape and size to a Palm Pilot. In contrast to the CardioMEMS sensor, the HeartPOD sensor has the ability to accurately measure and transmit direct LAP measurements to the monitoring physician, thus allowing the opportunity for early medical intervention prior to the onset of symptomatic pulmonary edema and acute decompenated heart failure. The successful implantation of the HeartPOD device in eight patients with heart failure (NYHA Class II–III) was recently reported in *Circulation*. Jay Ritzema, Iain C. Melton, A. Mark Richards, Ian G. Crozier, Chris Frampton, Robert N. Doughty, James Whiting, Saibal Kar, Neal Eigler, Henry Krum, William T. Abraham, and Richard W. Troughton Direct Left Atrial Pressure Monitoring in Ambulatory Heart Failure Patients: Initial Experience With a New Permanent Implantable Device Circulation, December 18/25, 2007;116:2952–2959. Implantation was performed and sensor accuracy was evaluated in a prospective, nonrandomized, open-labeled, feasibility clinical trial named, HemOdynaMically guidEd hOme Self-Therapy in Severe heart failure patientS (HOMEOSTASIS I). The HeartPOD LAP sensor comprises a monitoring lead with a sensor diaphragm on the distal tip coupled to a relatively small antenna coil. The procedure requires right femoral venous access below the inguinal ligament and an additional access site 1 cm above the inguinal ligament guided via a wire from the distal sheath. The sensor is implanted via a closed right femoral (via the suprainguinal ligament venous sheath) transseptal puncture with final sensor deployment on the left side of the atrial septum. After successful deployment of the distal sensor lead tip, the proximal end of the sensor lead is then connected to an antenna coil and placed in a small subcutaneous pocket above the right rectus abdominus sheath. Calibration of the HeartPOD sensor was performed using a Swan–Ganz PA catheter at time of implant and at 12 weeks for determination of sensor accuracy and device stability. Compared with the CardioMEMS implantable sensor, the HeartPOD requires a physician with experience, knowledge, and training in transeptal atrial puncture. Despite the differences in approach for implantation, no serious adverse events occurred in the HOMEOSTASIS I trial. The relative absence of adverse events in this small patient population is in concert with events reported with transseptal puncture during atrial fibrillation ablations and atrial septal closure device implantation [35].

Ongoing and future clinical investigations will elucidate any long-term complications from device implantation as well as assess overall accuracy. Furthermore, the HeartPOD sensor system is under evaluation for possible incorporation into CRT-D devices, which hold promise for reducing additional risks inherent in having a lower abdominal subcutaneous pocket with a chronic lead in the inferior vena cava, iliac, and femoral veins.

Peak Endocardial Acceleration

The Peak Endocardial Acceleration (PEA) sensor device analyzes the amplitude of the first heart sound (S1) using a more sophisticated accelerometer that can be attached to current pacemakers. Interestingly, the changes in PEA are reported to correlate with left ventricular Dp/dt in humans, a measure of left ventricular contractility [21]. Ongoing clinical trials as well as future large-scale clinical trials are warranted to determine the effectiveness and utility of this type of sensor in patients with chronic heart failure.

Remote monitoring integrated systems

Technological advances extending beyond device-based therapy (e.g. chronic resynchronization therapy and internal automated defibrillators) are emerging. For example, incorporation and integration of device-based therapies into out-patient management programs is now the focus of intense research. Specifically, diagnostic capabilities inherent in these implantable devices with the integration of wireless and remote monitoring capabilities provide for seamless and expeditious data transmission from patient to provider, adding an additional and potentially useful adjunct to the present outpatient heart failure management programs.

Biotronik home monitoring system

The Biotroniks Home Monitoring System (Figure 11.4) utilizes a series of radio frequency (RF) communication links that are incorporated into implantable pacemakers, ICDs, and CRT devices. Data automatically transmits critical data related to the patient's cardiac condition and the status of their device remotely to his or her physician.

The wireless system requires no active patient involvement and is completely mobile. This means that patients are free to maintain their normal routines,

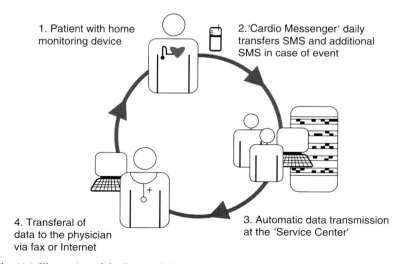

1. Patient with home monitoring device

2. 'Cardio Messenger' daily transfers SMS and additional SMS in case of event

4. Transferal of data to the physician via fax or Internet

3. Automatic data transmission at the 'Service Center'

Fig. 11.4 Illustration of the Biotronik Home Monitoring System.

whether they are home or away on vacation, while their implant maintains regular communication with the physician. This contrasts with other technologies touted as "remote monitoring," where patient intervention is necessary for coordinating appropriate transmission of data.

With the Biotronik system, the physician has the ability to set the device for home monitoring to "ON" prior to hospital discharge. In addition, the physician can program the device or sensor that will trigger thresholds upon which he or she would like to be alerted. If the patient's condition reaches one of these threshold points, a message is sent to the physician notifying them of such an occurrence. For example, if a patient has been in Atrial Fibrillation (AF) for 12 hours, the physician will be automatically notified. Furthermore, access to patient data transmissions is readily available via a secure Web-based server (Figure 11.5). The ability to set alert thresholds is a feature that is, for the most part, universal with current remote monitoring systems. [33,34]

Parameters measured with biotronik devices:

1 Battery status
2 Pace and shock lead impedance
3 Ventricular capture thresholds
4 Ventricular episode detection and therapy
5 A and V pacing percentages
6 Atrial burden statistics
7 Ventricular extra systoles (VES)

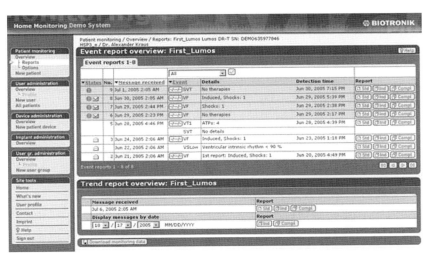

Fig. 11.5 Example of the Biotronik Web-based Server window demonstrating transmitted patient data for review, A. Highlights of the major advantages in the Biotronik Home Monitoring Diagnostics Online system, B.

...and patient status diagnostics for early intervention.

Seven Heart Failure Monitor™ Online diagnostics, transmitted on a daily basis, allow for proactive management of the heart failure status of your patients.

Heart Failure Monitor™ Online
• Clinical indicators for heart failure management
  – Heart Rate Variability
  – Mean Heart Rate
  – Mean Heart Rate at Rest
  – Percent CRT Pacing
  – Patient Activity
  – Atrial Arrhythmias
  – Ventricular Ectopy
• Automatic daily trending

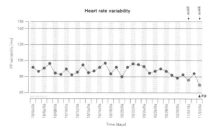

Heart Failure Monitor™ Online provides clinically significant diagnostics and alerts to assist you in achieving optimal outcomes.

Heart Failure Monitor™ Online
Event Triggers
  – Mean Heart Rate
  – Mean Heart Rate at Rest
  – Percent CRT Pacing
  – Atrial Burden
  – Ventricular Ectopy

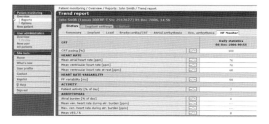

 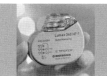 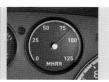

Fig. 11.5 (continued)

8 Heart rate variability
9 Daily activity level
10 Mean heart rate/heart rate-rest (24 hrs)

CARELINK™ Network by Medtronic

The CareLink Network by Medtronic is an Internet-based system, which provides complete device analysis and interrogation. CareLink provides an integrated data delivery and tracking system with the aim of improving heart failure disease management via remote monitoring of patient's symptoms and physiological parameters wirelessly. This monitoring of devices has the potential to better target the expanding heart failure population, the group of patients who are the true end-users of Medtronic's biventricular and combined CRT-D devices. This Network tracks and reports key physiological parameters, such as heart rate variability, patient activity, and night heart rate trends, coupled with intrathoracic impedance monitoring. For example, the INSYNC III® device monitors all of these, in addition to lead impedance, rhythm trends, and therapy delivered, all of which have important implications in identifying patients with a sudden decline in function. Unfortunately, unlike the Boston Scientific Latitude system discussed below, the Web-based data is accessible only to the electrophysiologist. The Network's applicability, efficiency, and both indirect and direct resource requirements have not yet been fully evaluated in the heart failure setting [22].

Latitude™ by Boston Scientific

Latitude™ is the remote monitoring system developed by Boston Scientific as an adjunctive diagnostic management program for all patients (Figure 11.6) who have their ICD or CRT-D devices (Figure 11.7). Specifically, the Latitude patient management system is intended to provide remote access or communication with compatible Guidant pulse generators via data transfer to a central database (Figure 11.8). Similar to the CareLink Network, Latitude uses a patient initiated

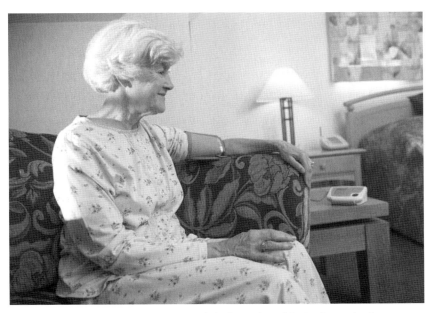

Fig. 11.6 A woman illustrating the use of the home-based Latitude monitoring system. (See color plate section).

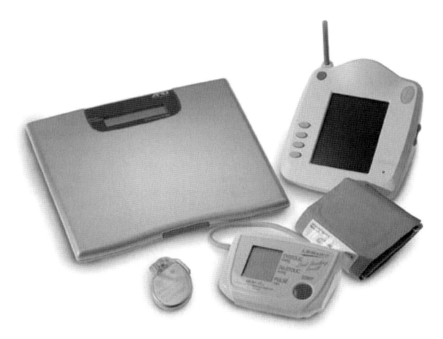

Fig. 11.7 The Latitude remote monitoring equipment for home-based transmission. Monitoring equipment includes a blood pressure cuff, weight scale, and a main unit that allows wireless transmission to a central Web-based server.

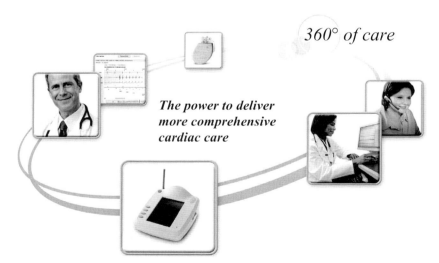

360° of care

The power to deliver more comprehensive cardiac care

Fig. 11.8 Illustration of the Latitude system and the relationship of the key aspects involved in successful data transmission and evaluation.

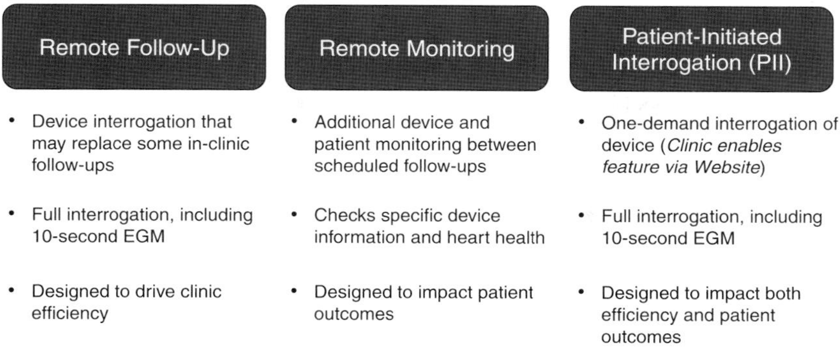

Remote Follow-Up	Remote Monitoring	Patient-Initiated Interrogation (PII)
• Device interrogation that may replace some in-clinic follow-ups	• Additional device and patient monitoring between scheduled follow-ups	• One-demand interrogation of device (*Clinic enables feature via Website*)
• Full interrogation, including 10-second EGM	• Checks specific device information and heart health	• Full interrogation, including 10-second EGM
• Designed to drive clinic efficiency	• Designed to impact patient outcomes	• Designed to impact both efficiency and patient outcomes

Fig. 11.9 Key aspects of the Latitude wireless remote monitoring system in outpatient management.

device interrogation with wireless remote monitoring via a web-based secure server (Table 11.2, Figure 11.9). In contrast to CareLink, LATITUDE divides incoming data transmissions into two categories: notifications appropriate for the "Device Managing Physician" or electrophysiologist and those directed to the "Health Following Physician" or heart failure specialist (Figure 11.10). Although both managing physicians have access to all transmitted data via a web-based central server, each physician receives only the alerts that are specific and clinically relevant to his or her role (Figure 11.9). For example, intrinsic device management issues including all arrhythmia alerts, battery status, and

Table 11.2 Comparison of CareLink™ & Latitude® remote monitoring systems

	CareLink™	Latitude®
Remote wireless Data Transmission?	YES	YES
Accessible to "Device Physician" or electrophysiologist?	DEVICE PHYSICIAN[†]	YES
Intrathoracic Impedance Monitoring?	YES	NO
Arrhythmia Alert Notification?	YES	YES
Electronic Vital Sign Transmission?	NO	YES[‡]

[†] not readily accessible to the heart failure physician.   [‡] Blood pressure (systemic) only.

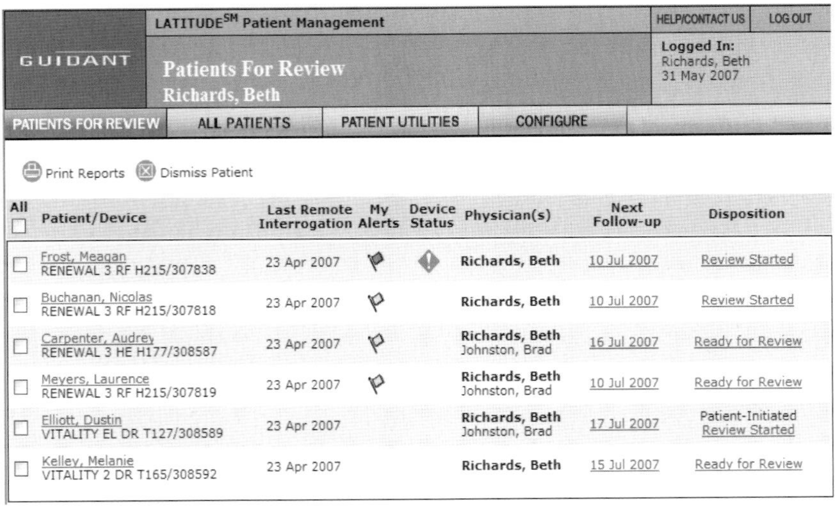

| LATITUDE^{SM} Patient Management | | | | | | HELP/CONTACT US | LOG OUT |

Fig. 11.10 Example of the Latitude Web-based Server window demonstrating transmitted patient data for review.

lead issues are directed to the Device Managing Physician, while weight change trends, systemic blood pressure, heart rate variability, and for patients and clinicians, cost, and required resources. Most likely, additional personnel will be necessary to monitor patient data and relay any clinical changes in medical management to the patient. In addition, another barrier to implementation must be recognized in determining clinic outpatient processes. This added hurdle directly results from the lack of interchangeable systems among device manufacturers. This is one of several challenges that will need to be overcome for successful clinical application and integration into disease management at outpatient clinics.

More recently, the ability to effectively treat and manage patients with chronic heart failure in an outpatient setting has become more of a challenge. The increased survival of patients with acute myocardial infarction, coronary artery disease, and improvements in secondary prevention likely contribute to higher acuity patients and an increasing population of patients with heart failure. Consequently, it is imperative that the medical community continues to adapt to the changing healthcare environment with the ability to remain ahead. In fact, evidence indicative of the significant outcome of mid-level care phone support systems on the risk of admissions for acute decompensated heart failure (risk differences estimated between 2% and 35%), likely a direct result of appropriate triage of patients by coordinator at the first sign of clinical decompensation, will become obsolete as the future demands increase with exhaustion of clinical resources [12–14].

To date, most trials on telemonitoring involved daily transmission of vital signs, weight, and subjective signs and symptoms to healthcare providers thus potentially leading to earlier detection and management of clinical deterioration by the patient and the managing healthcare provider [30]. Therefore, in an effort to remain efficient and effective in successfully managing the heart failure population now and in the future, remote monitoring in the outpatient setting is a viable option and is advantageous for improving on current management strategies for chronic heart failure patients [23]. The successful implementation of a disease management program in heart failure that incorporates device-based remote monitoring capabilities requires dedication and commitment to the patients from the device manufacturers. More specifically, a lack of uniformity and cross platform utility in the present available programs is discouraging.

In fact, any future success in implementing advanced technology will depend on the ability of device manufacturers to successfully collaborate with the goal of creating a single and universal remote monitoring system that is transparent no matter what device a patient has. Furthermore, validation, via further clinical trials, of physiological parameters, such as heart rate variability, heart rate, and activity trends among others, is required in order to demonstrate the clinical efficacy and evidenced-based interpretation in order to determine appropriate applicability in the clinical setting and patient outcomes.

Despite the potential for the practical application of device-based heart failure monitoring in the outpatient setting, many issues remain that must be resolved for these novel ideas to come to fruition. Therefore, the addition of wireless and remote monitoring technology using device based management programs for chronic heart failure will necessitate scientific evidence demonstrating efficiency, cost effectiveness, and improvement on current phone support systems.

Economic and outcome measures

Although few studies have examined economic outcomes, studies on telephone support suggest that the interventions are cost effective [25,26]. Moreover, with the increasing demand on accountability of healthcare systems and their providers, accurate and risk-adjusted attributes of statistical models used for publicly reported outcomes is necessary. Furthermore, an accurate assessment of quality of care and the promotion of reporting of healthcare provider outcomes to the public will ensure the validity of rankings used by various organizations in defining institutional outcomes and further maximize reimbursement [27–29].

Remote monitoring offers a potentially feasible option for better resource utilization and management of the growing population of patients with chronic heart failure. However, economic burden and examination of resource utilization in addition to other barriers to successful implementation is yet to be defined.

Outpatient management decisions in nonresponders

Approximately 30% of patients with heart failure who receive CRT devices are classified as "nonresponders". Specifically, nonresponders are patients who fail to demonstrate an objective or subjective improvement usually within a 6-month, post implant period [31]. Different studies evaluating CRT-D devices report varying criteria for who is classified as a responder versus a nonresponder. For example, nonresponders according to Diaz-Infante et al. [35] are those patients who do not show a benefit of >10% in 6-minute walk distance, death from heart failure, or cardiac transplantation in a 6-month follow-up period after initial CRT implantation. On the other hand, Lellouche et al. [32] classify nonresponders as patients who survived 6 months after implantation, no hospitalization for heart failure decompensation, and improvement of one or more grades in the NYHA classification.

In general, once a patient is evaluated by their physician or heart failure specialist and is deemed an appropriate candidate for CRT-D therapy, the patient is promptly referred to electrophysiology specialists for further evaluation, assessment, and device implantation. Once a patient receives a CRT device, regular and routine follow-up in the outpatient heart failure clinic for ongoing disease management continues.

Most patients that receive CRT-D for advanced heart failure management will attain some benefit in cardiac structure and function and improved quality of life. Unfortunately, the natural course of end-stage heart failure is often unpredictable and depends on a multitude of variables all of which play a vital role in determining an individual's appropriateness for advanced heart failure therapy. Common procedures available at most tertiary centers include advanced imaging modalities, advanced cardiac electrophysiology procedures, such as ablation for atrial and ventricular arrhythmias, percutaneous coronary and valvular interventional procedures, coronary artery bypass graft surgery, and left ventricular reconstruction surgery. In addition, centers with expertise and experience in advanced heart failure management can provide patients with aggressive medical management including, but not limited to, hemodynamically tailored-therapy using single or multiple inotropic, lusitropic, and diuretic intravenous agents. The overall goal in this approach is establishing euvolemia with successful conversion from intravenous therapy to optimal oral medications in order to maintain adequate cardiac output and end-organ perfusion.

Many patients at this stage are inotropic dependent and should be considered for cardiac transplantation. Patients who are referred early in their disease process before the onset of end-organ damage, such as hepatic failure, chronic renal failure with baseline creatinine usually above 2.0, mg/dl, right heart dysfunction, and/or failure with irreversible pulmonary hypertension, often do well overall. With the advancement of mechanical circulatory support (MCS), many options are available that can "buy time" and essentially save lives for many patients with end-stage cardiomyopathy who fail conventional therapy, including CRT-D. Today, with the advancement of MCS, patients who are acutely decompensating have a much better chance of survival to transplant with a left ventricular assist device or LVAD, Total Artificial Heart (TAH-t), right ventricular assist device or RVAD, cardiopulmonary support, or one of the percutaneous ventricular assist devices such as the tandem heart or PVAD. In those patients who do not meet criteria for cardiac transplantation, MCS remains a viable option as destination therapy.

Despite the positive and dramatic impact of CRT-D treatment in the heart failure patient population, overall disease progression often necessitates a multidisciplinary team approach to patient care. Moreover, the incorporation of hospice specialists as part of the multidisciplinary heart failure team continues to play an important and significant role in end-of-life decisions and patient management. Although advances in the past decade in the treatment of the advanced heart failure patient has positively impacted patient care and overall quality of life, advanced heart failure therapies are often necessary even in those patients deemed to be "responders."

References

1. Hunt SA, Abraham WT, Chin MH, et al. ACC/AHA 2005 guideline update for the diagnosis and management of chronic heart failure in the adult: a report of the American College of Cardiology/American Heart Association Task Force on Practice Guidelines (Committee to Update the 2001 Guidelines for the Evaluation and Management of Heart Failure). *J Am Coll Cardiol*. 2005;46:1116–43.
2. O'Connell JB, Bristow M. Economic impact of heart failure in the United States: time for a different approach. *J Heart Lung Transplant*. 1993;13:S107–S112.
3. Heart Disease and Stroke Statistics-2008 Update: A Report From the American Heart Association Statistics Committee and Stroke Statistics Subcommittee. Wayne Rosamond, Katherine Flegal, Karen Furie, Alan Go, Kurt Greenlund, Nancy Haase, Susan M. Hailpern, Michael Ho, Virginia Howard, Bret Kissela, Steven Kittner, Donald Lloyd-Jones, Mary McDermott, James Meigs, Claudia Moy, Graham Nichol, Christopher O'Donnell, Veronique Roger, Paul Sorlie, Julia Steinberger, Thomas Thom, Matt Wilson, Yuling Hong for the American Heart Association Statistics Committee and Stroke Statistics Subcommittee.
4. Kannel WB, Belanger AJ. Epidemiology of heart failure. *Am Heart J*. 1991;121:951–7.
5. Kannel WB. Epidemiology and prevention of cardiac failure: Framingham Study insights. *Eur Heart J*. 1987;8 Suppl F:23–26.
6. Massie BM, Shah NB. Evolving trends in the epidemiologic factors of heart failure: rationale for preventive strategies and comprehensive disease management. *Am Heart J*. 1997;133:703–12.

7. Anderson C, Deepak BV, Amoateng-Adjepong Y, Zarich S. Benefits of comprehensive inpatient education and discharge planning combined with outpatient support in elderly patients with congestive heart failure. *Congest Heart Fail.* 2005;6: 315–21.

8. Phillips CO, Wright SM, Kern DE, Singa RM, Shepperd S, Rubin HR. Comprehensive discharge planning with postdischarge support for older patients with congestive heart failure: a meta-analysis. *JAMA.* 2004; Mar 17;291(11):1358–67. Erratum in: *JAMA.* 2004; Sep 1;292(9):1022.

9. Krumholz HM, Amatruda J, Smith GL, Mattera JA, Roumanis SA, Radford MJ, Crombie P, Vaccarino V. Randomized trial of an education and support intervention to prevent readmission of patients with heart failure. *JACC.* 2002:83–9.

10. *Health Care Financing Administration,* Department of Statistics, 1997.

11. Wolinsky FD, Smith DM, Stump TE, Overhage JM, Lubitz RM. The sequelae of hospitalization for congestive heart failure among older adults. *J Am Geriatr Soc.* 1997; May;45(5):558–63.

12. Fisher ES, Wennberg JE, Stukel TA, Sharp SM. Hospital readmission rates for cohorts of Medicare beneficiaries in Boston and New Haven. *N Engl J Med.* 1994; Oct 13;331(15):989–95.

13. Luepker RV, Michael JR, Warbasse JR. Transthoracic electrical impedance; quantitative evaluation of a non-invasive measure of thoracic fluid volume. *Am Heart J.* 1973; Jan;85(1):83–93.

14. Van de Water JM, Mount BE, Barela JR, Schuster R, Leacock FS. Monitoring the chest with impedance. *Chest.* 1973; Nov;64(5):597–603.

15. Wang L. Fundamentals of intrathoracic impedance monitoring in heart failure. *Am J Cardiol.* 2007; May 21;99(10A):3G–10G.

16. Yu CM, Wang L, Chau E, Chan RH, Kong SL, Tang MO, et al. Intrathoracic impedance monitoring in patients with heart failure: correlation with fluid status and feasibility of early warning preceding hospitalization. *Circulation.* 2005; Aug 9;112(6):841–8.

17. Steinhaus D, Reynolds DW, Gadler F, Kay GN, Hess MF, Bennett T. Implant experience with an implantable hemodynamic monitor for the management of symptomatic heart failure. *Pacing Clin Electrophysiol.* 2005; Aug;28(8):747–53.

18. Rajagopal V, Yadav JS. Management of carotid artery disease in the high-risk patient with emphasis on the SAPPHIRE study. *Curr Cardiol Rep.* 2007; Mar;9(1):20–4.

19. Verdejo HE, Castro PF, Concepcion R, Ferrada MA, Alfaro MA, Alcaino ME, et al. Comparison of a radiofrequency-based wireless pressure sensor to Swan–Ganz catheter and echocardiography for ambulatory assessment of pulmonary artery pressure in heart failure. *J Am Coll Cardiol.* 2007; Dec 18;50(25):2375–82.

20. Binanay C, Califf RM, Hasselblad V, O'Connor CM, Shah MR, Sopko G, et al. Evaluation study of congestive heart failure and pulmonary artery catheterization effectiveness: the ESCAPE trial. *JAMA.* 2005; Oct 5;294(13):1625–33.

21. Rickards AF, Bombardini T, Corbucci G, Plicchi G. An implantable intracardiac accelerometer for monitoring myocardial contractility. The Multicenter PEA Study Group. *Pacing Clin Electrophysiol.* 1996; Dec;19(12 Pt 1):2066–71.

22. Schoenfeld MH, Compton SJ, Mead RH, Weiss DN, Sherfesee L, Englund J, et al. Remote monitoring of implantable cardioverter defibrillators: a prospective analysis. *Pacing Clin Electrophysiol.* 2004; Jun;27(6 Pt 1):757–63.

23. Saxon LA, Boehmer JP, Neuman S, Mullin CM. Remote Active Monitoring in Patients with Heart Failure (RAPID-RF): design and rationale. *J Card Fail*. 2007; May;13(4):241–6.

24. Ara S. A literature review of cardiovascular disease management programs in managed care populations. *J Manag Care Pharm*. 2004;10(4):326–44.

25. Riegel B, Naylor M, Stewart S, McMurray JJ, Rich MW. Interventions to prevent readmission for congestive heart failure. *JAMA*. 2004; Jun; 16;291(23):2816; author reply 2816–7.

26. Rich MW. Heart failure in the elderly: strategies to optimize outpatient control and reduce hospitalizations. *Am J Geriatr Cardiol*. 2003; Jan–Feb;12(1):19–24.

27. Krumholz HM, Brindis RG, Brush JE, Cohen DJ, Epstein AJ, Furie K, Howard G, Peterson ED, Rathore SS, Smith SC Jr, Spertus JA, Wang Y, Normand SL; American Heart Association; Quality of Care and Outcomes Research Interdisciplinary Writing Group; Council on Epidemiology and Prevention; Stroke Council; American College of Cardiology Foundation. Standards for statistical models used for public reporting of health outcomes: an American Heart Association Scientific Statement from the Quality of Care and Outcomes Research Interdisciplinary Writing Group: cosponsored by the Council on Epidemiology and Prevention and the Stroke Council. Endorsed by the American College of Cardiology Foundation. *Circulation*. 2006; Jan 24;113(3): 456-62.

28. Radford MJ, Arnold JM, Bennett SJ, Cinquegrani MP, Cleland JG, Havranek EP, et al. ACC/AHA key data elements and definitions for measuring the clinical management and outcomes of patients with chronic heart failure: a report of the American College of Cardiology/American Heart Association Task Force on Clinical Data Standards (Writing Committee to Develop Heart Failure Clinical Data Standards): developed in collaboration with the American College of Chest Physicians and the International Society for Heart and Lung Transplantation: endorsed by the Heart Failure Society of America. *Circulation*. 2005 Sep 20;112(12):1888-916.

29. Strickberger SA, Conti J, Daoud EG, Havranek E, Mehra MR, Pina IL, et al. Patient selection for cardiac resynchronization therapy: from the Council on Clinical Cardiology Subcommittee on Electrocardiography and Arrhythmias and the Quality of Care and Outcomes Research Interdisciplinary Working Group, in collaboration with the Heart Rhythm Society. *Circulation*. 2005; Apr 26;111(16):2146-50.

30. Clark RA, Inglis SC, McAlister FA, Cleland JG, Stewart S. Telemonitoring or structured telephone support programmes for patients with chronic heart failure: systematic review and meta-analysis. *BMJ*. 2007;334(7600):942.

31. Bax JJ, Abraham T, Barold SS, Breithardt OA, Fung JW, Garrigue S, Gorcsan J, 3rd, Hayes DL, Kass DA, Knuuti J, Leclercq C, Linde C, Mark DB, Monaghan MJ, Nihoyannopoulos P, Schalij MJ, Stellbrink C, Yu CM. Cardiac resynchronization therapy: Part 2–issues during and after device implantation and unresolved questions. *J Am Coll Cardiol*. 2005;46(12):2168-2182

32. Nicolas Lellouche M.D., Carlos De Diego M.D., Marmar Vaseghi M.D., Eric Buch M.D., David A. Cesario M.D., Ph.D., Aman Mahajan M.D., Ph.D., Isaac Wiener M.D., Gregg C Fonarow M.D., Noel G. Boyle M.D., Ph.D., Kalyanam Shivkumar M.D., Ph.D. (2007) Cardiac Resynchronization Therapy Response is Associated with Shorter Duration of Atrial Fibrillation. *Pacing and Clinical Electrophysiology*. 30 (11), 1363–1368

33. Weretka S, Nagornova E, Bauer B, Karle C, Hardt S, Katus H, and Becker R. CP27: Initial Experience With A Home Monitoring System In Implantable Cardioverter Defibrillator Recipients. *Europace.* 7: 293.

34. Wildau H. Wireless remote monitoring for patients with atrial tachyarrhythmias. *J Electrocardiology*, 2004 October 1; (37):53-54.

35. Ernesto Díaz-Infante, Lluís Mont, Juan Leal, Ignacio García-Bolao, Ignacio Fernández-Lozano, Antonio Hernández-Madrid, Nicasio Pérez-Castellano, Marta Sitges, Ricardo Pavón-Jiménez, Joaquín Barba, Miguel A. Cavero, José L. Moya, Leopoldo Pérez-Isla, Josep Brugada, SCARS Investigators. Predictors of Lack of Response to Resynchronization Therapy. *Am J Cardiology.* 2005; June 15; 95(12):1436–40.

Chapter 12

Future directions in pacing to support the failing heart

Angelo Auricchio and Kenneth A. Ellenbogen

Key Points

1. Optimal timing of CRT implantation is an important clinical research area. Early promising results have been achieved in patients with NYHA functional class II. If confirmed by large ongoing randomized trials, a major breakthrough for device therapy in heart failure patients is expected.

2. Several multicenter prospective randomized trials including patients with traditional pacemaker indication are ongoing and will test the efficacy of CRT.

3. Reliable echocardiographic parameter(s) for studying mechanical dyssynchrony does not yet exist .

4. In the near future, magnetic resonance imaging and computerized tomography will play a key role for routinely assessing mechanical dyssynchrony, viable myocardium and coronary vein anatomy.

5. Multimodality imaging techniques for assisting in device implantation may play an increasing role for guiding LV lead placement.

6. Novel robotic-assisted implantation techniques are currently being investigated, but it is unclear is their use in routine device implantation.

7. Reliable prediction(s) of functional, volumetric, and survival outcome is still missing.

8. Definition of non-responder(s) to device therapy requires refinement.

9. Leadless pacing and endocardial pacing is just entering clinical investigation and may represent a revolutionary approach for CRT delivery.

10. Several novel sensor technologies are currently being investigated which should help in heart failure management, and prediction of both heart failure-related and non-heart failure related cardiac events.

Pacing to Support the Failing Heart, 1st edition. Edited by K. Ellenbogen and A. Auricchio.
© 2008 American Heart Association, ISBN: 978-1-4051-7534-0

Introduction

Since the clinical introduction of cardiac resynchronization therapy (CRT) in 1998, patient selection criteria have already expanded and therapy delivery has been significantly optimized. There is no doubt that understanding of the pathobiology of mechanical dyssynchrony has aided in both patient selection and therapy optimization. Moreover, our recently gained knowledge of the pathophysiology of mechanical dyssynchrony has opened up several intense areas of investigation including mode of therapy delivery, the role of different diagnostic imaging techniques, and device selection. Also novel sensor technologies for monitoring heart failure status and its evolution have been developed. In this chapter, we review some future directions in pacing to support the failing heart with particular focus to CRT.

Diagnostic Imaging

As already discussed in chapters 4 and 5, echocardiography is, at the present time, considered to be the most useful technique in clinical practice to assess cardiac dyssynchrony. However, in the light of the results of the PROSPECT [1] and RethinQ [2] trials, the most reliable echocardiographic parameter(s) for studying mechanical dyssynchrony is still a work in progress. More recently, various nonechocardiographic techniques have also been shown to provide an assessment of dyssynchrony in addition to information about myocardial viability and extent and location of scar tissue. Substantial attention has been focused on defining the size of the target region for left ventricular pacing lead implantation and assessment of cardiac venous anatomy. These techniques include nuclear imaging techniques, magnetic resonance imaging (MRI), and computed tomography (CT). With the exception only of MRI, routine use of both CT and nuclear imaging techniques may be limited by concern about the biological effects of ionizing radiation.

Nuclear imaging techniques

Nuclear imaging techniques have been used in the selection of CRT candidates and evaluation of CRT effects, and include radionuclide angiography, single photon emission computed tomography (SPECT), and position emission tomography (PET). Radionuclide angiography has been extensively used for the assessment of left and right ventricular ejection fraction, and by implementing Fourier analysis, precise quantification of inter-ventricular and intraventricular dyssynchrony with high reproducibility [3]. PET is the only imaging technique that allows quantitative assessment of myocardial blood flow and metabolism, and eventually cardiac innervation. This technique has been used in various research studies to evaluate the effect of CRT on myocardial blood flow and metabolism [4, 5], but its routine application is questionable. One major limitation is the lack of visualization of coronary sinus and coronary veins. At the present time, one may say that routine use of radionuclide angiography, PET, and SPECT is limited to those patients who are undergoing a nuclear imaging examination for other, nonpacing reasons.

Magnetic resonance imaging

The use of MRI for assessment of cardiac dyssynchrony is growing. Several novel techniques inclusive of strain-encoded MRI, harmonic phase analysis, and velocity encoded MRI's are being tested for their ability to measure mechanical dyssynchrony, with the hope that this may further enhance the patient selection process. Recent studies by Helm et al. [6] have shown the feasibility of MRI-based evaluation techniques in a dyssynchronous animal model, but more importantly have shown that cardiac dyssynchrony analysis may be more predictive of clinical response to CRT by using circumferential rather than longitudinal strain maps. This is particularly relevant when considering that most of the currently used echocardiographic dyssynchrony assessment parameters are usually collected in longitudinal view. On the other hand, recent data by Westenberg et al. [7] showed an excellent agreement between velocity-encoded MRI and Tissue doppler imaging with 95% of patients classified identically.

Similar to nuclear imaging, MRI is well-suited to the assessment of viability and scar tissue. In particular, contrast-enhanced MRI allows for the precise delineation of scar tissue. Shortly after intravenous injection of gadolinium-based contrast agents, the region with scar tissue shows increased image intensity (hyperenhanced). The major advantage of contrast-enhanced cardiac MRI over other imaging techniques is the excellent spatial resolution, making differentiation between transmural and subendocardial scar possible. The MRI approach is likely to further optimize selection of patients for CRT by excluding patients with a large scar in the target region for left ventricular lead positioning or such an extensive scar that improvement in left ventricular function is limited (Figure 12.1). Several investigators have recently pointed out that patients with a large area of scar tissue, particularly in the posterolateral region, do not respond or respond less well to CRT [8–10]. Scar burden of less than 15% seemed to be predictive of response to CRT. Notably, scar burden and scar distribution has also been an important factor predicting ventricular arrhythmias in patients with heart failure [11, 12]. Therefore, it is conceivable that the indication to undergo implantation of a CRT device (CRT-P or CRT-D) may be selected based upon scar burden, scar distribution, and myocardial viability.

Three-dimensional, whole-heart imaging of the coronary venous system is possible and enhanced by the use of an intravascular contrast agent [13]. However, there is limited data on the role of MRI in prospectively assessing the coronary sinus and venous anatomy. Recent work evaluating the coronary sinus ostium with MRI used cardiac-gated free-breathing T1-weighted spin-echo echo-planar images with sensitivity encoding, demonstrated considerable

(a)

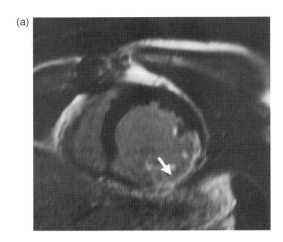

(b)

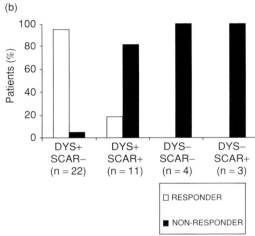

Fig. 12.1 Short-axis MRI image using contrast-enhanced imaging. An incomplete, non-transmural scar tissue is present in the inferolateral region. Percentage of responders to CRT for four different patient categories based on the presence or absece of transmural posterolateral scar tissue (SCAR+ or SCAR−) in combination with presence or absence of baseline LV dyssynchrony (DYS+/DYS−). Patients without scar and with LV dyssynchrony are most likely respond to CRT. (Adapted with permission from Bleeker et al. [8].)

individual variability depending on the cardiac substrate and ejection fraction [14]. Even though MRI images offer good resolution for the CS and its first-degree tributaries there is limited visualization of second-order and third-order tributaries. Early work has suggested that it may be useful to assess the angulations and take–off of the main branches.

One major limitation of all MRI-based studies is that they have included a relatively small number of patients with standard ECG criteria for CRT; thus, validation in larger patient cohorts and assessment in the "less traditional" CRT patient population is needed. Moreover, MRI technique has additional limitations, such as cost, data acquisition, and analysis, are time-consuming, and repeat analysis after CRT implantation may not be possible.

Computed tomography

Computed tomography is, at the present time, the best noninvasive visualization technique for venous anatomy in both candidates for CRT [15, 16] or in those in whom lead replacement is necessary [17]. To date, all studies reporting the value of electron beam CT or multislice CT in visualizing coronary veins have been primarily designed to assess the degree of coronary artery disease, which may have, in turn, had an impact on the accuracy of CT in directly evaluating the coronary veins and in particular second-order or third-order branches. Suboptimal enhancement of the coronary venous system, particularly of the second-order and third-order venous side branches, which have a smaller diameter, may be of great relevance in some patients and diagnostic inaccuracy may lead to an inappropriate decision in the implantation strategy. Segmentation of the distal part of the coronary veins can be a major issue due to the minimal density difference between the myocardium and coronary veins. Several factors including operator experience in performing the scanning procedure (administration of test bolus and/or precise detection of the time of coronary sinus opacification), patient's hemodynamic status, and operator experience in segmenting coronary veins may have a significant impact on the quality of acquisition and reconstruction of cardiac coronary veins.

CT has the potential to provide important information pertinent to enabling the development of a preprocedural implant strategy, such as follows: (1) assessment of patency of the venous system, (2) evaluation of proximity to the phrenic nerve [18], (3) measurement of luminal diameter of a suitable vein, and (4) analysis of concordance of the venous branch with the segment of dyssynchrony (Figure 12.2). The role of prospectively performing CT in patients scheduled to undergo CRT implants is not yet well-defined. At the present time, this imaging technique should be still considered to be experimental. Using CT in screening CRT candidates with suitable anatomy for the transvenous approach may be limited in patients with atrial fibrillation, high intrinsic heart rates, and frequent ectopic beats, all of which are often seen in this group of sick patients. Another major concern related to the use of CT is the relatively high radiation dose exposure reaching 15–20 mSv per scan. Recently, however new detection and reconstruction algorithms have allowed cardiac CT scanning with dose exposure in the range of 1 to 5 mSv.

Finally, assessment of dyssynchrony has been another major limitation in the use of CT. However recently, Truongh et al. [19] have demonstrated the

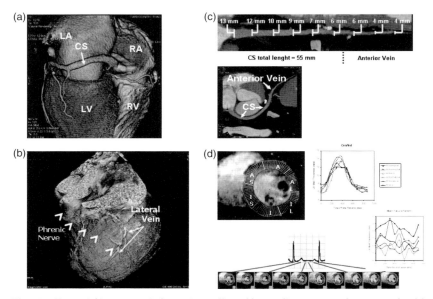

Fig. 12.2 Potential important information collected by cardiac computed tomography. (a) The importance of the assessment of patency of the venous system. (b) Visualization of the phrenic nerve and its distance from a possible target vein. In this patient, the phrenic nerve crossed over the target vein (lateral vein). (c) Measurement of luminal diameter of a vein, which may help in lead selection. (d) Assessment of mechanical dyssynchrony in control patient and in one heart failure patient with left bundle branch block. (See color plate section).

proof-of-principle that cardiac dyssynchrony can be assessed by the latest generation of CT scanner[19]. These authors have shown, in a relative small group of CRT patients, a high correlation between dyssynchrony assessment by CT with three-dimensional echocardiographic evaluation (time to minimum volume).

Multimodality imaging techniques

Considering the strength and the relative limitation of each noninvasive imaging technique, it is very likely that a combination of diagnostic imaging techniques will be used in the near future for the selection of a CRT candidate and for optimization of CRT delivery [20]. There are several potential advantages when considering how to merge different imaging modalities, such as Doppler echocardiography, and intracardiac three-dimensional and four-dimensional echocardiography to CT imaging or MRI imaging. Moreover, combination of advanced techniques of fusion between fluoroscopy and CT or MRI dataset (cardiac venous tree) may be of great help in guiding CRT delivery. Indeed, registering CT imaging or MRI anatomical data into the fluoroscopic system may help guide coronary sinus and vein cannulation, thereby reducing the implantation time and the intraprocedural dye-load. Currently, this approach is under intense study.

Selection of pacing site

Several reports have emphasized the importance of pacing site optimization for improving hemodynamic and short-term outcome of CRT. There is consistent evidence that, in both animal model and patients with left bundle branch block, pacing at the free wall of the left ventricle significantly increases left ventricular function compared to any other left ventricular sites. Nevertheless, 30–40% of seemingly appropriate patients in whom CRT was apparently properly delivered do not show significant short-term and long-term benefits. Among the other issues, such as presence and magnitude of mechanical dyssynchrony, and scar burden, optimization of therapy application, improvement in pacing site selection, may play a role.

Multisite pacing

One important question is whether adding more pacing sites in the left and/or right ventricle could improve outcome. Indeed, it seems feasible that placement of multiple pacing leads at different ventricular sites would create multiple waves of electrical activation, thus further reducing asynchrony in case of ventricular conduction delay. A few recent observational studies in heart failure patients have attempted simultaneous pacing at two sites within the same left ventricular region, a few case reports appeared about pacing at two different sites within the left ventricle, and some studies have evaluated two simultaneous pacing sites within the right ventricle along with one left ventricular pacing site. Although the results of these small, single-center observational studies showed a large individual variability, triple ventricular pacing sites, no matter whether on right or left ventricle, resulted in a larger hemodynamic improvement compared to conventional biventricular pacing. More recently, the first randomized, prospective multicenter trial (TRIP-HF) comparing triple site stimulation—two epicardial transvenous leads placed on anterior and lateral or posterolateral left lateral wall and one right ventricular lead—to conventional biventricular pacing has been reported [21]. The TRIP-HF study enrolled a highly selected, yet small group of severe heart failure patients presenting with slow ventricular rate during atrial fibrillation. The study showed that, compared to dual site biventricular pacing, triple site ventricular pacing promoted further left ventricular reverse remodeling as assessed by left ventricular end-systolic and end-diastolic volumes and ejection fraction at the 3-month follow-up. One important question related to the intriguing results of the TRIP-HF is the observation from detailed electrical activation mapping studies that the anterior wall is activated early during intrinsic rhythm in heart failure patients with left bundle branch block and pacing from a single left ventricular pacing site [22]. Moreover, the number of nonresponders was shown to be higher using anterior rather than a posterolateral left ventricular lead placement [23]. In addition, animal studies showed that no additional improvement can be expected when adding more left ventricular pacing sites to a well chosen one [24]. The finding that adding anterior LV pacing to postero-lateral wall stimulation seems to improve CRT is, therefore, not trivial and deserves further experimental and clinical investigation. One possible explanation for the beneficial effect observed during triple pacing site is the technical approach used by the investigators (i.e. the second left ventricular lead was connected to the atrial port) and was stimulated 25 ms before the right ventricular and the first left ventricular lead. Consequently, in the triple site stimulation mode, CRT is not truly simultaneous but sequential with moderate left ventricular pre-excitation. It is known from both animal studies and patient research that on average, left ventricular pre-excitation provides a better effect than simultaneous biventricular pacing. Thus, part of the benefit of the triple site pacing in the TRIP-HF study might be explained by the sequential ventricular pacing.

Endocardial and leadless pacing

Recent three-dimensional electroanatomical mapping in humans has indicated that, in patients with heart failure and ventricular conduction disturbance, the transmural activation time is often abnormal [22]. This abnormal transmural activation may be not corrected by conventional biventricular pacing. Indeed, during conventional biventricular pacing LV activation sequence starts at the epicardium and is slowly conducted (cell-to-cell conduction) over the epicardium and toward the endocardium. This direction is opposite to natural conduction. Endocardial biventricular pacing has been recently proven to improve LV pump function more than epicardial biventricular pacing, and the increase in LV function seems to be less pacing site dependent and less dependent on proper timing of stimulation [25]. This may indicate that full restoration of transmural activation sequence is of key importance. A very limited experience exists with endocardial pacing in CRT patients [26, 27]. The data have been mostly collected in patients in whom transvenous epicardial pacing failed so that a head-to-head comparison in the same patient is not possible. However, there are limited hemodynamic data in humans showing improved mechanical function during endocardial pacing compared to epicardial pacing. Endocardial stimulation is however technically challenging and may carry additional morbidity and mortality. Novel microtechnologies and nanotechnologies may enable the construction of implantable leadless "vectors," which may permit continuous endocardial pacing. In a series of recent investigations, acoustic energy was received by an ultrasound transducer in the heart and converted to electrical energy. Safety testing of this system has been performed in pigs showing that ultrasound energy results in no damage to the myocardium. Proof of this concept was demonstrated in patients undergoing electrophysiology studies showing that acute pacing thresholds in multiple right atrial, right ventricular, and left ventricular sites are comparable to those found with a temporary pacing catheter. An implantable device system that is currently under development will incorporate a leadless intracardiac electrode and a sub-cutaneous implanted transmitter [28, 29]. Moreover, future studies are required to determine whether endocardial CRT can turn nonresponders to conventional CRT into responders when using endocardial CRT.

In about 8–14% of patients from various studies, placement of an LV lead is difficult or impossible. In CARE-HF, only 86% of patients underwent successful LV lead implantation at the first implantation attempt. Inability to cannulate the coronary sinus is rare, but inability to obtain a stable left ventricular lead position occurred in at least 3–5% of patients in some recent studies. Additional causes of failure to place an LV lead include unsuitable cardiac veins, increased pacing thresholds over time and phrenic nerve stimulation. The ability to manipulate the LV lead in the coronary sinus using Stereotaxis™ has been reported [30]. This system uses a magnetic field of 0.08 Tesla created by two large permanent magnets (neodymium boron iron) placed close to the patient's chest (Figure 12.3). The LV pacing wire is directed over a magnet tipped 0.014-inch guide

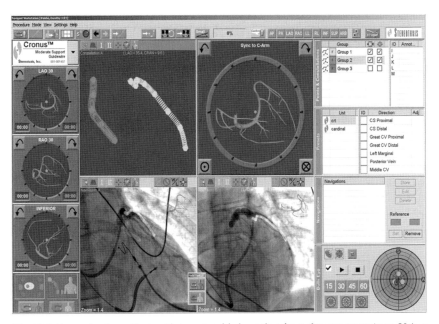

Fig. 12.3 Example of a patient with two sizeable branches from the coronary sinus. Using the Stereotaxis™ system, the two branch vessels are reconstructed and the system soft-ware helps to calculate appropriate vectors for the cannulation of each branch with the magnetic angioplasty wire. (See color plate section).

wire (Cronus™ Stereotaxis, St. Louis, MO, USA) and then magnetically directed through the venous system. The left ventricular over the wire leads are then manipulated over the guide wire. After an initial operator learning curve, the LV lead could potentially be positioned more quickly. Prior to directing the wire, a venogram is performed in two views, separated by at least 20 degrees. Computer software is used to reconstruct the coronary sinus and its branches, and the movement of the angioplasty wire through the coronary sinus can be performed remotely and endoscopically by changing the vector of the magnetic field. Potential advantages of this approach include the ability to easily map multiple sites through the venous system. Limitations to this approach include, difficulty manipulating the lead over the wire, and the need to have the magnets within inches of the patients' thorax, thus limiting the ability of the operator to be close to the patient.

Timing of therapy delivery

An important area of clinical research is the optimal timing of CRT implantation. At the present time, CRT therapy is reserved for patients with NYHA Class III or Class IV heart failure while on optimal medical therapy. A small number of patients with NYHA functional Class II CHF were included in CONTAK CD [31] and MIRACLE ICD [32] trials. A number of trials that include patients with less severe degrees of heart failure are in progress. These trials include: REVERSE, MADIT-CRT, RAFT, BLOCK-HF, BioPace and PACE [33]. Both BioPace and PACE include patients with a normal ejection fraction and a conventional indication for pacing.

The results from the REVERSE (Resynchonization reverses remodeling in systolic left ventricular dysfunction) trial were presented in March 2008 [34]. The purpose of this randomized double blind, parallel controlled clinical trial was to determine the effects of CRT on disease progression over 12 months in patients with asymptomatic and mildly symptomatic heart failure and ventricular dyssynchrony. Patients were enrolled in NYHA functional Class I (previously symptomatic) or in NYHA functional Class II, all without a clinical indication for permanent pacing. A total of 610 patients were enrolled, with CRT off in 191 and CRT on in 419 patients. The primary endpoint was a heart failure composite clinical endpoint and showed a trend toward improvement in this endpoint (composite of all cause mortality, CHF hospitalizations, crossover due to worsening CHF, NYHA class, and a double blind patient global assessment), while secondary endpoints of LVESV, LVEF, and LVEDV all showed statistical improvement. The time to first CHF hospitalization was prolonged in the CRT patients, but Minnesota Living with Heart Failure index and 6 minute walk test did not show a significant improvement.

MADIT CRT will enroll approximately 1,800 ischemic cardiomyopathy patients undergoing primary prevention ICD implantation comparing patients with NYHA Class I or Class II heart failure [33]. BLOCK-HF is a randomized double blind trial comparing CRT in patients with a wide range of functional NYHA class (I-III) and with an ejection fraction ≤50% who require pacing for AV block [33]. The primary endpoints of BLOCK HF are LV function, emergency admissions, and mortality. The Resynchronization/Defibrillation for Ambulatory Heart Failure Trial will assess 1,500 patients receiving a CRT-D device to determine mortality and hospitalization of a 5 year period [33]. Patients with NYHA Class II CHF will be enrolled. This trial will also include patients with atrial fibrillation. BioPace (Biventricular pacing to prevent cardiac desynchronization) and PACE (Pacing to avoid cardiac enlargement) are both trials that compare CRT to RV pacing in patients with well-preserved systolic function [33]. The endpoints for BioPace are survival, quality of life, and the 6-minute hall walk distance with follow-up for up to 5 years. For PACE, the primary endpoints will include echocardiographic parameters, as well as exercise capacity, quality of life, and clinical events [33].

Novel sensor technologies

Echocardiographic technique for optimization may not be readily available for every cardiologist for a variety of reasons. A device-based automatic optimization algorithm or hemodynamic sensor to adjust AV and/or VV intervals may have obvious clinical advantages.

The peak endocardial acceleration (PEA) can now be measured by a right ventricular lead equipped with a microaccelerometer located at the lead tip. Signals measured by the sensor are based on the amplitude of the first heart sound vibrations and identified as the variation of the PEA at each systole. By temporarily occluding the pulmonary artery in an animal model, Rickards et al. [35] demonstrated that the PEA signals variations remained highly correlated to the LV dP/dt_{max} rather than to the RV dP/dt_{max}[35]. Variations of the LV dP/dt_{max} in heart failure patients and comparison to PEA variations have also been studied. The first results seem to be promising, having exhibited a high correlation between variations of the LVdP/dt_{max} and PEA at different combinations of atrio-ventricular delay and at different right and left ventricular pacing sites.

Noninvasive optimization techniques

As pointed out in Chapter 7, the proportion of nonresponders is likely to be reduced by optimization of therapy application (tuning of atrio-ventricular and intraventricular delays). Several different echocardiographic methods have been employed for noninvasive optimization of atrio-ventricular and interventricular delay including the so-called Ritter's method, mitral inflow method, maximal left ventricular filling time, mitral and aortic velocity-time integral, and iterative method. Although echocardiographic approaches have shown value in the optimization of CRT devices, simpler and more rapid methods to routinely optimize devices are warranted. At the present time, there are five different techniques for noninvasive optimization of atrio-ventricular and inter-ventricular delay: (1) photoplethysmography [36], (2) impedance cardiography [37], (3) ultrasonic continuous-wave Doppler [38], (4) acoustic cardiography [39], and (5) continuous, noninvasive finger arterial pressure [40, 41]. Each method has intrinsic limitations and a head-to-head comparison has not been done yet, so that it is not possible to make a definite statement about reliability and accuracy of each method and comparison to each other.

Before discussing in greater details different methods of noninvasive optimization, it is important to briefly review some physiological concepts related to effect of atrio-ventricular and inter-ventricular timing optimization. The atrio-ventricular interval that maximizes resting cardiac output during dual-chamber pacing varies widely among patients. This is even truer for patients with depressed left ventricular ejection fraction. As discussed elsewhere in this book, the atrio-ventricular interval strongly influences ventricular preload and thereby stroke volume in patients with reduced left ventricular systolic function. However, during CRT, the atrioventricular interval also affects ventricular pump function by modifying ventricular synchrony. The largest improvement in LV dP/dt_{max} has been found to occur at the point of transition from noncapture to complete pacing capture; the best left ventricular pump function is obtained with use of a relatively short atrioventricular intervals, which allow complete activation of the ventricles from two pacing sites [42]. This atrioventricular interval may be different from the one resulting in optimized preload. Data from the PATH-CHF studies showed that in one-half of heart failure patients, the atrioventricular interval for optimal preload is usually longer that the one for optimal synchrony [41]; henceforth, it is no surprise that the mean difference between the two atrioventricular intervals is close to zero. To date, no clinical data are available to help sort through the relative importance of optimizing synchrony and optimizing preload. However, considering that asynchrony is the key determinant for depressed ventricular function in CRT patients, one may postulate that synchrony optimization should be preferred to optimization based on ventricular inflow. Finally, examination and calculation of cardiac output with Doppler echocardiography or most other noninvasive methods, as is easily and frequently performed in patients with dual-chamber pacemakers, is more problematic in heart failure patients with low cardiac output. In the latter patients, the value of the effect of pacing may be near the magnitude of variability of the measurement method. Thus, the number of repetitions required to obtain a clinically meaningful and reproducible approximation of the optimal atrioventricular interval makes this method, as a single assessment, almost impractical for patients with depressed ejection fraction. In future, semi automatic or fully automatic closed-loop (implantable device/noninvasive optimization device) optimization systems should probably be developed in order to reliably and reproducibly perform atrioventricular and/or interventricular optimization.

Photoplethysmography

Plethysmography can easily and automatically calculate variations in cardiac output [36]. The optimal delay should result in the highest cardiac output value recorded. Finger photoplethysmography correctly identified positive aortic pulse pressure responses with 71% sensitivity and 90% specificity, and negative aortic pulse pressure responses with 57% sensitivity and 96% specificity. The magnitude of plethysmographic changes was strongly correlated with positive aortic pulse pressure changes but less well-correlated with negative aortic pulse pressure changes. Plethysmography selected 78% of the patients having positive aortic pulse pressure changes to CRT and identified the AV delay giving maximum aortic pulse pressure change in all selected patients. Accordingly, plethysmography can provide a simple noninvasive method for identifying significant changes in aortic pulse pressure in CRT patients and the optimal atrioventricular delay giving the maximum aortic pulse pressure.

Impedance cardiography

The measurement of cardiac output can also be done by impedance cardiography [37]. Paired dual sensor pads are placed on both sides of the neck and both sides of the lower thorax at the level of xiphoid region. A low-voltage, high-amplitude alternating current of a known voltage is introduced through the outermost sensors. The conducted voltage is sensed through the innermost sensor pads and the drop in voltage is used to determine impedance to the current. Impedance changes over time during systole and diastole are measured and recorded as impedance waveform. Cardiac output and other hemodynamic parameters are also calculated by preset algorithms. The optimal atrioventricular interval is adjusted to achieve the highest cardiac output.

Ultrasonic continuous-wave Doppler

Another noninvasive method used to assess cardiac output is an ultrasonic, continuous-wave Doppler cardiac output monitoring device [38]. From the suprasternal notch, the ultrasound beam is directed toward the aortic outflow and gradually adjusted until the highest audio frequencies corresponding to the visual display of the highest velocities are achieved. Minute distance is the distance a blood cell travels in meters per minute and is a surrogate of cardiac output. In a small study, the minute distance measured was in good agreement with atrioventricular delay determined by the Ritter's and aortic velocity time integral methods.

Acoustic cardiography

A new technique called acoustic cardiography permits acquisition of detailed information about systolic and diastolic left ventricular function through dual-purpose sensors that simultaneously acquire ECG and sound data from precordial locations [39]. Several studies have shown that acoustic cardiography is a reliable, fast and cost-efficient alternative to echocardiographic methods. Acoustic cardiography parameters correlate well with established measures of LV systolic function, and that the optimization of pacing delays using acoustic cardiography not only improves the systolic function in CRT patients but also yields improvements in exercise tolerance, and therefore improves the quality of life in those patients. The algorithmic interpretation and trending of the results for various AV and VV delay settings is automated and allows optimization of the AV and VV intervals in a patient within 10–15 minutes as part of a regular CRT follow-up visit. Besides the optimization of CRT, its clinical applications include the evaluation of patients with suspected heart failure, ischemia, and cardiac arrhythmias. It can be used in a wide variety of diagnostic and monitoring applications in the hospital and office setting, and, in within the near future, the ambulatory monitoring of patients at home.

Continuous noninvasive finger arterial pressure

Noninvasive measurement of pressure waveform analysis uses a compact and simple cuff on the finger [40]. Then, the algorithm computes beat-to-beat cardiac output from radial artery pressure by simulating a three-element model of aortic input impedance, and includes nonlinear aortic mechanical properties and a self-adapting systematic vascular resistance. Monitored parameters include systolic, diastolic, and true mean pressure as well as heart rate. Additional derived hemodynamic parameters include stroke volume, systolic vascular resistance, and first derivative of pressure (dP/dt) in real-time. Usually optimization is based on the maximization of dP/dt and stroke volume data. Although the background of this technology is well validated, there is limited clinical experience. Future comparative studies are required in order to confirm the reliability and reproducibility of this novel technique for atrioventricular and inter-ventricular optimization.

Conclusions

Technological advances and better understanding of the pathobiology of CRT will likely results in further changes in both the timing of therapy delivery (less symptomatic patients) and the mode of therapy delivery (endocardial and multisite pacing). In a similar manner, diagnostic imaging modality may allow better dyssynchrony characterization and quantification, which will results in optimization of patient selection and more reliably prediction of functional, volumetric, and survival outcomes. Finally, new sensor technology may enable reliable, automatic noninvasive built-in device or external optimization will all represent major upcoming areas of investigation leading to further expansion of the clinical role of CRT and eventually leading to further improvement of clinical benefits by CRT.

References

1. Results of the Predictors of Response to CRT (PROS-PECT) trial. Available at: http://www.escardio.org/knowledge/congresses/CongressReports/2007/hl-ctu/3222-linde-hotline2.htm. Accessed December 27, 2007.

2. Beshai JF, Grimm RA, Nagueh SF, et al. Cardiac-resynchronization therapy in heart failure with narrow QRS complexes. *N Engl J Med*. 2007;357:2461–7.

3. Botvinick EH. Scintigraphic blood pool and phase image analysis: the optimal tool for the evaluation of resynchronization therapy. *J Nucl Cardiol*. 2005;12:424–8.

4. Knaapen P, van Campen LM, de Cock CC, et al. Effects of cardiac resynchronization therapy on myocardial perfusion reserve. *Circulation*. 2004;110:646–51.

5. Lindner O, Vogt J; Kammeier A, et al. Effect of cardiac resynchronization therapy on global and regional oxygen consumption and myocardial blood flow in patients with non-ischemic and ischemic cardiomyopathy. *Eur Heart J*. 2005;26:70-6.

6. Helm RH, Byrne M, Helm PA, Daya SK, Osman N, Tunin R, Halperin HR, Berger RD, Kass DA, Lardo AC. Three-dimensional mapping of optimal left ventricular pacing site for cardiac resynchronization. *Circulation*. 2007;115:1–9.

7. Westenberg JJ, Lamb HJ, van der Geest RJ, Bleeker GB, Holman ER, Schalij MJ, de Roos A, van der Wall EE, Reiber JH, Bax JJ. Assessment of left ventricular dyssynchrony in patients with conduction delay and idiopathic dilated cardiomyopathy: head-to-head comparison between tissue doppler imaging and velocity-encoded magnetic resonance imaging. *J Am Coll Cardiol*. 2006;47:2042–8.

8. Bleeker GB, Kaandorp TA, Lamb HJ, et al. Effect of posterolateral scar tissue on clinical and echocardiographic improvement after cardiac resynchronization therapy. *Circulation*. 2006;113:969–76.

9. Bleeker GB, Schalij MJ, Van Der Wall EE, Bax JJ. Postero-lateral scar tissue resulting in non-response to cardiac resynchronization therapy. *J Cardiovasc Electrophysiol*. 2006;17:899–901.

10. Chalil S, Stegemann B, Muhyaldeen SA, Khadjooi K, Foley PW, Smith RE, Leyva F. Effect of posterolateral left ventricular scar on mortality and morbidity following cardiac resynchronization therapy. *Pacing Clin Electrophysiol*. 2007;30:1201–9.

11. Assomull RG, Prasad SK, Lyne J, et al. Cardiovascular magnetic resonance, fibrosis, and prognosis in dilated cardiomyopathy. *J Am Coll Cardiol*. 2006;48:1977–85.

12. Bello D, Fieno DS, Kim RJ, et al. Infarct morphology identifies patients with substrate for sustained ventricular tachycardia. *J Am Coll Cardiol*. 2005;45:1104–8.

13. Rasche V, Binner L, Cavagna F, et al. Whole-heart coronary vein imaging: a comparison between non-contrast-agent- and contrast-agent-enhanced visualization of the coronary venous system. *Magn Reson Med*. 2007;57:1019–26.

14. Wijetunga M, Cuoco F, Ravi ND, Fuisz A, Strickberger SA. Characterization of the coronary sinus ostium by cardiac magnetic resonance imaging. *Am J Cardiol*. 2006;98:1400–2.

15. Van de Veire NR, Schuijf JD, De Sutter J, et al. Non-invasive visualization of the cardiac venous system in coronary artery disease patients using 64-slice computed tomography. *J Am Coll Cardiol*. 2006;48:1832–8.

16. Tada H, Kurosaki K, Naito S, et al. Three-dimensional visualization of the coronary venous system using multidetector row computed tomography. *Circ J*. 2005;69: 165–70.

17. Auricchio A, Sorgente A, Singh JP, et al. Role of Multislice Computed Tomography for Preprocedural Evaluation Prior to Revision of a Chronically Implanted Transvenous Left Ventricular Lead. *Am J Cardiol*. 2007;100:1566–70.

18. Matsumoto Y, Krishnan S, Fowler SJ, et al. Detection of phrenic nerve and their relation to cardiac anatomy using 64-slice multidetector computed tomography. *Am J Cardiol*. 2007;100: 133–7.

19. Truong QA, Singh JP, Cannon CP, Sarwar A, Nasir K, Auricchio A, Faletra FF, Sorgente A, Conca C, Moccetti T, Handschumacher M, Brady TJ, Hoffmann U. Novel method for assessing intraventricular dyssynchrony using quantitative analysis of regional wall thickness by multi-detector computed tomography. *J Am Coll Cardiol*. 2008;51:Suppl A:A20 (abstract).

20. Goiten O, Lacomis JM, Gorsan J III, et al. Left ventricular pacing lead implantaiton: potential utility of multimodal image integration. *Heart Rhythm*. 2006;1:91–4.

21. Leclercq C, Gadler F, Kranig W, et al. (for the Triple Resynchronization In Paced Heart Failure Patients (TRIP-HF) study group). A randomized comparison of triple versus dual site ventricular stimulation in patients with congestive heart failure. *J Am Coll Cardiol*. 2008; in press.

22. A. Auricchio, C. Fantoni, F. Regoli, et al.: Characterization of left ventricular activation in patients with heart failure and left bundle branch block. *Circulation*. 2004;109:1133–9.

23. Butter C, Auricchio A, Stellbrink C, et al; Pacing Therapy for Chronic Heart Failure II Study Group. Effect of resynchronization therapy stimulation site on the systolic function of heart failure patients. *Circulation*. 2001;104:3026–9.

24. Peschar M, de Swart H, Michels KJ, et al. Left ventricular septal and apex pacing for optimal pump function in canine hearts. *J Am Coll Cardiol*. 2003;41:1218–26.

25. Van Deursen C, Van Hunnik A, Kuiper M, et al. Endocardial Left Ventricular Pacing Improves Cardiac Resynchronization Therapy In Canine LBBB Hearts. *Circulation*. 2007;116 Supplement II: 2515 (abstract).

26. Van Gelder BM, Scheffer MG, Meijer A, Bracke FA. Transseptal endocardial left ventricular pacing: an alternative technique for coronary sinus lead placement in cardiac resynchronization therapy. *Heart Rhythm*. 2007,4:454–60.

27. Garrigue S, Jaïs P, Espil G, et al. Comparison of chronic biventricular pacing between epicardial and endocardial left ventricular stimulation using Doppler tissue imaging in patients with heart failure. *Am J Cardiol*. 2001;88:858–62.

28. Echt DS, Cowan MW, Riley RE, Brisken AG. Feasibility and safety of a novel technology for pacing without leads. *Heart Rhythm*. 2006;3:1202–6.

29. Lee KL, Lau C-P, Tse H-F, Echt DS, Heaven D, Smith W, Hood M. First human demonstration of cardiac stimulation with transcutaneous ultrasound energy delivery: Implication for wireless pacing with implantable devices. *J Am Coll Cardiol*. 2007;50:877–83.

30. Gallagher PL, Martin L, Angel L, Tomassoni G. Initial clinical experience with cardiac resynchronization therapy utilizing a magnetic navigation system. *J Cardiovas Electrophysiol.*. 2007;18:174–80.

31. Lozano I, Bocchiardo M, Achtelik M, et al. Impact of biventricular pacing on mortality in a randomized crossover study of patients with heart failure and ventricular arrhythmias. *Pacing Clin Electrophysiol.* 2000;23:1711–12.

32. Abraham WT, Young JB, León AR, et al. Effects of cardiac resynchronization on disease progression in patients with left ventricular systolic dysfunction, an indication for an implantable cardioverter-defibrillator, and mildly symptomatic chronic heart failure. *Circulation.* 2004;110:2864–8.

33. Hayes DL, Yu CM. Ongoing trial to further shape the future of CRT. In: *Cardiac resynchronization therapy*, 2nd edition. CM Yu, DL Hayes, A Auricchio, eds., 2008;290–300.

34. Linde C, Abraham W, Daubert JC. Late breaking clinical trial. *J Am CollCardiol.* 2008. in press.

35. Rickards AF, Bombardini T, Vorbucci G et al. An implantable intracardiac accelerometer for monitoring myocardial contractility. *Pacing Clin Electrophysiol.* 1996;19:2066–71.

36. Butter C, Stellbrink C, Belacazar A et al. Cardiac resynchronization therapy optimization by finger plethysmography. *Heart Rhythm.* 2004;1:568–73.

37. Zhang Q, Fung JW, Chan YS, et al. The role of repeating optimization of atrioventricular interval during interim and long-term follow-up after cardiac resynchronization therapy. *Int J Cardiol.* 2007; April 16: Epub ahead of print.

38. Siu CW, Tse HF, Lee K, et al. Cardiac resynchronization therapy optimization by cardiac output monitoring (USCOM device). PACE. *Pacing Clin Electrophysiol.* 2007;30:50–55.

39. Toggweiler S, Zuber M, Kobza R, et al. Improved response to cardiac resychronization therapy through optimization of atrioventricular and interventricular delays using acoustic cardiography: a pilot study. *J Cardiac Failure.* 2007;13:637–42.

40. Models of brachial to finger wave distortion and pressure decrement. *Cardiovasc Res.* 1997; 33: 698–705.

41. Jansen JRC, Schreuder JJ, Mulier JP, Smith NT, Settels JJ, Wesseling KH. A comparison of cardiac output derived from the arterial pressure wave against thermodilution in cardiac surgery patients. *Br J Anaesthesia.* 2001;87:212–22.

42. Auricchio A, Ding J, Spinelli JC, et al. Cardiac resynchronization therapy restores optimal atrioventricular mechanical timing in heart failure patients with ventricular conduction delay. *J Am Coll Cardiol.* 2002;39:1163–69.

Index

Page numbers followed by *f* indicate a figure; by *t* a table.

(Author Disclosure Table)

Working group member	Employment	Research grant	Other research support	Speakers bureau/ honoraria	Expert witness	Ownership interest	Consultant/ advisory board	Other
Blendea	Massachusetts General Hospital	None	None	None	None	None	None	None
Borggrefe	Universitätsklinikum Mannheim	None	None	None	None	None	None	None
Burkhoff	Columbia University/ Impulse Dynamics	None	None	None	None	Impulse Dynamics – participate in company option plan*	None	None
Butter	Heart Center Brandenburg in Bernau		Impulse Dynamics*	Impulse Dynamics*				
Chakir	Johns Hopkins University	None	None	None	None	None	None	None
Fisher	Intermountain Medical Center	Novartis*, Roche*, XDx*, PARACOR*, Medtronic*, Guidant*, Boston Scientific*	None	None	None	None	Boston Scientific*	None

Working group member	Employment	Research grant	Other research support	Speakers bureau/honoraria	Expert witness	Ownership interest	Consultant/advisory board	Other
Grimm	Cleveland Clinic	Medtronic*	None	Boston Scientific*, Medtronic*	None	None	GE St Jude Medical*	None
Helm	Johns Hopkins University	None	None	None	None	None	None	None
Herweg	None	None	None	Cryocath*	None	None	None	Medtronic+
Illercil	University of South Florida	None	None	None	None	None	None	None
Israel	J. W. Goethe University	None	St. Jude Medical+, Medtronic+	St. Jude Medical (speakers bureau)*, Medtronic*, Biotronik*, Boston-Scientific*, St. Jude Medical (honoraria)*, Medtronic (honoraria)*	None	None	Sorin Group*, Medtronic*	None

Kass	Johns Hopkins University Medical Institutions	None	None	None	None	None	Boston Scientific+	None
Kfoury	Intermountain Medical Center	Novartis*, Roche*, XDx*, PARACOR*, Medtronic*, Guidant*, Boston Scientific*	None	None	None	None	XDx*	None
Kocovic	Lankenau Medical	Medtronic+, St. Jude+, Boston Scientific+	None	Medtronic*, St. Jude*, Boston Scientific* (speakers bureau), Medtronic*, St. Jude*, Boston Scientific* (honoraria)	None	None	Medtronic*, St. Jude*, Boston Scientific*	None

Working group member	Employment	Research grant	Other research support	Speakers bureau/ honoraria	Expert witness	Ownership interest	Consultant/ advisory board	Other
Metra	University of Brescia	None	None	Myogem*, Corthera*, Servier*, Otsuka*, Merck*	None	None	None	None
Mika	Impulse Dynamics	None	None	None	None	None	None	None
Perloff		None	None	None	None	None	None	None
Renlund	Intermountain Healthcare, USA	Novartis*, Roche*, XDx*, Medtronic*, Boston Scientific*	None	None	None	None	None	None
Singh	Massachusetts General Hospital	Biotronik+, Boston Scientific+, Medtronic+, St. Jude Medical+	None	Biotronik*, Boston Scientific*, Medtronic*, Sorin*, St. Jude Medical*	None	None	Biotronik*, Boston Scientific*, Medtronic*, St. Jude Medical*	None

Name	Institution							
Spragg	John Hopkins Hospital	None	None	None	None	None	None	None
Stein	Weill Medical College of Cornell University	Medtronic*, Boston Scientific*, St. Jude Medical*	None	Medtronic+, Boston Scientific*, St. Jude Medical*	None	Medtronic*, Boston Scientific*, St. Jude Medical*	None	Medtronic*, Boston Scientific*, St. Jude Medical*
Sticherling	University Hospital Basel, Switzerland	Guidant (Boston)*	None	Medtronic*, Boston Scientific*	None	Biotronik+	None	None

*Modest
+Significant

This table represents the relationships of writing group members that may be perceived as actual or reasonably perceived conflicts of interest as reported on the Disclosure Questionnaire which all writing group members are required to complete and submit. A relationship is considered to be "Significant" if (a) the person receives $10,000 or more during any 12 month period, or 5% or more of the person's gross income; or (b) the person owns 5% or more of the voting stock or share of the entity, or owns $10,000 or more of the fair market value of the entity. A relationship is considered to be "Modest" if it is less than "Significant" under the preceding definition.

The AHA Clinical Series

SERIES EDITOR • ELLIOTT ANTMAN

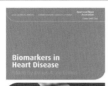
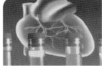

Biomarkers in Heart Disease
James A. de Lemos
9781405175715

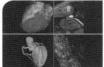

Novel Techniques for Imaging the Heart
Marcelo Di Carli & Raymond Kwong
9781405175333

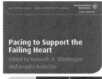
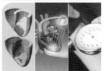

Pacing to Support the Failing Heart
Kenneth A. Ellenbogen
& Angelo Auricchio
9781405175340

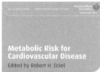
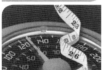

Metabolic Risk for Cardiovascular Disease
Robert H. Eckel
9781405181044

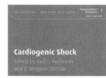
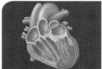

Cardiogenic Shock
Judith Hochman
& E. Magnus Ohman
9781405179263

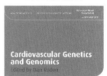
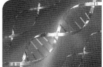

Cardiovascular Genetics and Genomics
Dan Roden
9781405175401

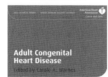
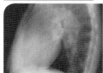

Adult Congenital Heart Disease
Carole A. Warnes
9781405178204

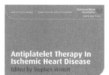
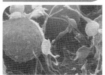

Antiplatelet Therapy In Ischemic Heart Disease
Stephen Wiviott
9781405176262

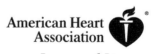